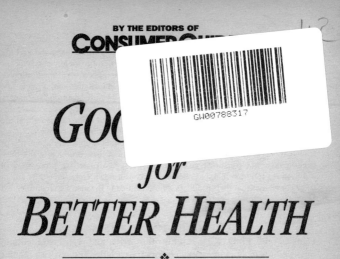

BY THE EDITORS OF
CONSUMER GUIDE

GOOD

for

BETTER HEALTH

❖

Densie Webb, Ph.D., R.D.

Susan Male Smith, M.A., R.D.

PUBLICATIONS INTERNATIONAL, LTD.

CONTRIBUTING WRITERS

Densie Webb, Ph.D., R.D., is a nutrition writer and registered dietitian. She is editor of *Environmental Nutrition* newsletter and writes a regular health column for *Woman's Day* magazine. She has written several nutrition-counter books and contributes to consumer magazines such as *American Health, Eating Well, Men's Fitness,* and *Cooking Light.* Dr. Webb has also served as health editor of *McCall's* magazine.

Susan Male Smith, M.A., R.D., is a registered dietitian and nutrition consultant who frequently writes for both professional and consumer publications. Her writing credits include such magazines as *Family Circle, Redbook, McCall's, American Health,* and *Woman's Health Adviser.* Her consulting work includes advising corporations and public relations firms on a variety of nutrition issues. Ms. Smith is assistant editor of *Environmental Nutrition* newsletter.

CONSULTANTS

J. B. Anderson, Ph.D., is professor of nutrition at the University of North Carolina at Chapel Hill. He serves on the editorial board of several professional journals and is a fellow of the American College of Nutrition. Dr. Anderson received his Ph.D. from Cornell University.

Merrill J. Christensen, Ph.D., is associate professor of nutrition at Brigham Young University. Dr. Christensen received his Ph.D. from the Massachusetts Institute of Technology and further training in molecular biology and oncology from the University of Wisconsin at Madison.

Kay B. Franz, Ph.D., is associate professor of nutrition at Brigham Young University. She received her Ph.D. from the University of California at Berkeley and is a fellow of the American College of Nutrition.

Contents

Contents

PART III: HEALTH-WISE EATING 228

PART IV: FOODS FOR HEALTHIER LIVING 275

Contents

INTRODUCTION

Listen to the popular media, and you'd think there was nothing good left to eat. That's because newspapers, magazines, and the nightly news look for sound bites. You know, those easy-to-package, better-if-they're-negative nuggets of sensational information. They'd rather not tell the whole story, because frankly, it takes too long. But we would. It's here in this book.

In these pages, we've strived to give you the theories, the for-sures, and the I-don't-knows of nutrition, as well as the basics about food and how to put it all into practice.

But this book is far more than just a collection of facts. We've devoted a major portion of the book to detailing the what, why, and how of healthy foods. And because we don't want to leave you scratching your head at the checkout counter, we've given you plenty of mouth-watering recipes as well. Go ahead—enjoy the colors, flavors, and tastes of the healthy diversity of foods here.

Twenty years ago, a "1984" Orwellian fantasy of what we'd be eating today might have had us dialing up dosages of nutrition pellets from a vending machine. Luckily for us, the visions of that frightful dinner scenario never came to be.

Skip ahead ten years. Fish Oils. Oat bran. These are just two of the fizzles from the "downer decade." That's how we've dubbed the 1980s, because it seems we got off track somewhere along the line. We began to think of food in isolation, trying to find that miracle cure. Today we're back to thinking of whole foods, but with a healthy '90s twist. We're yearning to eat right—and to enjoy eating.

To get started, check out Part I, The Essential Nutrients. Here we bring you the vital "stats" on the major and minor nutrients that keep you alive. You'll find out some pretty amazing facts about how they interact—in both good ways and bad.

We've even highlighted some food sources of the important nutrients.

Not to offend you vegetarians, but Part II, Diet and Disease, is the "meat" of the matter. It goes to the heart of *why* we want to eat healthy. Living longer isn't really the point—living *better* is. So, in this section, we shine the spotlight on dozens of health problems that appear to have a link to nutrition. The focus is on preventing diseases that debilitate, such as cancer and heart disease, as well as finding ways to soothe life's minor annoyances, such as constipation and flatulence.

Then it's on to Part III, Health-Wise Eating, or how to put it all to work for you. Here's what you need to know to marry the basics from Part I to the ideas in Part II. We'll tell you why there's no need to be paranoid about eating right.

Aaahhh...Part IV, Foods for Healthier Living, our favorite section. Sit back, relax, and revel in the abundance of fruits, vegetables, grains, and protein sources we've collected for you. These are our top food choices for a healthy diet. Here you'll find tips for choosing, preparing, and serving, as well as those tasty recipes we mentioned. Once you explore this section, you'll realize how truly enjoyable a healthy diet can be.

THE ESSENTIAL NUTRIENTS

Talk of protein, carbohydrates, and RDAs can be a yawner. But you wouldn't have bought this book if you weren't interested in eating healthfully. And you can't completely appreciate what it means to eat a healthy diet without first having a basic understanding of the nutrients in the foods you eat and your body's requirements for those nutrients.

Nutrition is an ever-evolving, ever-changing science. Anyone who tells you they have all the answers is either a liar or a fool. Barely a week goes by that you don't hear of new research findings relating to what we eat and how it affects our health. What is accepted as fact today may tomorrow be questioned or even disproved. It's hard to know exactly what to eat and what the makeup of your diet means to your health.

Still, based on what researchers know today, experts have made specific recommendations for several nutrients. The most commonly used guide is the Recommended Dietary Allowances (RDAs). The RDAs specify recommended intakes of protein, 11 vitamins, and 7 minerals (but not of carbohydrate, fat, or fiber). The recommended allowances differ by age groups. The RDAs are not requirements nor are they minimum intakes. They are exactly as they say—recommended allowances. These recommended allowances, or dietary recommendations, are set high enough to ensure that almost everyone, even those who have higher-than-average requirements, get enough nutrients. But the National Academy of Sciences' Food and Nutrition Board, which sets the RDAs, emphasizes that the RDAs are designed to measure the nutritional adequacy of a population's diet, not an individual's diet.

It is best to leave the RDAs of specific nutrients to the scientists. Most of us simply want to know what foods we should be including in our diets and why; we want to know what

9

foods or combinations of foods would be best for us in order to get the nutrients we need. Fortunately, guidelines for food intake have been developed that provide this information. The Food Guide Pyramid (see Part III) is one such set of guidelines. The recently developed Pyramid gives recommendations about the number of servings from different food groups that we should have each day. If we all followed these guidelines, we would be eating a variety of foods. And most of us would be eating more fruits, vegetables, and whole grains—the foods that, more and more, are stealing the spotlight in terms of helping us stay healthy and fight disease.

The next few chapters lay out for you why eating healthy foods is such a smart thing to do. You'll find out how it's the balance of nutrients in foods—from proteins, fats, and carbohydrates to the wide array of vitamins and minerals—that make some eating styles better for you than others. No food should be off-limits. As always, moderation is the key. But it only makes sense that some foods benefit your health more than others. Once you understand the complexities of the nutrients in the foods you eat, you can appreciate why moderation and variety are, indeed, the smartest approach to healthy eating.

WATER AND OTHER FLUIDS

You may not think of it as a vital nutrient, but that's exactly what water is. In fact, it's probably the most vital nutrient in your diet. You can go without food for weeks, but without water, you won't survive more than a few days.

How important is it? If you're a woman, more than half your body weight is water; two-thirds if you're a man. That's because water is a partner in nearly every process your body performs. It helps you digest food, absorb nutrients, circulate blood, and excrete waste. Water carries nutrients throughout your body and carries away your body's waste products. (It also helps prevent constipation.) One of water's most critical functions is to maintain your body's normal temperature—about 98.6 degrees Fahrenheit. Without it, your temperature would soar.

But the water that's in your body doesn't just sit there. It constantly needs replacing. You lose water each time you breathe and when you sweat (you perspire even when you're sitting comfortably in a chair). You also lose it through bowel and kidney functions. All told, you lose about 2½ quarts of water a day.

Because the body doesn't store water like it does some vitamins and minerals, water must constantly be replaced. Six to eight glasses of fluid (including water and other beverages) every day is generally recommended, whether you're thirsty or not. Your need for fluids increases at high altitudes where the air is cool and dry. When you exercise intensely and are sweating, you should drink four to six ounces of water every 10 to 15 minutes.

When the water in your body drops by as little as one percent of your body weight, or by one to two pounds (not unusual during an hour of exercise), dehydration begins and you become thirsty. Though thirst is an important regulator of fluid intake, it is often not an accurate indicator of your real needs, especially during exercise or illness or in very hot, humid weather. Older people and young children, in particular, shouldn't rely on thirst to indicate their true fluid needs.

Your best bets for replacing lost fluids are water, unsweetened plain or flavored seltzer, or club soda. Because of their sugar content, sweetened drinks such as colas or fruit juices are not absorbed as rapidly as water. When replenishing fluids, avoid caffeinated coffee, soft drinks, and tea. Caffeine causes you to produce more urine, so you may lose more fluid than you gain.

Is the Water Safe?

Despite the fact that water is vital to life, or perhaps because of it, most of us are anxious about the safety of the water we drink. You may hear about contaminants in tap water that can make you sick.

The thousands of illnesses that occur each year from contaminated drinking water are caused mainly by parasites and bacteria growing in water that has not been properly purified. Still, most of the headlines and scare stories are about chlorine, fluoride, and lead. Here's the lowdown on what you need to know to keep yourself and your family safe:

Chlorine

One recent report found that people who drink chlorinated water have a significantly higher risk of bladder and rectal cancer than those who don't. That report was based on a reanalysis of studies from the past 25 years. While the findings are no reason to stop drinking chlorinated water, they do indicate a need for closer scrutiny of the way we purify water. The most important point to remember is that any risk of cancer that chlorination may pose is greatly outweighed by its benefits. For example, you can thank chlorination for the virtual elimination of two potentially deadly diseases, cholera and typhoid, in the United States.

Fluoride

For more than 40 years, scientists have known that fluoride is important for building and maintaining strong teeth and bones. Since that discovery, many water supplies in the United States have been fluoridated. But concerns have been raised over and over again that fluoride causes cancer. So, is fluoride good or bad? In most areas with fluoridated water supplies, people consume only about one-hundredth of one percent of the level of fluoride that has been shown to cause cancer in animals. One estimate is that a person would have to drink 20,000 gallons of fluoridated water a day to get a cancer-promoting dose of fluoride. In addition, the U.S. Public Health Service has stated that a recent year-long study found no evidence establishing an association between fluoride and cancer.

Nothing seems to take fluoride's place in preventing tooth decay. Studies consistently show that children who drink fluoridated water have less than half the number of cavities of those who drink unfluoridated water. The American Dental Association has endorsed fluoridation of water for the last 40 years.

Lead

Lead in water is a legitimate and growing health concern, especially among infants and young children. Not all water supplies are contaminated with lead, but several around the country have tested positive for high levels of lead. Over time, lead builds up in the body, causing brain and nerve damage in young children and causing high blood pressure, headaches, nausea, and vomiting in adults. The Environmental Protection Agency has mandated that water systems everywhere clean up their act and "get the lead out" by setting tougher limits on lead levels. However, the deadline for revamping these systems is the year 2014. To minimize your exposure until then, take these simple precautions:

• Never use the first water drawn in the morning. Let it run for at least three minutes before use.

• Use cold tap water instead of hot, especially to reconstitute powdered infant formula. Hot water allows lead in pipes to leach into the water.

• Let the water run until it is cold any time you use it.

• Don't boil water any longer than necessary—five minutes is enough. Boiling concentrates contaminants in water, including lead.

CALORIES

Just as a car needs gasoline to run, your body needs fuel to make it through the day. That fuel, of course, comes from food. The fuel that food supplies is measured in units called kilocalories, or simply calories. Though we think of food as containing calories, the truth is, it does not. Your body produces energy, measured as calories, when it burns the proteins, fats, and carbohydrates in foods.

A gram of carbohydrate provides four calories, as does a gram of protein. But watch out for fat—one gram of fat packs nine calories. Alcohol also provides calories—about seven per gram. Because fat has more than twice as many calories as does carbohydrate or protein, and because it's more easily deposited as body fat (see Fat), it's not hard to see why eating too many fatty foods can lead to a flabby body.

How should total calorie intake break down? Many experts recommend 30 percent or less from fat and 12 to 15 percent from protein, with the rest coming from carbohydrate. That means that carbohydrate would make up from 55 percent to 78 percent of calories.

Because carbohydrate, protein, and fat can be burned to provide calories, we need to eat a lot of them every day, with carbohydrate providing the largest portion. Vitamins and minerals are also very important, but we need only small amounts of them to build bone and other tissue and to regulate body processes.

The way your body obtains energy from its fuel generally goes something like this: Protein, fat, and carbohydrate in food are broken down into smaller, more simple compounds. The process produces energy, or calories, and small pieces of the original materials. The energy obtained during the process makes it possible for you to expend energy in walking, running, and other activities. Some energy simply escapes as heat;

this release of heat cools your body and helps to keep its temperature constant. Fat and protein that aren't needed to produce energy are used to build new compounds, such as fat and muscle tissue.

For most of us, only one-third of our calorie requirements is used for daily activities—dressing, walking, sitting, exercising. The other two-thirds support more important behind-the-scenes dramas: keeping our body temperature constant, repairing internal organs and skin, keeping our heart beating and lungs breathing, and maintaining the proper chemical balance inside and outside our body's cells.

The number of calories your body requires depends on your gender, your weight, and your activity level. The longer you do an activity and the harder it is, the more calories it requires. A woman generally requires fewer calories per pound than a man, in part, because women have more body fat than men (muscle burns more calories).

In general, you can figure how many calories you need each day using one of the following equations:

For men:
900 + (10 × your weight*) × 1.2 (little activity)
                          1.4 (moderate activity)
                          1.6 (regular exercise or manual labor)

For women:
800 + (7 × your weight*) × 1.2 (little activity)
                          1.4 (moderate activity)
                          1.6 (regular exercise or manual labor)

   * In pounds

If you don't need calories right away, your body conveniently stores the energy-providing nutrients for later. If you need carbohydrate that same day, it is available as glycogen in your liver. Excess carbohydrate, fat, and protein are stored as fat—your evolutionary insurance against starvation. Of course, if you store too much fat, you gain weight.

Counting Calories

"How many calories does it contain?" That's a common question when you're worried about your weight. But obsessive calorie counting is not the way to lose weight. If you follow the guidelines for healthy eating—replacing fatty foods with those high in complex carbohydrates—you'll find that your calorie intake automatically drops. Both human and animal studies have proven this.

As you count your calories, keep in mind that if you cut back on calories too much, your metabolism becomes sluggish and you may retain more water. You'll also stop losing weight because your body will try to protect itself from what it perceives as starvation. Keep your calorie intake at a reasonable level for a slow, steady weight loss.

HOW MANY CALORIES DO YOU BURN?

	Weight (in pounds)					
	100	130	150	170	190	210
	Calories Burned Per Hour*					
Basketball	414	486	564	636	714	786
Card playing	78	90	102	114	132	144
Cycling, leisurely	192	228	264	294	330	354
Eating	72	84	96	108	120	132
Fishing	186	222	252	288	318	354
Running (11.5 minutes per mile)	408	480	552	630	702	774
Tennis	330	384	444	504	564	624
Walking, normal pace	240	282	324	372	414	456

*These are estimates; the actual number of calories you burn during these activities may vary.

Once you know the daily calorie level you need to keep your present weight, you can lose weight by taking in fewer calories each day than you need. Specifically, to lose one pound of fat a week, you should consume about 3,500 calories less per week than you need, either by eating less or being more active (see "How Many Calories Do You Burn?"). But it's best not to go below 1,200 calories per day.

At first glance, a weight loss of only one pound a week seems like very little, especially when you're tempted by diets promising weight losses of a pound a day. But remember, on those pound-a-day diets, you lose mostly water, not fat. And past experience shows that even if you lose more, it won't last. If you want successful, permanent weight loss, the slow, steady approach is your best and most nutritionally sound course. Add an exercise program, and you can lose an additional pound or two a month.

Changing Calorie Needs

Age

Your calorie needs are greatest as an infant. Pound for pound, you require more calories than you ever will as an adult. But this high calorie requirement drops during childhood and continues to decline in adult life by about two percent each decade.

Weather

Generally, your calorie needs are affected very little by the temperature outside. But, there are a few exceptions. The energy cost of being active is slightly greater in temperatures below 22 degrees Fahrenheit than in a warm climate. Some of the extra calories burned are simply due to the extra weight of cold-weather clothing and footwear. In addition, because bulky winter clothing makes you "hobble," your clumsy movements burn more calories. If exposure to cold air or water causes your body to cool much below its fairly steady 98.6 degrees Fahrenheit, your body responds by shivering and increasing its metabolism, burning even more calories.

Your energy needs also are greater if you're active in temperatures of 99 degrees Fahrenheit or higher. Your body temperature and metabolic rate increase, requiring extra energy to maintain a constant temperature.

PROTEIN

Do you get enough protein? Chances are, you do. Anyone who eats a variety of foods gets plenty. In fact, most of us consume quite a bit more protein than we need, and that includes athletes and bodybuilders. So, should you worry about getting too much? Probably not. Unless you have kidney disease, you're unlikely to suffer from an overindulgence in protein.

All foods, with the exception of pure fats or pure sugars, contain at least a little protein. If you're like most Americans, your protein intake averages about 16 to 18 percent of the total calories you take in each day. That translates into about 63 grams a day for a woman and about 90 grams a day for a man. The Recommended Dietary Allowance (RDA) of protein for women over the age of 25 is 50 grams, and for their male counterparts, 63 grams. To put that into food terms: A fast-food burger provides about 14 grams; 3½ ounces of cooked rib-eye steak provides about 20 grams; 3½ ounces of broiled cod fish, 26 grams. But don't forget all the smaller amounts of protein you get from almost everything you eat.

Not counting water, protein makes up about three-quarters of the weight of your body's tissues. Hair, skin, nails, and muscle are mostly protein. Even bone contains a significant amount of protein. In addition, the enzymes in your body—which perform the chemical reactions that produce energy and manufacture the thousands of different molecules that make up your muscle, bone, skin, hair, and organs—are also protein compounds.

What Is Protein?

Proteins are complex compounds composed of smaller chemical units called amino acids. Unlike carbohydrate and fat, these amino acids contain nitrogen. There are 20 different amino acids that can be combined in a seemingly infinite number of ways to make up the thousands of different proteins that are found in your body. Your body is able to manufacture all but nine of these amino acids—histidine, isoleucine, leucine, lysine, methionine, phenylalanine, threonine, tryptophan, and valine. These nine are called the "essential amino acids."

The protein in your diet must supply these nine "gotta-have-'em" amino acids. If you don't get enough, your body cannot function. If your diet lacks even one of these amino acids, you can't produce enough new protein, and your body's tissues begin to break down.

Animal products, which contain so-called "complete proteins," are generally rich in all nine essential amino acids. This includes meat, fish, poultry, eggs, milk, and cheese. Proteins that come from plant sources such as wheat or oats are generally low in one or more of the essential amino acids (soybeans are an exception—their protein is considered "complete"), and so you must combine different protein sources to make up for these shortages. For example, peanut butter and bread combined are a complete protein source. So, too, are rice and beans. Such combinations are called "complementary proteins." But it's not necessary to eat them at the same meal; eating them the same day is usually enough. Even if you eat vegetarian-style, you needn't worry about a delicate balancing act of complementing proteins at each meal. As long as you eat a wide variety of foods, the right combination of amino acids will fall into place.

THE TRYPTOPHAN TRAUMA

In the late 1980s, L-tryptophan supplements were a popular home remedy for insomnia sufferers, and some psychiatrists prescribed it to treat depression. By many accounts, it worked. But in 1989, reports started popping up of a rare and dangerous muscle disorder called eosinophilia myalgia syndrome (EMS). By early 1990, several thousand cases and some 20 deaths had been reported. In response to the ever-increasing numbers of tryptophan-takers who were identified as having EMS, the Food and Drug Administration banned sale of the supplement in the United States. Though it isn't known for sure what caused the sometimes deadly reaction to tryptophan, it's generally believed to have been caused by a contaminant introduced during manufacturing of the supplements, rather than being a toxic reaction to the amino acid itself.

Protein Digestion

When you eat any protein-containing food, your digestive system uncoils the protein molecules in that food and breaks them into smaller strings of amino acids, or even into individual amino acids. These are absorbed into the bloodstream and transported to all the cells in the body. Enzymes and other molecules inside cells reassemble the amino acids into the specific proteins that the cells need. It may seem illogical to break the protein molecules apart, only to build them back again, but this allows your cells to make the specific proteins they need.

Getting enough protein is essential for growth and development. That includes the growth of a fetus, the production of human milk, the growth of children, the healing of a wound, and the growth of hair and nails. Not as visible, but just as important, is the need for amino acids to replace and maintain your body's tissues, such as muscles, blood, skin, body organs, and connective tissue, which are constantly being broken down and rebuilt in a never-ending process called protein turnover.

In addition to forming major body tissues, amino acids are needed in much smaller amounts to manufacture the enzymes and some of the hormones that regulate the body's processes. For example, the hormone insulin is actually a protein that regulates the level of sugar in the blood. All of the enzymes in the body are proteins. They regulate thousands of chemical reactions constantly taking place in your body, from the release of energy to the production of brain chemicals.

Proteins are also critical components of the disease-fighting immune system. Antibodies, the substances manufactured by your immune system to fight off infections and invading viruses, are proteins. Hemoglobin, an iron-containing protein in the blood, contains hundreds of amino acids that carry oxygen from the lungs to all of your body tissues. Protein-containing complexes called lipoproteins carry fats and cholesterol in the blood.

Although carbohydrates and fats are used far more efficiently, in a pinch protein can also be used for energy. If your diet does not contain enough carbohydrate and fat to meet calorie needs, proteins are stripped of their nitrogen and burned for energy instead of being used for other vital functions. For example, on a very-low-calorie diet, the body's priorities change, forcing dietary protein to be used for energy. That's why it's important to eat enough protein, to prevent the tissues in your body from being broken down and used for energy.

Picking Protein Sources

Your body isn't able to store significant amounts of amino acids, so you have to eat protein regularly. Meat is one of the richest sources of dietary protein. So, too, are dairy products.

Beans, nuts, and cereal grains are also good dietary sources of protein.

Though meat is one of the best protein sources, it is also the biggest source of fat in the U.S. diet, so choose other protein foods, too. Whitefish are delicious low-fat sources of protein that can replace some of the beef and pork you may currently be eating.

The Myth of Protein as a Power Food

In recent years, protein has acquired a reputation as a super nutrient—a substance that can improve athletic performance, aid in weight-reduction programs, and enhance overall health. And it's been assumed that if a moderate amount of protein is good, then more protein must be even better.

The myths surrounding protein have led athletes, especially bodybuilders, to follow high-protein diets or take large amounts of protein or amino-acid powders and pills in the belief that the supplements will help develop muscles and keep them in peak physical condition. While it's true that some athletes, such as bodybuilders, weight lifters, and endurance athletes, may require more protein than recommended in the RDA, mainly because they are building muscle, their needs are easily met by the typical American diet. There is no need for a high-protein diet or protein supplements of any kind.

The regular consumption of amino-acid supplements is a potentially dangerous fad. And because of the potential toxicity of large doses of single amino acids, the Food and Drug Administration (FDA) no longer recognizes them as safe.

CARBOHYDRATES

Carbohydrates—much maligned and too long ignored—are now center-stage attractions in a healthy diet. Many health experts recommend that between 55 percent and 78 percent of the calories you eat every day come from carbohydrates.

You'll find carbohydrates in an amazing array of foods, from those with a healthy image (whole-grain cereals, pasta, and bread) to those dismissed as so-called "junk food" (cookies, cakes, and candy). All carbohydrates have one thing in common, however; they provide a readily available supply of energy to the body.

Nutritionists categorize carbohydrates as either simple or complex. Complex carbohydrates can be further categorized as either digestible (starches) or indigestible (fiber), depending on their chemical composition. But all carbohydrates are made of the three elements carbon, hydrogen, and oxygen arranged in rings. These rings may stand alone or be strung into chains that are two rings to hundreds of rings long. The longer the chain, the more complex the carbohydrate.

Simple Carbohydrates

Glucose, sucrose, fructose, maltose, and lactose are common simple carbohydrates, or simple sugars. Your body is able to convert any of these sugars directly into energy, or it can store them as fat. Glucose and fructose, which are single-ring sugars, are called monosaccharides. These simplest of sugars are primarily found in honey and fruit.

The sugars sucrose, maltose, and lactose contain two rings and are called disaccharides. When the body digests any of these sugars, it first splits them into simpler single-ring monosaccharides. Sucrose, made of one ring of glucose hooked to one ring of fructose, is what you know as table sugar. It is also found in molasses, maple syrup, and fruits. Maltose, made of two single glucose rings hooked together, is found in sprouting grains, malted milk, malted cereals, and some corn syrups. Lactose, or milk sugar, is made of a single ring of glucose hooked to one ring of another monosaccharide, galactose. A large percentage of the population lacks the enzyme needed to break these two rings apart. This condition is called lactose intolerance. (See Lactose Intolerance in Part II.)

Sucrose and fructose are the sugars most commonly added during food processing. Corn syrup, which is used in many baked goods, gets its sweetness from glucose and maltose. In recent years, food processors have learned how to make inexpensive high-fructose corn syrups by rearranging the glucose ring to make fructose. High-fructose syrups now replace most of the sucrose in sodas.

Complex Carbohydrates

Starches, made of hundreds of glucose rings and called polysaccharides, are the major source of energy in the human diet. Grains, beans, and some fruits and vegetables are rich sources of starch.

In the digestive system, large starch molecules are broken down, or digested, into individual glucose molecules. It is these individual glucose molecules, not the original starch molecule, that are absorbed from the digestive tract into the bloodstream. When a person says they have "high blood sugar," they are talking about having too much glucose in their bloodstream; that glucose can come from sucrose or starches.

Fiber is a complex mixture of many indigestible substances that make up the structural material of plants. (See Fiber.) The main difference between fiber and starch is that the body is able to digest starch but not fiber.

Carbohydrates as Fuel

Carbohydrates are like high-octane fuel for your body. When you eat carbohydrates, complex or simple, your body converts them to fuel in the form of glucose. Glucose is the form of carbohydrate the body uses directly for energy; it is the preferred fuel for the brain and central nervous system. The body's delicate regulatory system automatically maintains close control over the level of glucose, or sugar, in your blood, because if it goes too high or too low, it can quickly prove harmful or even fatal.

If all carbohydrates are converted to glucose in the body, why is there such a push to choose unrefined foods such as oatmeal over refined sugars like hard candy? After all, by the time a cell metabolizes glucose, it doesn't seem to matter what source it originally came from. There are several good reasons.

SMART CHOICES FOR COMPLEX CARBS

Bagels	Pasta
Beans	Peas
Corn	Rice
Crackers	Rolls
French bread	Sandwich bread
Low-sugar cereals	Sweet potatoes
Oat bran	Wheat germ
Oatmeal	White potatoes

The type of carbohydrate you eat greatly influences how fast your body produces the much-needed fuel. Basically, if you eat complex carbohydrates like bread, rice, oats, or beans, blood sugar forms in a slow, steady, gentle way, and you produce only a small amount of insulin. (Insulin is the hormone that regulates blood-sugar level; a high concentration of sugar in the blood stimulates the secretion of insulin.) If, on the other hand, you consume mostly simple sugars, your body converts them right away into blood sugar, boosting insulin quickly. Such a sudden boost in insulin can cause blood sugar to drop just as suddenly, stimulating hunger prematurely.

A diet that consists of mostly simple sugars tends to cause these out-of-control peaks and valleys in blood-sugar levels. In contrast, complex carbohydrates that are high in fiber are absorbed more slowly and, as a result, tend to give you the steady-as-she-goes energy you need for the long haul. (The total amount and type of food eaten along with carbohydrate also influences how quickly blood sugar rises.)

Unrefined complex carbohydrates offer a wide assortment of vitamins and minerals in addition to calories. And many starchy foods contain dietary fiber, unless they have been processed to remove it. In contrast, foods high in refined sugar tend to be low in fiber and most other nutrients.

Despite the obvious advantages to eating starchy foods, there have been significant shifts in the types of carbohydrates Americans typically put on their plates. As we have been transformed from a mostly rural society to a more affluent, industrialized one, we eat fewer complex carbohydrates while eating more sugars, particularly corn syrup and other sweeteners hidden in processed foods.

Cereal grains contain an average of 75 percent carbohydrate; vegetables are about 10 to 15 percent carbohydrate. Animal foods, on the other hand, contain a mere one percent carbohydrate. With the exception of lactose (which comes from milk), most dietary sugars come from plants. Plants use some of their carbohydrate for their own needs; the rest is stored in seeds, leaves, stalks, roots, and tubers.

The biochemistry of plants explains why some starchy vegetables become less sweet after they are harvested. The carbohydrate that is initially stored in the plant in the form of sugar gradually converts to starch. This is why corn that is right off the stalk is sweetest, and why carrots grow tougher and more bitter as their freshness wanes. Most fruits, on the other hand, tend to become sweeter as they ripen—as their starch reserves are converted to sugar.

Is Sugar a Poison?

Sugar is not a poison, nor is it addictive, despite what some people claim. Although there has been some speculation that it's possible to become dependent on carbohydrates in general, there is no evidence that you can become addicted to sugar. However, sugar provides no nutrients (other than calories), and eating too many sugary foods can lead to poor nutrition by crowding out more nutrient-dense foods from your diet.

Do Carbohydrates Make You Fat?

Although many Americans shun carbohydrates such as bread and rice as fattening, nothing could be further from the truth. In reality, carbohydrate calories are your best bet when you're trying to lose weight or when you're just trying to eat more healthy foods. But you do need to watch what you pile on top of those carbs. (See "Carb Spoilers" to see how much fat damage common toppings can cause.)

Carbohydrates provide only four calories per gram. Starchy foods also offer the advantage of being filling due to their bulk while being relatively high in nutrients. Studies show that the body may actually be less efficient at converting carbohydrates to body fat than it is at converting dietary fat into body fat.

CARB SPOILERS

Piling these toppings on carbohydrates, such as bread or potatoes, can turn these healthful foods into fat- and calorie-laden monsters.

Spoiler	Serving	Fat (grams)
Butter	1 tbsp	12
Margarine	1 tbsp	11
Mayonnaise	1 tbsp	11
Cream cheese	1 oz	10
Tartar sauce	1 tbsp	8
Cheese spread	1 oz	4-7

Moreover, the process of digesting carbohydrates burns more calories than does the process of digesting an equivalent amount of fats. Studies at the University of Massachusetts indicate that the body uses up to 25 percent of excess carbohydrate calories to convert the carbohydrate to body fat—leaving only 75 percent of the extra carbohydrate calories for actual fat storage. By comparison, 97 percent of excess fat calories are stored as body fat.

Carbohydrates and Cavities

Any fermentable carbohydrate food can contribute to tooth decay if you don't brush your teeth soon after eating. Given enough time, enzymes in saliva break starch down to sugar right in the mouth. Bacteria normally present then ferment the sugar, producing acid that eats through the tooth enamel and causes cavities. Residue from sticky-sweet snacks (including "natural" ones such as raisins and honey-sweetened granola bars) may cling to tooth enamel just as tightly as foods you normally consider sugary treats, giving the sugar time to be fermented to acid. You may be surprised to learn that research shows crackers are one of the worst offenders in terms of promoting cavities. (See Dental Disease in Part II for more information on diet and cavities.)

Sugar and Diabetes

Sugar cannot cause you to develop diabetes, although sugar can make matters worse if you already have the disease. (See Diabetes in Part II for more information.)

Hyperactivity

Sugar does not cause hyperactivity in children. Most experts agree that sugar does not cause changes in a child's behavior. In pointing a finger at sugar, parents often fail to consider the potent effect of a child's surroundings. Children usually consume sweets at birthday parties or during holiday get-togethers, when they are likely to be excited anyway. The charged atmosphere, not the sugar, may cause what some people label hyperactive behavior.

FAT

Fat. Just the mention of the word conjures up unpleasant images of fat bodies, heart disease, and cancer. But fat is not inherently bad. In fact, it is a vital part of your body's makeup. Only when you overindulge does fat become the dietary bad guy everyone loves to hate.

Fats are actually just one of several members of the lipid family. Lipids also include hormones and cholesterol. Like carbohydrates, fats are made of the elements carbon, hydrogen, and oxygen, but their structure is considerably different. Each cell in your body contains lipids that are responsible for critical functions such as storing energy, supporting the structure of each of the millions of the body's cells, and storing or transporting the fat-soluble vitamins A, D, E, and K.

Fat in the food you eat is made up of fatty acids, which fall into one of three categories: saturated fatty acids, monounsaturated fatty acids, and polyunsaturated fatty acids. It may come as a surprise to learn that all foods contain mixtures of the three. A fat is referred to simply as saturated, monounsaturated, or polyunsaturated according to which type of fatty acid predominates.

Animal fats, such as those in meat and dairy products, are high in saturated fatty acids and are usually referred to as being "saturated." The only plant oils that are saturated are coconut oil, palm oil, and palm kernel oil.

In general, the more solid a fat is at room temperature, the more saturated it is. This is a helpful clue when you're in the store trying to decide between fats. Stick margarine, for example, is more saturated than margarine in tubs.

Saturated fats are frowned on because most of them tend to raise blood cholesterol and increase the risk of heart disease. Scientists suspect that these saturated fatty acids somehow interfere with the removal of artery-clogging cholesterol in the blood. As a result, cholesterol accumulates and eventually deposits itself in arteries.

Monounsaturated fatty acids are found in such foods as avocados, nuts, peanut butter, and canola and olive oils. Monounsaturated oils are liquid at room temperature but tend to turn cloudy in the refrigerator.

Your body can make saturated fatty acids, but it cannot produce all of the polyunsaturated fatty acids you need. That's why you must get these polyunsaturated fatty acids in your diet. The so-called "essential fatty acids"—linolenic and linoleic—should make up about three percent of your daily calories. Polyunsaturated fatty acids are abundant in most vegetable and fish oils.

These essential fatty acids play a role in normal cholesterol metabolism, in keeping all the cells of your body in top shape and in the production of vital cell regulators such as prostaglandins. Prostaglandins are hormonelike compounds involved in several body processes, including regulation of blood pressure and blood coagulation.

Feeding Off the Fat of the Land

Most Americans consume too much fat. Unfortunately, we evolved in conditions of scarcity, so our bodies adapted and developed the ability to store endless quantities of fat. We're saving up for the next famine, which is unlikely to come.

When your body burns fat, it produces more than twice the number of calories than when it burns proteins or carbohydrate. A gram of fat yields about nine calories, compared to four from a gram of protein or carbohydrate. But fat carries a double whammy. Not only does it provide more calories per gram, but each calorie is more determined to be stored as body fat than are protein calories or calories from carbohydrates. That is why, calorie for calorie, fat is more "fattening" than carbohydrate or protein. When we eat dietary fat, we tend to store it as body fat. It makes perfect sense then, that in order to lose weight or maintain normal weight, limiting fat is the number one dietary action to take. (It is important to note, however, that infants and children under the age of two years should not have their fat intake restricted, since they need a higher intake of calories from fat for normal growth and development.)

The Truth About *Trans* Fatty Acids

Recent evidence strongly suggests that *trans* fatty acids—formed when polyunsaturated and monounsaturated fats are hydrogenated to make them more solid—can raise blood cholesterol, possibly as much as saturated fat. Actually, studies began suggesting this as early as the 1950s, but no one paid much attention until recently when Dutch researchers found that hydrogenated oils had unhealthy effects on blood lipids. People who consumed large amounts of hydrogenated fats had higher levels of low-density lipoproteins, or LDLs (the "bad" cholesterol that increases risk of heart disease), and reduced levels of high-density lipoproteins, or HDLs (the "good" cholesterol that protects against heart disease). More recent findings from the long-running Nurses' Health Study analyzed the diet of more than 85,000 nurses over eight years and found that those who ate a lot of margarine, cookies, biscuits, and cakes—all foods high in *trans* fatty acids—had a higher risk of heart disease than those who ate little.

How to spot *trans* fatty acids? You know a product contains at least some *trans* fatty acids when the label lists "partially hydrogenated oil" as an ingredient. What to do about *trans* fatty acids: Don't switch from margarine to butter. The key is to use as little fat as possible overall. Do that, and *trans* fatty acids in your diet drop automatically.

Clearing Up Cholesterol Confusion

Cholesterol has been the object of more than its fair share of confusion, leaving a lot of questions unanswered. Is cholesterol a fat? (No. It's a hormonelike compound which is a member of the lipid family.) Does fat contain cholesterol? (Again, the answer is no. Many high-fat foods are also high in cholesterol. But even some low-fat foods, like skinless chicken breast or shellfish, contain cholesterol.) Does the cholesterol in the food you eat go directly to your arteries? (Yes and no. The process is very complex; it depends on how much cholesterol you consume and how efficiently it is absorbed, as well as on your genes, your weight, and your intake of other nutrients.)

Dietary cholesterol, by itself, has a smaller impact on blood-cholesterol levels than saturated fats or *trans* fatty acids in your diet do. Still, the American Heart Association (AHA) recommends limiting your cholesterol intake to less than 300 milligrams a day. Dietary cholesterol is found only in foods derived from animals, such as meat, poultry, fish, eggs, and dairy products. You won't find it in any plant-based food. One egg yolk contains approximately 213 milligrams of cholesterol. The AHA has given the green light to four egg yolks (all the cholesterol resides in the yolk) a week, but that includes yolks used in cooking and in processed foods.

Your body does need some cholesterol for synthesis of sex hormones, bile acids, and vitamin D, and it is an important constituent of all the cells in your body. Because your body can make it, it is not an essential nutrient. When everything works in concert, your body's production of cholesterol drops as your blood cholesterol begins to rise, thus keeping the blood level from rising too high. But sometimes this feedback mechanism doesn't work normally, and blood-cholesterol levels rise and remain elevated.

Cholesterol travels back and forth from the liver to your body's cells by way of the bloodstream. But, because it cannot move through the bloodstream on its own, it must be carried.

The cholesterol carriers are called lipoproteins. Lipoproteins, like cholesterol, are produced in the liver. HDLs carry the most cholesterol out of cells and deliver it to the liver for processing. LDLs either deliver their cholesterol to cells or leave some behind in arteries. Thus the designations of "good" HDL cholesterol, the kind processed in your liver, and "bad" LDL cholesterol, which is left behind in the arteries.

Fat and Heart Disease

Studies in the United States and abroad have established a clear association between high blood-cholesterol levels and heart disease. Other studies show that people who eat too much fat, particularly saturated fat, have higher total cholesterol and LDL-cholesterol levels than people who eat diets that are relatively low in fat. (See Heart Disease in Part II.)

Fat and Cancer

Eating a diet high in fat may increase the risk of developing cancer, particularly cancers of the colon and breast. None of the research is as conclusive as that linking high-fat diets to heart disease. In fact, the link between fat and breast cancer has come under increasing scrutiny in the last few years because of new research showing little or no association between the two. So the jury is still out on the connection between fat and breast cancer.

Fat Recommendations

Most scientists believe that fat is the single most important nutrient to limit if you want to reduce your risk of chronic disease. Try to keep your fat intake to less than 30 percent of your total calories. Some experts even go so far as to recommend cutting down to 25 percent or 20 percent of calories. Of the fat you put on your plate, less than one-third should be saturated (the less, the better), less than one-third polyunsaturated, and the rest monounsaturated.

There is another camp of cholesterol researchers that says you don't need to lower your fat intake drastically to reduce your blood-cholesterol and LDL levels. Rather, they say, just reduce your intake of saturated fatty acids and replace them with carbohydrates and vegetable oils rich in monounsaturated fats such as olive and canola oils.

Which is better? That remains to be proven. But current research suggests that monounsaturates do have a healthy edge. While all unsaturated fats help lower total blood cholesterol when they replace saturated fats in the diet, there is some evidence that monounsaturated fats may be less likely to lower beneficial HDL cholesterol in the process.

Furthermore, monounsaturated fats may be safer. Polyunsaturated fats are naturally less stable than monounsaturated

---

CALCULATING THE FAT

Most health experts recommend you limit fat intake to 30 percent or less of the day's total calories. You can either choose foods with no more than three grams of fat per 100 calories (fat provides nine calories per gram) or limit your daily fat intake as follows:

If your total daily calories are:	Limit your daily fat grams to:
1,000	33
1,200	40
1,500	50
1,800	60
2,100	70
2,400	80
2,700	90

fats and are more likely to combine with oxygen to form free radicals, which damage tissues, and, ultimately, place you at higher risk for diseases such as arthritis, cataracts, and cancer. Furthermore, polyunsaturated fats may impair the immune system. The net effect of polyunsaturated fats is far from established. But it's a concern that makes the move to monounsaturated fats a smart one.

Olive and canola oils, containing primarily monounsaturated fats, may have the nutrition edge, but a healthy diet can include such cooking oils as soybean oil, sesame oil, walnut oil, hazelnut oil, sunflower oil, corn oil, and safflower oil. It can also include margarine, especially the less-saturated soft margarines (tub margarines), and diet margarines, which have more water and less fat. The key is to go easy on all types of oils and margarine.

Cutting Back on Fat

If you eat a typical high-fat American diet, your goal should be to reduce the amount of fat you consume overall. This means eating about a third less fat. (If you are already consuming a diet that is lower in fat than the typical American diet, keep up the good work.) Choose mainly low-fat food, cook with little or no fat, and add as little fat as possible to prepared foods.

Foods naturally low in fat such as fruits, vegetables, and whole-grain products form the foundation of a healthy diet. Replacing high-fat foods with these nutritious foods is as important as reducing the amount of fat you eat. The fiber and nutrients in fruits, vegetables, and whole grains are vital to staying healthy and reducing your risk of cancer. Just remember not to cover them with high-fat toppings (See "Carb Spoilers" in the carbohydrates chapter).

To take in less fat, you'll need to choose smaller and fewer portions of high-fat foods. The following is a shopping guide for ferreting out fat.

Meats

• Choose leaner cuts of meat. Look for beef cuts with "loin" or "round" in the name, such as sirloin, tenderloin, or eye of round.

• Another clue to the fat content of a piece of meat is its grade. "Prime" beef, because it is heavily marbled, has the highest fat content. Prime is followed by "choice" and "select." Choice cuts contain about one-third less fat than prime cuts. The fat content of select cuts is about half that of prime.

• For leaner pork, look for cuts with "loin" or "leg" in the name. Boiled ham and Canadian bacon are also lean choices.

• Trim all the fat you can see off of meat before you cook it.

• Limit your meat servings to no more than six ounces a day; a three-ounce portion of meat is about the size of a deck of playing cards.

• Buy extra-lean ground beef, or ask your butcher to freshly grind a leaner cut.

• Opt for skinless chicken or turkey breast. It's low in fat, saturated fat, and cholesterol. White meat is leaner than dark meat.

• Choose more fish and shellfish. Even the fattiest fish have only about as much fat as the leanest meats. But skip the breaded or batter-dipped varieties. Fish and shellfish are comparable to lean meat and poultry in cholesterol content, but they supply less saturated and total fat.

Dairy

• Choose skim milk or one-percent milk over whole milk.

• Try evaporated skim milk as a substitute for cream in recipes or in your coffee.

• Shop for reduced-fat cheeses or cheese made with part-skim milk. Look for ones that provide no more than five grams of fat per ounce.

• Try plain, low-fat yogurt instead of sour cream in dips and sauces.

• Try reduced-calorie cream cheeses and margarines.

SEEKING OUT SATURATED FATS

Food	Saturated Fat (grams)
Chicken breast, skinless (3 oz, roasted)	0.9
Half & half (1 tbsp)	1
Pork, tenderloin (3 oz, cooked)	1.4
Beef, eye of round (3 oz, cooked)	1.5
Egg, large (1 egg)	1.5
Chicken leg, skinless (3 oz, roasted)	2
Beef, top sirloin (3 oz, cooked)	2.4
Pork, loin chop (3 oz, cooked)	2.5
Chicken thigh, skinless (3 oz, roasted)	2.6
Pork, sirloin roast (3 oz, cooked)	3.1
Ice milk, 5.1% butterfat (1 cup)	3.7
Beef, flank (3 oz, cooked)	3.7
Milk, whole (1 cup)	4.7
Cheddar cheese (1 oz)	5
Ice cream, regular, 10% butterfat (1 cup)	7.8
Ground beef, 85% lean (3 oz, broiled)	12
Ground turkey (3 oz, broiled)	12
Ice cream, premium, 16% butterfat (1 cup)	13.1
Ground beef, 80% lean (3 oz, broiled)	15

Produce

• Eat more fresh fruits and vegetables. They're virtually fat-free.

• Avoid frozen vegetables smothered in butter or cheese sauces.

• Make vegetables, rather than meat, the focus of your meal.

Breads and Cereals

• Eat more whole-grain breads and cereals.

• Some low-fat breads include French bread, Italian bread, pita bread, English muffins, bagels, and corn tortillas. Though they're not high in fiber, they are good sources of complex carbohydrates.

• Stay away from high-fat fare such as croissants, crescent rolls, biscuits, scones, sweet rolls, Danish pastries, and donuts.

• Opt for low-fat crackers such as saltines, matzo, melba toast, rye crisp, and oyster crackers. Limit cheese- or butter-flavored crackers.

FIBER

What Is Fiber?

By definition, fiber is the part of plants that your body can't digest. You'll find at least some fiber in all fruits, vegetables, whole grains, and legumes, but never in animal products, like milk, meat, or eggs.

Because fiber passes right through your system undisturbed, it provides no calories or energy. But its presence in the intestines can have a dramatic effect on your health, depending on the type of fiber.

There are six distinct types of fiber: cellulose, hemicellulose, lignin, gums, mucilages, and pectin. All except one—lignin—are complex carbohydrates, but because your body lacks the enzymes needed to break them down, they can't be absorbed and used for energy.

To simplify matters, think of the different fibers as either soluble or insoluble, depending upon whether they dissolve in water. This will help you understand why all fibers are not created equal.

High-fiber foods generally contain both soluble and insoluble fibers, but are often considered a source only of the one they are richest in. Because soluble and insoluble fibers have some very different health effects, it's important to include both types in your diet.

But don't rely on a crunchy sound or texture as your clue to the fiber content of foods. You may get fooled. For instance, celery looks and sounds like it contains a lot of fiber, but it really has very little. Read on to discover where to get the fiber you need.

Insoluble Fiber

This is the type of fiber that probably comes to mind first—the stuff in bran cereals that you eat "to keep things moving." Insoluble fiber is like a sponge, soaking in up to 15 times its weight in water. Your bowel contents expand when you eat insoluble fiber, such as wheat bran. This swelling makes your stools softer and bulkier. The bulk increases pressure against the intestinal wall, stimulating it to contract and speeding the contents through your system. This makes insoluble fiber a natural for preventing constipation and other conditions, such as hemorrhoids, that are aggravated by stagnating stool. (See Part II for more information on the role of fiber in preventing and treating constipation and hemorrhoids.)

FOODS HIGH IN INSOLUBLE FIBER

Bran cereals
Brown rice
Corn and popcorn
Fruits, especially apples, berries, pears
Vegetables, especially asparagus, beets, carrots, kale, okra,
    peas, potatoes (white and sweet), spinach
Whole-wheat breads and pastas

A softer stool eliminates the wear and tear that a hard stool can have on the intestinal wall and limits the amount of time it comes into contact with the wall. These effects may decrease the risk of colon and rectal cancers.

Soluble Fiber

This type of fiber doesn't absorb water; it dissolves in it, forming gummy or gel-like substances. It comes in very handy in the fight to prevent heart disease and treat diabetes. The resulting gums and gels tie up carbohydrates and bile acids, lowering both blood-sugar and blood-cholesterol levels.

FOODS HIGH IN SOLUBLE FIBER

Barley
Dried beans and peas
Fruits, especially apples, apricots, figs, mangos, oranges,
     peaches, plums, rhubarb, strawberries
Lentils
Oats/oatmeal (oat bran)
Vegetables, especially broccoli, brussels sprouts, cabbage,
     carrots, okra, potatoes (white and sweet), turnips

Fiber's Disease-Prevention Powers

Twenty years ago, researchers began to prove what Sylvester Graham (of graham cracker fame) preached 100 years ago, that fiber can help prevent disease. Here's what we know today:

Gastrointestinal Disease

Because insoluble fiber softens stools and speeds their passage, it's the time-honored cure—and prevention—for constipation (just add water and exercise). A high-fiber diet promotes intestinal-muscle tone, which harsh laxatives often destroy. Likewise, softer stools help prevent hemorrhoids, which can form or be aggravated by straining.

Fiber is also believed to prevent diverticular disease, a condition where outpouchings develop on the intestinal wall, possibly as a result of inadequate muscle tone. There's also evidence suggesting that people who eat lots of fiber are less likely to suffer gallstones, duodenal ulcers, hiatal hernia, irritable bowel, and varicose veins.

Cancer

Although not all the evidence is unanimous or incontrovertible, there's a heap of data to suggest that eating a high-fiber diet reduces your risk for colon and rectal cancers. The original tip-off came from studying the diet of Africans who eat tremendous amounts of fiber and in whom colorectal cancer is virtually nonexistent. Studies of other cultures have found a similar link between low fiber intake and colorectal cancer.

Here's how experts think fiber works to protect your colon:

• By moving your bowel contents along faster, fiber shortens the amount of time that potentially harmful substances spend in contact with the intestinal wall.

• By creating a larger stool, it helps dilute carcinogens (cancer-causing agents).

• By influencing the type of bacteria in the intestines, it discourages toxic substances from forming (some bacteria form toxins as byproducts of their own metabolism).

• By binding with toxins, it helps to flush out carcinogens.

Diabetes

Soluble fiber, like that found in oatmeal and fruit, is the hero here. Because it slows the digestion and absorption of carbohydrates, soluble fiber can stabilize blood-sugar levels and may reduce or eliminate the need for oral medication in some individuals with diabetes.

Heart Disease

The brief love affair Americans had with oat bran in the 1980s was the result of research that showed it lowered blood-cholesterol levels. Unfortunately, oat bran was treated as a miracle cure. Still, the subsequent downfall of oat bran in the public's eye was just as unfortunate. Oat bran lost respect as a result of misreporting of a study that, not surprisingly, found that oat bran did not benefit healthy people with normal blood-cholesterol levels.

In fact, oat bran and other soluble fibers, particularly beans and barley, have consistently shown an ability to modestly lower blood cholesterol levels in those whose blood cholesterol levels were already high. Conveniently, the benefit seems to be greatest for those individuals who have the highest blood cholesterol levels.

How does it work? Researchers think the gums and gels bind with substances called bile acids in the intestines, preventing them from being reabsorbed into the body and forcing their excretion. This obliges the body to make more bile acids, which requires cholesterol. Voilà—this lowers the amount of cholesterol circulating in your blood.

Weight Control

Fiber adds bulk to your diet, filling up the stomach and delaying emptying so you feel full longer. And high-fiber foods can rarely be eaten fast, forcing you to take more time to eat and allowing you time to realize you're full. All of this is helpful when you're trying to lose weight.

How Much Fiber Should You Get?

If you're typical, you probably eat only about 10 to 15 grams of fiber a day right now. Experts recommend you double that, at least, to 20 to 35 grams a day, with about one-quarter of that (five to nine grams) being soluble fiber, and the rest insoluble.

Do you have to calculate all this? Certainly not. That's the beauty of eating a varied diet. If you concentrate on eating a variety of whole foods, such as fruits, vegetables, legumes, and whole grains, you will automatically be set. Just don't do it all of a sudden. Give your body time to adjust to the new fiber routine, otherwise you might experience bloating, gas, and intestinal pain.

Too Much of a Good Thing?

Theoretically, you can get too much fiber. But the reality is that few people come close to what's considered too much (more than 50 grams of fiber a day) to make it a significant problem.

The most common side effect from adding insoluble fiber to the diet is gas and bloating, but that's only a problem if you add fiber too fast. You can easily prevent gastrointestinal trouble by adding fiber to your diet gradually, over six to eight weeks. The most serious problem that can result from a high-fiber diet—intestinal blockage—results from not drinking enough fluids. Because insoluble fiber soaks up any available water, you must increase your fluid intake along with your fiber intake to prevent this problem.

What about the warnings that too much fiber interferes with mineral absorption? It's true that insoluble fiber can bind with minerals—especially calcium—but losses are probably not of importance until you're eating more than 35 grams of fiber a day.

If you're eating a mixed-fiber diet, the mineral problem may not matter. That's because soluble fiber, notably pectin, actually improves your absorption of minerals—all except calcium—so it's a trade-off. Too much soluble fiber has also been linked to increased colon cancer. But the evidence is scanty and comes mostly from animal studies. Including a variety of soluble and insoluble fibers in the diet is probably the best defense.

What about children? It's good to get kids used to eating whole grains and fresh fruits and vegetables when they are young. But be sure you don't overdo it. High-fiber foods fill them up quickly, and they may not take in enough calories for their growing bodies' needs.

What About Fiber Supplements?

It may be tempting to think you can get all the fiber that your body needs from a pill that you buy at the store or order from a catalog. But it's not that easy. Fiber supplements sold for weight loss are a gimmick. The fiber in supplements has been ground up so small as to be worthless to your body. Real foods are much more effective, but the same thing happens to them, too, if you start altering their structure. Eat an apple whole and you'll get more fiber than if you eat it as applesauce. You get even less benefit when you reduce that fiber-rich apple to apple cider or apple juice.

VITAMINS

If you reach for a bottle of vitamins whenever you start to feel a little tired, run-down, or out of sorts, then you have a basic misunderstanding of what vitamins are and what they can do for you.

Yes, vitamins are important. They get their name because they are vital to life. Take in too little, and you will eventually develop a deficiency, which can kill you if it's not corrected.

Now that vitamins have your respect, here's what they can't do. They provide no calories, which means they do not, by themselves, provide energy. However, vitamins are an integral part of processing carbohydrates, proteins, and fats, all of which do provide calories. Only in this sense do they affect your energy level.

By its nature, a little bit of a vitamin goes a long way. That is, it takes only a tiny amount to sustain life—the grand total of all the vitamins you need could fit into an eighth of a teaspoon. But, tantalizing new research suggests that, for some vitamins, amounts larger than what is required to simply keep you functioning may help protect against some chronic diseases.

The following is a vitamin-by-vitamin guide to good health.

FAT-SOLUBLE VITAMINS

Fat-soluble vitamins can be stored away in your body, so deficiencies are unlikely (unless the vitamin is missing from the diet for a long time), but toxicity is a possibility. Vitamin D and vitamin A are toxic at high doses; vitamins E and K are not known to be toxic.

Vitamin A (retinol)/Beta-carotene (carotene)

Vitamin A is a good news/bad news nutrient. That is, as a vitamin, it's necessary for life, but it's easy to get too much. "Preformed" vitamin A is found in animal foods, such as milk, butter, cheese, egg yolks, and liver.

But the double billing above is warranted because beta-carotene fulfills your vitamin A needs without the risk of overdose. Even better, as an antioxidant, it may fight heart disease and cancer. So it's more than a good substitute; it's actually superior.

There are other plant-derived carotenoids that can be converted to vitamin A in the body, but beta-carotene is the most abundant and best known. Beta-carotene is converted to vitamin A only when your body needs it, so there's no excess to pile up in toxic amounts in the liver.

Carotenoids are the red, orange, and yellow pigments in plants—like pumpkin, carrots, red peppers, and mangos. In general, the deeper the color, the more carotene present in the plant.

If you eat a lot of foods rich in beta-carotene, the worst that will happen is your skin may look orange, but there's absolutely no danger from this—just embarrassment. Many a new mother has rushed her seemingly jaundiced baby to the doctor, only to find that the child has simply "overdosed" on strained carrots.

But color is not a foolproof guide to the carotene content of foods. In some carotenoid-rich foods, for example, the chlorophyll overwhelms the red-orange-yellow hues, so green predominates; such is the case with kale, spinach, and broccoli. And a few orange foods—such as oranges, for instance—are not rich in carotenes. It seems that Mother Nature likes to keep us guessing.

In order to get the best absorption of vitamin A or beta-carotene from foods, eat a food that contains fat in the same meal.

Functions: Growth, infection resistance, night vision, bone and tooth development, and antioxidant protection

Deficiency: Rare in the United States. Symptoms include night blindness (you may remember your mother telling you over and over again to eat your carrots for good vision), dry scaly skin, tooth decay, abnormal bone development, loss of appetite, and diarrhea.

---

17 SOURCES OF BETA-CAROTENE

Apricot nectar	Papayas
Apricots	Persimmons
Cantaloupe	Pumpkins
Carrot juice	Soups and stews with
Carrots	carrots
Greens (beet, collard,	Spinach
mustard, turnip)	Sweet potatoes
Kale	Tomato juice
Mangos	Winter squash
Nectarines	

Toxicity: Vitamin A is toxic at doses greater than 50,000 International Units (IU) in adults and greater than 20,000 IU in children.

Beta-carotene is not known to be toxic. Symptoms of vitamin A toxicity include blurred vision, hair loss, irritability, aching bones, nausea, and vomiting.

Vitamin D (calciferol)

This is one of three vitamins with a unique characteristic: You don't have to get it in your diet. (The others are vitamin K and biotin.) That's because the body has a complex mechanism by which it can synthesize vitamin D when the skin is exposed to sunlight.

While the synthesis mechanism is complex, vitamin D is the easiest vitamin to obtain. Experts say you only need to expose your face and hands to the sun for 10 to 15 minutes. Because sunscreens will block the sun's intended effect, you must expose unprotected skin. Try the early morning or late afternoon hours, to avoid the possibility of sunburn. If you burn easily, five minutes may be all you need to generate enough vitamin D. Don't worry if you don't catch some rays every day. Two or three times a week is enough, because your body can store vitamin D. If you live in a perennially cloudy climate (say, Seattle or London), you may not be able to rely on the sun, and you'll need to stock up on dietary sources.

That's easier said than done. Until 1992, you might have felt secure if you drank milk, because milk has been fortified with vitamin D since the 1930s, to prevent rickets—the deficiency disease caused by lack of vitamin D. But a survey of East Coast dairies revealed milk to be a shockingly unreliable source of vitamin D. Some milk labeled as containing the vitamin actually had none at all. In all, 62 percent of the milks were underfortified. Ten percent were overfortified.

Vitamin D's role in calcium absorption is legendary. Without it, children get rickets—with the classic bowed legs—and adults get osteomalacia—a similar softening of the bones. A new theory has emerged that vitamin D and calcium also offer important protection from colon cancer. That could be why people who live in sunny Florida experience much less colon cancer than those living up North.

But vitamin D is another good news/bad news nutrient—not one to fool around with. It is the most toxic vitamin; symptoms appear at just five times the recommended amount (the RDA of vitamin D for men and women ages 1 year through 24 years is 10 micrograms; after age 24, it's 5 micrograms). Therefore, supplements of vitamin D—other than a multivitamin that provides no more than 100 percent of the RDA—are a bad idea.

Functions: Bone formation and strength, calcium absorption, tooth strength, and proper functioning of nervous system

Deficiency: Rickets in children; osteomalacia in adults (rare). Breast-fed infants may not get enough vitamin D, unless exposed to sunlight or given a supplement. As you age, your skin is less able to convert sunlight to vitamin D. Symptoms include poor growth, deformed bone growth (bowed legs, malformed joints), poor tooth development, bone pain, muscle weakness, brittle bones, and nervous-system sensitivity.

Major Food Sources: Egg yolk, canned herring, liver, milk (1% fortified with vitamin D), sardines, and yogurt made from fortified

Toxicity: Overdosing on vitamin D can cause dangerously high blood-calcium levels, especially in children. The toxic level is only five times the RDA. Check to be sure you aren't doubling up on vitamin D in a multivitamin and a calcium supplement that contains vitamin D. Symptoms include nausea, vomiting, abdominal pain, excessive urination, and weight loss.

Vitamin E (tocopherol)

It used to be that vitamin E was a wallflower nutrient. It wasn't associated with a dramatic deficiency disease and it was relatively easy to get in the diet. But that's all changed, in a big way. Now, vitamin E is hailed as one of the most valuable antioxidant nutrients. The debate these days is over whether to supplement, and if so, how much.

There's no need to look past your diet to prevent a deficiency. Vitamin E is plentiful, concentrated mostly in fats and oils. But there's no way to get 800 International Units—about 50 times the RDA—from foods. That's the amount traditionally used in studies to show significantly lowered risk of heart disease, cancer, and infection. But newer research is racking up results with "only" 100 IU—still more than you could realistically get from foods, because most food sources of the vitamin are high in fat.

Many nutrition experts have never been closer to recommending a single supplement than they are for vitamin E. But your final decision about a supplement will have to be one that you and your doctor make after a thorough discussion of the possible risks and benefits to you.

Functions: Protects red blood cells, muscle, and other vitamins from oxidation

Deficiency: No classic deficiency disease, except in premature infants. Rarely, in adults, may cause anemia, muscle weakness, and inability to concentrate.

Major Food Sources: Kale, nuts, spinach, sunflower seeds, sweet potatoes, vegetables oils, and wheat germ

Toxicity: Not known to be toxic. Demonstrated to be safe in amounts up to 1,000 IU. But high doses can deplete vitamin A stores, alter hormone metabolism, and prolong bleeding. Do not take vitamin E if you also take anticoagulant medication (for example, Coumadin, or warfarin), or are deficient in vitamin K.

Vitamin K

You won't find it in supplements, because this is a nutrient with which few people have problems. It's essential for blood clotting, or *koagulation* in Dutch—a hint as to why it's called vitamin K. Dietary sources aren't really needed, because your body manufactures vitamin K from bacteria in your intestines.

Function: Blood clotting

Deficiency: Rare. Breast-fed babies may not receive adequate vitamin K. Most babies are given an injection within the first few days after birth. The primary symptom is excessive bleeding due to defective blood coagulation.

Toxicity: High doses can cause skin irritation, rash, and itching.

Major Food Sources: Green, leafy vegetables are the best dietary sources; root vegetables, fruits, dairy products, meats, and eggs contain smaller but significant amounts.

WATER-SOLUBLE VITAMINS

Because your body doesn't store water-soluble vitamins, your diet must provide them regularly. For that very reason, it has always been assumed that overdosing was impossible and that any excess that was consumed would be excreted in the urine. We now know that side effects can occur with megadoses of some water-soluble vitamins.

Vitamin C (ascorbic acid)

Vitamin C is the only water-soluble vitamin that's not in the B family, so we'll start with it. Besides, as an antioxidant, it has special importance. (See the special section entitled "Antioxidants—What's all the Fuss?" at the end of this chapter.) Today, we're long past preventing scurvy, the disease that results from a deficiency of vitamin C, and into reducing the risk of chronic diseases, such as cancer, heart disease, and cataracts. (See the profiles for these diseases in Part II.)

17 SOURCES OF VITAMIN C

Broccoli	Mangos
Brussels sprouts	Orange juice
Cantaloupes	Oranges
Cauliflower	Peppers, sweet, red or
Grapefruit juice	green
Grapefruits	Potatoes
Greens, collard	Spinach
Kale	Strawberries
Kiwifruit	Tomatoes

And what about that seemingly endless controversy regarding vitamin C and the common cold? Here's the latest on the "common cold controversy": Most studies have failed to show that megadoses of vitamin C can prevent colds, as asserted by Linus Pauling. But, some research seems to suggest that, if started soon enough after getting a cold, 500 to 1,000 milligrams of vitamin C a day may shorten a cold's duration and lessen its symptoms.

Functions: Wound and bone healing, infection resistance, collagen and blood-vessel strengthening, aiding iron absorption, formation of brain-chemical messengers, and antioxidant protection

Deficiency: Scurvy. Almost unheard of today, because it's so simple to prevent (it only takes a paltry ten milligrams, or less than two ounces of orange juice a day). But what are optimal levels is hotly debated. There's agreement that smokers need about twice the vitamin C of nonsmokers, at least 100 milligrams. Alcoholics may have increased needs also. Symptoms of deficiency include bruising easily, swollen and bleeding gums, tooth decay, slowly healing wounds, nosebleeds, aching joints, fatigue, muscle weakness, shortness of breath, and frequent infections.

Toxicity: At very high doses, over 1,000 milligrams, it may cause diarrhea. There have been scattered reports of abdominal cramps, headaches, sleep disturbances, nausea, and vomiting. Chewable supplements of vitamin C can eat away at the enamel coating of your teeth. Large doses of vitamin C have been reported to interfere with copper levels.

Vitamin B1 (thiamin)

This is one of the ubiquitous B vitamin trio. Many processed foods are enriched with thiamin (and riboflavin and niacin), so there's no longer a threat of deficiency.

Functions: Helps convert sugar and starches into energy and promotes normal appetite, nerve function, growth, and muscle tone.

Deficiency: Beriberi. Rare in the United States, due to enrichment of flour, but still seen in alcoholics and in other countries that eat nonenriched polished white rice as a staple food. Deficiency symptoms can develop in as few as two to three weeks. Early signs of deficiency are wasting of muscles, mental confusion, fluid retention, loss of appetite, and fatigue. The condition progresses to one of two different forms of deficiency. "Wet" beriberi involves fluid accumulation and heart disturbances. "Dry" beriberi involves nerve and muscle problems.

Toxicity: No reports of toxicity from oral supplements

---

10 SOURCES OF THIAMIN

Beans, dried	Fish
Bread, whole wheat or enriched	Nuts
	Pasta, enriched
Brewer's yeast	Pork
Cereals, whole grain or enriched	Sunflower seeds
	Wheat germ

Vitamin B₂ (riboflavin)

Part of the B-complex trio of "enriched stars," riboflavin is considered a "marker" nutrient. If your riboflavin intake is good, it's likely you are getting your fill of the other B vitamins, too. Likewise, if you're deficient in riboflavin, you may be lacking in the others as well. Riboflavin may also be an antioxidant.

Functions: Needed to release energy from carbohydrates, proteins, and fats; promotes good vision and healthy skin

Deficiency: Deficiency of thiamin is not too common in the United States, but it may be seen in strict vegans who eat no dairy products and in alcoholics. Athletes may have increased needs for the vitamin. Children who don't drink milk may not be getting enough. Symptoms of thiamin

---

15 SOURCES OF RIBOFLAVIN

Almonds	Chicken, dark meat
Asparagus	Mackerel
Beef	Milk, skim or 1%
Bread, enriched	Pork
Broccoli	Spinach
Cereal, fortified	Turkey
Cheese, low fat	Wheat germ
(including cottage)	Yogurt, low fat

deficiency include sensitivity of the eyes to light, cracks in the corners of the mouth, and scaly skin.

Toxicity: There have been no reports of toxicity; the intestinal tract has a limited ability to absorb large amounts of this vitamin. However, supplements of riboflavin may interfere with some cancer chemotherapies.

Niacin

Deficiencies of this vitamin were all but wiped out when enrichment of grains began. Niacin is really a catch-all name for two similar substances: nicotinic acid and niacinamide (or nicotinamide). Both can prevent a niacin deficiency. The amino acid tryptophan can also prevent a deficiency, because your body can convert it to niacin.

Nicotinic acid has received a lot of attention in recent years for its role in treating high blood-cholesterol levels. But a lot of do-it-yourselfers have discovered a most disconcerting effect of too much of this form of niacin—called "niacin flush." It's an acute reaction that occurs within minutes of taking large doses. You may feel incredibly hot and itchy, and your face and chest may turn bright red.

15 SOURCES OF NIACIN

Beef	Peanut butter
Bread, enriched	Pork
Cereal, fortified	Sardines
Cheese, low fat*	Sunflower seeds
Chicken	Tuna
Eggs*	Turkey
Liver	Yogurt, low fat*
Milk, skim or 1%*	

*Not good sources of niacin, but provide tryptophan, which can be converted to niacin by the body.

This reaction to nicotinic acid—it doesn't happen with niacinamide—happens to everyone, but some people are more sensitive than others, reacting to as low a dose as 50 milligrams; others may not react unless they take a few hundred milligrams. Generally, if you keep taking it, the flush will become less intense each time. But at levels approaching 1,000 milligrams, other adverse effects can occur: headaches, nausea, hives, fatigue, and skin problems.

The point here is that you should not fool around with large doses of niacin on your own; at such high dosages, it acts more like a medication than a dietary supplement. If you have abnormally high blood-cholesterol levels and you want to try nicotinic acid instead of other medication, consult with your physician. If it's decided that nicotinic acid may be of benefit to you, then your physician will need to monitor your dosages and reactions.

Functions: Essential for processing carbohydrates, proteins, and fats into energy; promotes healthy skin, nerves, appetite, and digestion

Deficiency: Pellagra. Rare in the United States because of enrichment of grains. Still seen in alcoholics. Symptoms include fatigue, indigestion, irritability, loss of appetite, skin disorders, and dizziness.

Toxicity: No reports of toxicity to niacinamide. Nicotinic acid can produce flushing, itching, headache, cramps, nausea, diarrhea, and irritability. There is a danger to your liver with extremely high doses. Do not self-medicate; consult with a doctor first, especially if you have gout, diabetes, or liver disease.

Vitamin B6 (pyridoxine, pyridoxal, pyridoxamine)

There's been a lot of debate going on about what B6 can do, and how much is too much. It has been touted for treating everything from premenstrual syndrome (debatable) and carpal tunnel syndrome (not scientifically proven) to relieving symptoms of sickle cell anemia (promising). Supplement sales were brisk until 1983, when signs of overdosing started appearing. It seems B6 is more complicated than we thought. A lot of people are not getting enough B6—maybe partly because up to 50 percent of vitamin B6 is lost during food processing.

---

15 SOURCES OF VITAMIN B6

Bananas	Pork
Beans, dried	Potatoes
Bread, whole wheat	Rice, brown
Broccoli	Shellfish
Chicken	Sunflower seeds
Eggs	Tuna
Oatmeal	Walnuts
Peanut butter	

Functions: Aids immune-system functioning; carbo-hydrate, protein, and fat metabolism; sodium-potassium balance; red-blood-cell formation; conversion of tryptophan to niacin

Deficiency: Severe deficiency usually occurs along with deficiencies of other B vitamins. But suboptimal intakes are more common than with any other B vitamin, especially in older people. Women taking oral contraceptives may need more B6. Many drugs interfere with B6. Symptoms of deficiency include anemia, depression, confusion, irritability, muscle twitching, insomnia, and skin problems.

Toxicity: It used to be thought that B6 was nontoxic, until people started taking megadoses to treat various conditions. Reversible neurological side effects are to be expected at doses in the 2,000-milligram-and-above range. But nerve damage has also been reported at levels as "low" as 500 milligrams. Consult with your doctor before exceeding even 50 milli-grams, because 75 milligrams has caused mild effects. It can also interfere with the drug used to treat Parkinson's disease—L-Dopa (levodopa). Symptoms of toxicity include nausea, headache, fatigue, dizziness, skin rash, and rapid heartbeat. If severe, nerve damage of your extremities can result; it starts with a tingling sensation and progresses to numbness and loss of coordination. Once the excessive supplementation is stopped, the nerve problem reverses itself.

Vitamin B12 (cobalamin)

This is a most misunderstood vitamin. It's not unusual to hear someone say they need a B12 injection for a pick-me-up because they're tired. But B12 can only pep you up if you were deficient in the vitamin to begin with. And B12 deficiency is very rare. It takes 6 to 12 years of a dietary deficiency to de-plete your body's stores of the vitamin.

---

10 SOURCES OF VITAMIN B12

Beef	Milk, skim or 1%
Cheese, low fat	Oysters
Clams	Pork
Eggs	Salmon
Liver	Tuna

At any rate, you wouldn't need to get it by injection unless you have an inherited disorder in which you lack something called "intrinsic factor," which is needed to absorb B12, or you had a portion of your stomach surgically removed. In these cases, taking it by mouth would be useless, because it wouldn't be absorbed. But for everyone else, oral supplements are fine, though probably unnecessary.

Functions: Carbohydrate, protein, and fat metabolism; maintains healthy nerves; needed to form red blood cells

Deficiency: Pernicious anemia (see Anemia in Part II). Dietary deficiency is only likely in strict vegans, especially vegan children. But most deficiencies are due to inadequate absorption (see above). Alcoholics may have increased needs. Symptoms include anemia, nerve damage, weakness, nervousness, and sore tongue.

Toxicity: No toxicity has been reported, just allergic skin reactions and acne from high doses.

Folic Acid (folate)

Folate is a general term for folic acid and other substances chemically similar to folic acid. Folic acid made headlines recently for the discovery that, with supplementation before conception and during the first few weeks of pregnancy, women could significantly reduce the chance of giving birth to a baby with a neural-tube birth defect. It's not that huge amounts are needed, but many women are lacking in this nutrient, and supplementation assures an adequate blood level. (See Birth Defects in Part II.)

---

16 SOURCES OF FOLATE

Asparagus	Mushrooms
Beans, dried	Orange juice
Beets	Oranges
Broccoli	Peas, green or dried
Chicken liver	Rice, brown
Chickpeas	Spinach
Kale	Sweet potatoes
Lentils	Wheat germ

Low folic-acid blood levels have also been linked to a higher risk of cervical cancer. So it's especially disturbing that, although folate is widely distributed in foods, many of us, especially women, do not get recommended amounts in our diets. Perhaps it's because up to 50 percent of folate is destroyed during the processing, storage, and home preparation of foods.

Functions: Essential for growth, especially protein metabolism, red-blood-cell formation, and cell division

Deficiency: You may not show signs of deficiency even if your diet is low in folate. The need for folate doubles during pregnancy, and now we know that adequate folate intake is important before conception. Women taking oral contraceptives,

---

MINIMIZING VITAMIN LOSS WHEN COOKING VEGETABLES

Water-soluble nutrients can be lost from vegetables when you cook, because they leach out into the cooking water. And many vegetables are susceptible to loss of vitamins if they are exposed to heat and air, as well. Here's how to minimize this nutrient loss from your vegetables:

• Choose microwaving over steaming and steaming over boiling.
• Cook vegetables in as little water as possible, and cook with the cover on.
• Cook vegetables only until they are tender-crisp and still bright in color.

---

the elderly, smokers, and alcoholics may need more, too. Symptoms of deficiency include anemia, poor growth, diarrhea, reddening of the tongue, and weakness.

Major Food Sources: Legumes, green, leafy vegetables, and oranges

Toxicity: Still controversial. Too much folate may cause lower blood levels of zinc. Folate can interfere with the anticonvulsant drug phenytoin, triggering seizures in susceptible individuals. And there have been reports of allergic skin reactions. Finally, folate supplements can "mask" a vitamin B12 deficiency, allowing neurological damage to continue unnoticed. An upper limit of 400 micrograms is probably wise, although pregnant women may need more. Symptoms of toxicity include excitability, sleep disturbances, and impaired concentration.

Pantothenic Acid and Biotin

You don't hear about these two B vitamins because there are few problems obtaining them in the diet, and no one overdoses on them. They just quietly go about their business.

Like all B vitamins, pantothenic acid and biotin are involved in energy metabolism. Deficiencies are unlikely. In fact, biotin can be produced in the intestines. (Raw egg whites can produce a biotin deficiency, but only when eaten in large amounts.) Toxicities are equally unlikely, except for occasional diarrhea from taking supplemental pantothenic acid.

Antioxidants—What's all the Fuss?

If the 1980s was the fiber decade, the 1990s belongs to antioxidants. You hear about them in research...you see them touted in ads for supplements...you debate their benefits at cocktail parties ... ad nauseam.

So what are antioxidants? An antioxidant is any substance that protects the cells in your body from oxidation, the chemical process in which oxygen molecules attach to almost anything in their path, creating destroyer compounds called free radicals. Just like the student radicals of the 1960s, these radicals like to stir up trouble, waging a silent war against your cells. Free radicals aren't foreign invaders. They are normal inhabitants of your body, produced in response to everyday chemical reactions.

Your body has a built-in protection mechanism and can, to some extent, protect itself from the damaging chain reactions that free radicals set off. But sometimes free radicals get out of control, outpacing the body's natural repair system, such as when too many are produced in response to cigarette smoke, ultraviolet light, and environmental pollutants like smog, car exhaust, and ozone. Left unchecked, they run amok, altering the genetic makeup of normal cells in the body.

You can see evidence of a simple oxidation process when a car rusts, when butter turns rancid, and when a cut apple turns brown. But dip that apple in lemon juice and—voilà!—it remains white. What happened? The vitamin C in the lemon juice acted as an antioxidant, protecting the apple from oxidation. In essence, the same thing happens in your body. Antioxidants help prevent it all, by neutralizing free radicals.

A fairly new wave of free-radical thinking is that they may contribute to aging. Likewise, if antioxidants curb free radicals, then perhaps they can help to slow down the aging process. That doesn't mean we'll live forever, but diseases that are thought to be a normal consequence of aging—cancer, cataracts, heart disease—may not be so inevitable after all. That's the optimistic outlook that's furiously fueling further research and prompting calls for more antioxidants in our diets, to "rustproof" our bodies.

Only certain vitamins and minerals have antioxidant properties. Three vitamins have received the most attention: vitamin A (as beta-carotene), vitamin C, and vitamin E. The trace mineral selenium also plays a role in the antioxidant drama, not as an antioxidant itself but as an element of an antioxidant. Riboflavin, which is one of the B vitamins, and magnesium are being newly recognized as having antioxidant properties as well.

Where's the best place to get antioxidants? Not necessarily in a pill. Most of the evidence in support of the benefits from these antioxidants has come from studies that looked at consumption of fruits and vegetables, because that's the best place to obtain beta-carotene and vitamin C. (A possible exception is vitamin E; see the section on Vitamin E for more information on this.)

So think of antioxidants as a fancy excuse to be able to tell your kids to eat their fruits and vegetables.

MINERALS

So, you're in the market for a supplement. You check out the selection at the drugstore and look for one with all the vitamins you need. Then you notice some brands that give you minerals, too. Is that better? If you need them as much as vitamins, then why do they sell vitamins without minerals? Good question.

You'll find the answer in Part III, in the discussion of supplements. But first, it's helpful to know more about minerals and their roles in the body.

Minerals are more complex than vitamins in many ways, but they are just as vital. There are a lot more of them—60 in your body, 22 that are essential to life. Minerals interact with each other, making it all the more important to get just the right balance—not too much and not too little. With most minerals, the balancing act is a little harder than with vitamins. But what distinguishes minerals the most is that there's a lot we still don't know. Here's what we do know.

MACRO-MINERALS

A handful of the minerals essential to life are needed in large quantities—relatively speaking, anyway—much greater than the microscopic amounts recommended for vitamins. That's why they're called "macro"-minerals. We need to worry about getting more of only one or two of them—calcium and perhaps magnesium. For two others—phosphorus and sodium—we need to worry more about excess than deficiency.

Calcium

You'd have to be from another planet not to have heard all the calcium talk in recent years. But with the spotlight on the connection between calcium and the bone-thinning disease called osteoporosis, you may have missed pivotal findings linking calcium with lower blood pressure and reduced risk of colon cancer as well as the good news about kidney stones. (See the individual disease profiles in Part II.)

Most of us simply don't get enough calcium. You may think it's kid stuff, but it's vital for adults, too. You build your bone mass until age 35 or so. After that, you need calcium to main-

15 Sources of Calcium

Bok choy	Orange juice (calcium fortified)
Broccoli	
Cheese, low fat (except cottage)	Pudding (made with low-fat milk)
Greens (beet, collard, mustard, turnip)	Salmon (with bones)
	Sardines (with bones)
Herring	Soybeans
Ice milk	Tofu (if made with calcium sulfate)
Kale	
Milk, skim or 1%	Yogurt, low fat

tain your bones' health and, according to the latest research, to help moderate your blood pressure and to reduce your risk of colon cancer.

The hot debate these days: How much calcium is enough? The RDA for most age groups is 800 milligrams, but many experts think that's not enough; they'd rather have you set your sights at 1,200 or even 1,500 milligrams, especially if you're a woman.

Children these days are particularly at risk. They're more likely to drink soft drinks, instead of milk, with meals. Not only are they missing a golden calcium opportunity by skipping milk, they're adding more phosphorus to their diets. Calcium and phosphorus work together in the body; however, it's best if there's an equal balance of the two minerals or if there's more calcium. Fortunately, children seem to absorb calcium twice as well as adults do.

Milk offers a double bonus. Not only is it a great source of calcium, the lactose in dairy products seems to aid calcium absorption. If you don't consume dairy products, you have your work cut out for you. You may still be able to get enough calcium, but it'll be a very tough assignment. For example, some leafy green vegetables that are rich in calcium are also rich in oxalates, compounds that tie up most of the calcium, making it unavailable. Spinach is a perfect example. New research, however, shows that the calcium in other vegetables—such as bok choy, broccoli, and kale—and in soybeans is surprisingly well absorbed.

If you don't think you're getting the recommended amount of calcium, you may want to consider a supplement. If so, you'll need to choose a separate calcium supplement, because multivitamin/mineral tablets just don't provide enough. Adding 100 percent of the RDA for calcium, or any of the macro-minerals, would simply make the pill too large. (See Osteoporosis in Part II for what to consider when shopping for a calcium supplement.)

Functions: Strengthening of bones and teeth, heartbeat regulation, muscle and nerve functioning, and blood clotting

Deficiency: Osteoporosis, marked by fractures of brittle bones, "dowager's hump" in spine, and back and leg pains

Toxicity: Recent research has discovered that calcium does not trigger kidney-stone formation, as was once thought. But excessive calcium may interfere with the absorption of other minerals like iron and zinc.

Chloride

There are no major problems with this mineral. Don't worry about getting too much or not enough.

Functions: Fluid balance, acid-base balance, and aid to digestion

Deficiency: Dietary deficiency is not generally seen, although it can occur in bulimics who vomit frequently.

Toxicity: Can only occur in dehydration.

Major Food Sources: Table salt (sodium chloride), processed foods

Magnesium

This very underrated nutrient is needed for many body processes. Though you may not hear as much about it, it's just as important to bones and teeth as calcium. Get too little and you may develop high blood pressure and heart abnormalities.

---

15 Sources of Magnesium

Almonds	Peanut butter
Avocados	Peas, dried
Bananas	Pumpkin seeds
Beans, dried	Soybeans
Bread, whole wheat	Spinach
Cashews	Tofu
Lentils	Wheat germ
Oatmeal	

Functions: Strengthening of bones and teeth; acid-base balance; carbohydrate, protein, and fat metabolism; muscle and nerve function; heartbeat regulation

Deficiency: Dietary deficiency, per se, does not occur, because it is widely available in all foods (you'll also find it in some antacids and laxatives. But suboptimal levels can occur, especially in alcoholics, athletes, the elderly, diabetics, and dieters, all of whom may have increased needs. Symptoms include nausea, high blood pressure, heartbeat irregularities, muscle weakness, mental confusion, brittle bones, tremors, and blood clots.

Toxicity: Doesn't normally occur, unless brought on by magnesium-containing drugs; also seen in people with impaired kidney function. Although generally safe, it is possible to get too much from overuse of magnesium-containing laxatives and antacids.

Phosphorus

This mineral works in tandem with calcium; it's best if it's balanced equally or if there's more calcium. Phosphorus also plays very important roles in metabolism and energy utilization inside every cell of the body. There's no problem with obtaining phosphorus; our problem is more one of excess. We drink too many phosphorus-rich soft drinks and eat too many prepared foods containing phosphate food additives. Eating too much meat adds to the problem. But the excess of phosphorus is not serious if calcium and vitamin D intakes are adequate.

Functions: Bone and tooth development, energy metabolism, nutrient transport, and acid-base balance

Deficiency: Dietary deficiency does not occur, because phosphorus is available in nearly all foods. Exceptions are premature infants and those taking aluminum hydroxide antacids for a prolonged time (aluminum binds with phosphorus). Alcoholics may have increased needs. Symptoms include weakness, malaise, loss of appetite, and bone pain.

Toxicity: No real risk of toxicity. Too much, however, may lower the level of calcium in your blood and cause bone loss if your phosphorus intake exceeds your calcium intake by more than two to one. Too much phosphorus may interfere with iron absorption as well.

Major Food Sources: In almost all foods: milk, meat, poultry, fish, cereals and grains, and green vegetables.

Potassium

Most people get quite a bit of this mineral but seem to think they need more. They may be right, because recent research has linked higher intakes of potassium to lower blood pressure levels and reduced risk of stroke. Lucky for us it is present in almost all foods; it's most abundant in fruits and vegetables.

---

15 SOURCES OF POTASSIUM

Apricots	Oranges, orange juice
Avocados	Pork
Bananas	Potatoes
Beans, dried	Prunes, prune juice
Beef	Spinach
Chicken	Tomatoes, tomato juice
Lentils	Winter squash
Milk, skim or 1%	

This mineral is extremely important for maintaining your body's fluid balance and for regulating your heartbeat. Too much or too little potassium can trigger a heart attack.

Functions: Muscle contraction, nerve impulses, fluid balance, functioning of the heart and kidneys, and blood pressure regulation

Deficiency: Dietary deficiency does not ordinarily occur. Unusual losses—through prolonged sweating, vomiting, diarrhea, or laxative abuse—can trigger deficiency. Symptoms include weakness, loss of appetite, low blood pressure, irregular heartbeat, drowsiness, and irrational behavior.

Toxicity: Can be a problem for people who have kidney failure (people who are on dialysis), so these individuals are instructed to follow a low-potassium diet. Symptoms of toxicity include irregular heartbeat, which, if severe, can trigger a heart attack.

Sodium

Everyone knows the sodium story, or at least they think they do. It can be summed up fast: Many people eat far more than they need. But there is a lot of misunderstanding and controversy regarding its relationship to high blood pressure. (See High Blood Pressure in Part II.) It certainly can't hurt to cut back, but not everyone needs to be paranoid about their sodium intake.

Functions: Fluid regulation, acid-base balance, cellular transport, and kidney-hormone regulation

Deficiency: Dietary deficiency does not occur, even on a low-sodium diet, because all foods, both processed and unprocessed, contain some sodium. However, a deficiency can occur as the result of depletion from prolonged excessive sweating, chronic diarrhea, or kidney disease.

Your basic needs to sustain life amount to only 115 milligrams of sodium (or 300 mg of sodium chloride) a day. Contrary to what you may have heard, everyday heavy sweating isn't a call for extra sodium.

Toxicity: Generally, the kidney can excrete any excess. In susceptible people—about 20 percent of the U.S. population—it can lead to retention of fluid and high blood pressure.

Major Food Sources: Table salt, many processed foods

TRACE MINERALS

So-called because they are needed only in minute amounts, trace minerals have two traits in common: the unlikelihood of a serious deficiency, although the consequences of suboptimal levels are considerable, and the danger of toxicity in amounts not that much greater than requirements.

Boron

Although no human requirement has been set, boron is considered an essential nutrient. New evidence of its role in keeping bones strong has brought it to the forefront in the fight against osteoporosis.

Functions: Calcium and magnesium metabolism and cell-membrane functioning

Deficiency: Relatively little is known about what symptoms show up from a deficiency, but a probable indicator is low vitamin D in the blood.

Toxicity: Little information is available.

Major Food Sources: Apples, applesauce, dried beans, beet greens, broccoli, grape juice, grapes, lentils, nuts, peaches, pears, spinach

Chromium

Here's another nutrient that's enjoying new-found fame. By all accounts, most diets are too low in chromium—a particular problem as we age and our blood levels of chromium become even more depleted. Some experts have suggested this may be a chief reason why diabetes becomes more likely as you get older. That's because chromium is a critical partner of insulin, an all-important hormone that keeps blood sugar levels within a normal range. (See Diabetes in Part II.)

Until recently, the only biologically active form of chromium was in brewer's yeast. Now, there's chromium picolinate, a government-patented form of the mineral that's highly absorbable. Chromium picolinate supplements may improve the results you get from exercise, by increasing your muscle mass. For dieters who also exercise, chromium may assist their efforts somewhat. But popular claims that it will magically melt away pounds are highly exaggerated.

Other studies have hinted that chromium may help lower blood cholesterol levels. And, if you make the broad leap from rat studies, perhaps even prolong life.

Functions: Maintenance of blood sugar levels and insulin effectiveness

Deficiency: Most of us don't get even the minimum that experts suggest. Diets high in refined carbohydrates are most likely to be suboptimal. Severe deficiency is rare, but a borderline deficiency may contribute to a buildup of sugar in the blood. Symptoms include high blood sugar levels accompanied by frequent urination, excessive thirst, weight loss, urinary tract infections, and fatigue.

Toxicity: None known. However, do not take supplements without your doctor's OK if you have impaired glucose tolerance or diabetes. The additional chromium may alter your need for medication.

Major Food Sources: Beef, whole-wheat breads, brewer's yeast, broccoli, whole-grain or fortified cereals, American cheese, chicken, calf's liver, oyster, wheat germ

Copper
Now this is a potential problem nutrient. Most of us probably don't get enough, but no one is exactly sure just how

much is enough. And interference from megadoses of other nutrients—vitamin C and zinc in particular—can decrease copper's absorption. Quite a copper quandary.

Copper is part of the tongue-twisting enzyme superoxide dismutase (SOD), which some say may one day prove important in cancer prevention. But that's still speculation. Closer at hand is research on copper's possible connection to heart disease prevention. It's thought to reduce blood cholesterol and lower blood pressure.

Functions: Iron storage and use, red-blood-cell formation, nerve functioning, melanin (skin pigment) production, and heartbeat regulation

Deficiency: Menkes' "steely hair" disease is a rare but severe hereditary disorder that causes a failure to absorb copper normally. Dietary deficiencies have been reported in infants consuming only cow's milk, and deficiency can result from kidney disease or taking excessive supplements of vitamin C or zinc. Symptoms include anemia and brittle bones.

Toxicity: Toxicity from dietary sources is rare in the United States. As a supplement, it is generally only available in multivitamin/mineral preparations. Those with the rare genetic disorder called Wilson's disease (overaccumulation of copper) should avoid copper-containing supplements.

Major Food Sources: Apricots, dried beans, whole-wheat bread, whole-grain cereals, crabmeat, liver, lobster, nuts, oysters, potatoes

Fluoride

Technically, fluoride doesn't qualify as an essential nutrient, yet. A set requirement has not been determined, but we know it's beneficial to our health. There's no question it has prevented cavities in tens of thousands of children. It offers the most protection when given before eight years of age, but it may be beneficial even into adulthood. It also may help prevent osteoporosis in adults. (See Water in Part I for the safety concerns of fluoride in water; see Dental Disease in Part II for fluoride's role in cavity prevention.)

Function: Strengthening of bone and tooth enamel

Deficiency: Not a deficiency disease per se, but dental disease is likely to result if not enough fluoride is given, particularly in childhood

Toxicity: Mottling of teeth occurs at high doses. Fluoride is fatal in extremely large doses.

Major Food Sources: Mackerel, salmon (with bones), tea, tuna (with bones), water (fluoridated)

Iodine

You may have forgotten that this is a nutrient, but it is. It is present in soil and water, but levels vary greatly in different geographic areas. Deficiency in the United States has been virtually wiped out since iodine was first added to salt in 1924. People living in the Northwest and Great Lakes regions of the United States should use iodized salt. Those living in other areas of the country need not use iodized salt, as foods from these other regions contain adequate iodine.

Cassava and cruciferous vegetables—such as cabbage, cauliflower, and brussels sprouts—exert an unusual effect, blocking iodine use in the body. But this only presents a problem for people who eat large amounts of these vegetables, eat mostly locally grown produce but don't eat much fish, and do not use iodized salt.

Function: Part of the thyroid hormone, which regulates energy

Deficiency: Goiter, mental retardation (cretinism). Symptoms of deficiency include fatigue, weight gain, nervousness, and dry skin and hair.

Toxicity: Ironically, very high iodine intake can also cause goiter and can inflame the salivary glands. Amounts ingested in the United States are not a problem. Although the issue is debated, some people believe the iodine in iodized salt and in multivitamin/mineral supplements can aggravate acne.

Major Food Sources: Iodized salt, seafood, seaweed

Iron

No other mineral requirement is so hard to fill for so many people. Iron is needed to produce red blood cells. If you don't get enough iron, your blood can't carry oxygen to the rest of your body; that's why shortness of breath is a symptom of deficiency.

Iron depletion is much more common than iron deficiency anemia. But both conditions require careful diagnosis through multiple blood tests rather than just a routine check of hemoglobin level. A low hemoglobin level can also be a sign of other diseases. (See Anemia in Part II).

Besides the usual round-up of suspects who may be iron deficient (see Anemia), add the unusual case of athletes. They can have a unique and not-well-understood anemia. Although the cause may be rooted in a physiological problem, it's also been suggested that their overzealous carbo-loading omits key iron-rich foods.

Iron's availability in foods is not well understood. It's based on a complicated set of factors. The most important is that vitamin C improves iron absorption tremendously if eaten simultaneously with an iron-containing food. But there are many more components of foods that undermine iron's absorption, such as oxalates, phytates, and tannins. The most well-known blocker is tea; drink it with meals, and you may undo all your good iron intentions.

Another less common, but more serious, problem is iron overload, due to a genetic defect that affects 3 in every 1,000 people, usually men. As its name implies, the problem is excessive storage of iron as a result of excess absorption; eventually, the iron accumulates in other organs in addition to the liver (where iron is usually stored), including the heart, where it causes a variety of problems.

A terrible irony is that iron overload shows up as low hemoglobin in blood tests, just like iron depletion. This is the reason you should never self-medicate with iron supplements; they can be dangerous if you suffer overload. There's also been a surge of interest lately in the possibility that excess iron in the general population may contribute to heart disease—another reason to avoid indiscriminate iron supplementation. (See Heart Disease in Part II.)

Other concerns regarding iron: learning problems in children who are deficient, and sleep disturbances among those who have depleted levels.

---

16 SOURCES OF IRON

Apricots, dried	Peas, green
Beans, dried	Pork
Beef	Potatoes
Brewer's yeast	Prunes, prune juice
Cereals, fortified	Raisins
Liver	Sardines
Molasses, blackstrap	Tofu
Oysters	Wheat germ

Functions: Part of hemoglobin (in blood), myoglobin (in muscles), and enzymes

Deficiency: Iron depletion progressing to iron-deficiency anemia. Symptoms include fatigue, listlessness, pallor, irritability, and shortness of breath.

Toxicity: Iron overload, due to a genetic defect. Symptoms may not be noticed until irreversible damage has been done. Without treatment, it is fatal. It's a good reason why you should never take iron supplements without first getting a solid diagnosis of deficiency from a physician. Even a multivitamin with iron might be too much of a risk, unless you know for sure you don't carry the iron overload gene. Others who should avoid iron supplements include people with acute hepatitis or hemolytic anemia and anyone who has had a recent blood transfusion. Symptoms of toxicity include abdominal and joint pain, fatigue, and weight loss. Iron toxicity is the most common cause of childhood poisoning and can be fatal. The usual cause: accidental ingestion of iron supplements by small children. Take care to keep them out of reach of little hands. Childproof caps are a must.

Manganese

This is the quiet nutrient; you just don't hear much about it, even though it may be as important to bone structure as calcium and magnesium. (You may not even have realized until just now that it's not the same mineral as magnesium.) It's pretty much an even-keel nutrient—no problems with deficiency or excess. New research suggests it has disease-preventing antioxidant properties.

Functions: Bone strengthening, carbohydrate and fat metabolism, and enzyme activation necessary for sex-hormone production

Deficiency: Because it is so widely available in foods, dietary deficiency is never seen in humans. Absorption of manganese is blocked by large doses of calcium or iron and possibly magnesium and phosphorus. Symptoms include poor growth in children with suboptimal intakes, and poor muscle coordination.

Toxicity: Only observed in workers exposed to high concentrations of manganese dust. Excessive amounts in supplements may interfere with your ability to absorb iron.

Major Food Sources: Dried beans, whole-wheat bread, whole-grain cereals, cocoa powder, coffee (instant), nuts, tea

Molybdenum

Mysterious molybdenum is probably the least well known of the essential minerals, perhaps owing to its hard-to-pronounce name. Some research suggests a role for molybdenum in preventing cancer.

Function: Enzyme activation

Deficiency: Dietary deficiency is not seen.

Toxicity: Excess can interfere with copper levels and may cause gout-like syndrome. Do not exceed 500 micrograms of molybdenum a day.

Major Food Sources: Milk, legumes, breads, cereals, and leafy green vegetables (content varies according to region where vegetables are grown)

Selenium

Selenium is a relative newcomer to the nutrition scene. It was only recently accepted as an essential nutrient, when a deficiency disease in low-selenium areas of China was identified as Keshan's disease. Like iodine deficiency, selenium deficiency was more common in years past, when people ate only foods grown locally in soil that lacked selenium. But now, because we eat foods grown in many different regions, deficiencies are rare in the United States.

---

15 SOURCES OF SELENIUM

Bread, whole wheat	Fish
Brewer's yeast	Liver
Broccoli	Lobster
Cabbage	Mushrooms
Carrots	Oysters
Celery	Radishes
Cereal, whole grain	Shrimp
Garlic	

More of a worry is selenium toxicity, which can occur at amounts only ten times the requirement. So while you should seek foods rich in selenium, leave the selenium supplements on the shelf.

Functions: Selenium is an essential part of the enzyme glutathione peroxidase, which protects against oxidative damage (see "Antioxidants—What's all the Fuss" in Vitamins), and of the enzyme that converts thyroxine to its active form. It also helps maintain healthy hair, nails, and muscles; protects against toxic effects of other metals; and is an important factor in sperm production, immune system functioning, and maintaining a healthy heart muscle.

Deficiency: Keshan's disease. Symptoms include weakness, muscle pain, and heart abnormalities.

Toxicity: Toxic at the one-milligram level if taken regularly. Supplements of sodium selenite may interfere with vitamin C absorption if the two are taken together.

Zinc

Zinc may be last, but it is certainly not least. Though it is overexposed as a favorite media topic, its importance is hard to overhype. Zinc is essential to growth, immune system function, sensory perceptions, and sexual development. Experts say most of us don't get enough of this mineral.

Zinc is complex, because of its interactions with other minerals. Many other food components reduce the availability of zinc in foods. Among them are excessive fiber, phytate, iron, calcium, and phosphate. Protein, on the other hand, increases absorption.

15 SOURCES OF ZINC	
Beans, dried	Lobster
Beef	Oysters
Bread, whole wheat	Peas, dried
Brewer's yeast	Pork
Cereal, whole grain	Shrimp
Crabmeat	Turkey
Eggs	Wheat germ
Liver	

Some of the latest research suggests zinc can reduce the severity and length of colds and may help prevent macular degeneration (an eye disorder that causes blindness).

Functions: Growth and development, wound healing, immune-system function, carbohydrate and protein metabolism, reproductive-system development, bone development, and enzyme component

Deficiency: Serious deficiencies are uncommon in the United States, but a mild deficit is. It may be a particular problem for vegetarians, the elderly, dieters, alcoholics, and athletes. Symptoms include retarded growth and sexual development, increased infections, altered sense of taste and smell, loss of appetite, skin scaling, depression, fatigue, diarrhea, vision problems, delayed wound healing, and low sperm count.

Toxicity: Acute toxicity can cause vomiting and diarrhea. More common is supplementation that interferes with copper, selenium, and iron absorption. Too much can even trigger a copper deficiency or may lower HDL levels. Amounts over 15 milligrams a day are not advised.

DIET AND DISEASE

If ever we've turned the corner on the link between diet and disease, it's now. Sure, we've long known that vitamin C cures scurvy, and that fat seems to be a contributor to heart disease. But now it's not just mumbo-jumbo statistics being jammed down our throats. Finally, research seems to be moving in a direction that makes sense in terms of our everyday diet. More important, it's proving that our admonition to eat more fruits, vegetables, and whole grains is right on target.

Study after study has shown that people who eat an abundance of fruits and vegetables have a lower risk for many chronic diseases, including cancer, heart disease, high blood pressure, stroke, cataracts, diabetes, and obesity. Why? A diet high in fruits and vegetables, is, by its nature, low in fat, high in fiber, and high in two important antioxidants—beta-carotene and vitamin C.

Antioxidants have been the driving force behind the new realization that diet can help to prevent disease. For other conditions, it's the more-familiar refrain of less fat, more complex carbohydrates, and more fiber. And the prevention or treatment of quite a few maladies—including diabetes, obesity, osteoporosis, and constipation—involves a combination of exercise and diet.

But we don't want you to come away from all this thinking that the link between diet and disease is a simple cause-and-effect relationship. It's not. There are many other influencing factors, from genetics to environment, that are beyond the scope of this book. But we're light years beyond simply preventing deficiencies, which was the focus of nutrition only 50 years ago. Improving health is what we aim for now. And good nutrition can make a difference—from lowering blood cholesterol to helping prevent cavities.

In these days of ballooning health-care costs, dietary prevention brings more bang for your buck. It would be foolish not to investigate every angle, while preserving our scientific principles. We've already done that for you here, with an exhaustive listing of diet-related conditions you may encounter throughout your life, from anemia to ulcers. Each is explained, with an emphasis on what nutrition can do to prevent the condition, as well as relieve the symptoms.

We also answer those timeless questions, such as: Is there an arthritis diet? Why do I get more gas than everyone else? Can my cholesterol level be too low? Above all, we try to be practical, because what is most important about discovering the links between diet and disease is the way these discoveries can help us live healthier lives.

ANEMIA

Iron-poor blood—what every woman dreads, according to advertisers. Makers of iron supplements have gotten their message across so well, you may be tempted to blame a deficiency of iron every time you're the least bit tired.

But don't self-medicate with iron under the assumption that your lack of energy is due to iron deficiency. While fatigue is a symptom of anemia—indeed, the word anemia means listless and weak—you could also be tired simply from lack of sleep, stress, mononucleosis, or many other conditions.

Even though iron deficiency is often thought of as a synonym for anemia, iron deficiency induces problems in addition to anemia. And iron-deficiency anemia is only one type of anemia. There are many types. It is essential that a physician test your blood for several components before you are diagnosed. Even then, anemia is not a diagnosis; it is simply a symptom of an underlying problem.

Being anemic means your blood is unable to carry enough oxygen to cells in your body. This shows up as a deficiency of hemoglobin, the protein in red blood cells that carries the oxygen and gives blood its color. A decrease in red blood cells is why severely anemic people look pale.

There are several nutritionally related anemias, but a lack of only three nutrients—iron, folic acid, and vitamin B_{12}—are the cause of most nutrition-related anemias.

Iron-Deficiency Anemia

Iron-deficiency anemia is the most common nutritional anemia; in fact, iron deficiency is the most common nutritional deficiency, period. Some say iron deficiency is the most common chronic disease in the world. In the United States alone, it is estimated that 18 million people are iron deficient.

Despite widespread iron deficiency, anemia is probably overdiagnosed. Simply having a low hemoglobin level and a low hematocrit (a measure of the volume of red cells in the blood) doesn't tell you enough. These could be due to a deficiency of iron, folate, or vitamin B_{12}. Ironically, they can even be a sign of iron overload.

If your doctor suspects iron-deficiency anemia, your blood should also be tested for serum ferritin; it is a measure of the

amount of iron you have stored in your body. In true iron deficiency, serum ferritin will also be low; in iron overload, it's
high. Another test that can confirm your diagnosis of iron deficiency is transferrin saturation. If low, it indicates a lack of
iron being carried by transferrin (a blood protein) to the parts
of the body where it's needed.

True iron-deficiency anemia only develops if you are deficient in iron over a long period and your body's stores are depleted. The symptoms —fatigue, headaches, tingling in your
hands and feet, irritability, and pica (cravings for unusual substances, like clay, ice, or starch)—appear slowly. The people
who should be concerned about this are those who lose blood
(menstruating women, those who have a bleeding ulcer),
those experiencing extraordinary growth (children six months
to four years, adolescents, and pregnant women), and dedicated athletes.

It's hard to get enough iron in your diet. It's not that there
aren't enough iron-rich foods; there are. But the iron that's
there isn't absorbed very well by the body. And there are ob-
stacles to iron's absorption everywhere you turn.

On average, only ten percent of the iron you eat is absorbed. So you must eat ten times your actual requirement to
be sure you get enough (the RDAs are calculated with this in
mind.) Prior to menopause, women need almost twice as
much iron as men do, because of the blood they lose every
month. During pregnancy, women need even more iron. (If
you are pregnant, be sure to discuss the need for iron supplementation with your doctor.)

But your body is incredibly smart when it comes to iron.
The less iron you eat, the more your body absorbs. But this
adaptability only goes so far.

Pumping Iron

If iron is so hard to get, why not just take iron supplements?
If you are iron deficient, you probably do need supplements to

re-establish your iron stores. But what seems like an obvious solution is not the automatic answer for everyone. Certainly, you must be accurately diagnosed as having iron-deficiency anemia before taking iron pills. Keep in mind that extra iron is dangerous if you have undiagnosed iron-overload syndrome.

If your body stores are adequate, you can probably rely on dietary sources to prevent a deficiency. While meat is high in iron, it's not essential. Vegetarians do not seem to have higher rates of anemia.

In general, there are two forms of iron—heme and nonheme; their characteristics affect how well they are absorbed. As much as 20 or 30 percent of heme iron is absorbed, compared to only about three to five percent of nonheme iron. About 40 percent of the iron in animal tissues is heme iron; about 60 percent is nonheme. However, all of the iron in plant foods is nonheme.

You can improve nonheme iron absorption. Eating just a little meat, fish, or poultry with your meals improves the absorption of all the iron in that meal, due to some unknown substance dubbed the "meat factor." Or you can include foods rich in vitamin C with your meal, which will greatly improve nonheme-iron absorption (the acidity of vitamin C actually seems to liberate iron). If a meal includes more than 75 milligrams of vitamin C, it boosts the availability of nonheme iron to the point that it rivals heme iron.

But take care to avoid consuming foods that interfere with iron absorption—such as tea, coffee, and wheat bran—during an iron-rich meal. These foods contain tannins, phytates, phosphates, or other substances that prevent absorption of nonheme iron.

Cooking in cast-iron pots and pans is an easy way to add iron to your diet. The iron in the pan leaches into the food, particularly if it is an acidic food cooked for a long time, like the tomatoes in spaghetti sauce.

FINDING HARD-TO-GET IRON

Foods Rich in Iron
Apricots, dried
Beans, dried (kidney, lima, white)
Beef
Brewer's yeast
Cereals (fortified ready-to-eat and fortified hot cereals)
Lentils
Liver, all types
Molasses, blackstrap
Oysters
Peas, green
Pork
Potatoes
Prunes, prune juice
Raisins
Sardines
Tofu
Wheat germ

Iron Boosters*
Vitamin C (rich sources include citrus fruits, cantaloupe,
    sweet peppers, broccoli, cauliflower, and kale)
Meat
Fish
Poultry
Acidic foods (sauerkraut, citrus fruits, white wine)

*Will only boost iron absorption if ingested at the same time as iron-containing foods.

Iron Blockers
Antacids	Tea
Coffee	Wheat bran

Megaloblastic Anemia

This anemia can be caused by a deficiency of vitamin B_{12} (pernicious anemia) or folic acid, or both. Folate supplementation can "mask" pernicious anemia—by correcting the anemia but allowing irreversible nerve damage to continue. So both causes should be considered before you are treated. A B_{12} deficiency actually causes a folate deficiency, because B_{12} is needed to activate folate.

Vitamin B_{12} Deficiency

Most pernicious anemia is caused by a deficiency of a substance in the stomach called "intrinsic factor," which is needed to absorb vitamin B_{12}. People who have had most of their stomach removed can't produce intrinsic factor. Also, people who have undergone surgery to remove the latter portion of their small intestines may be unable to absorb B_{12}. These people must be treated with B_{12} for life. It is usually given by injection, but some people are able to take a pill that contains B_{12} with intrinsic factor.

It's difficult to create a dietary B_{12} deficiency. It takes six to ten years of a diet that lacks B_{12} in order to produce symptoms, because the body stores B_{12} so efficiently. Still, strict vegans—vegetarians who eat no meat or milk—can eventually develop a B_{12} deficiency unless they get supplemental B_{12}.

Folate Deficiency

It's much easier to become deficient in folate than in B_{12}. Many of us don't eat enough folate-rich foods. Pregnant women have increased needs and must get enough in the first weeks of pregnancy; otherwise, the fetus may have a neural-tube birth defect, in which the skull or spinal cord does not close properly. (See Birth Defects for more information on the women's need for folate in the childbearing years.) Alcoholics are almost always deficient in folate.

ARTHRITIS

It's a mainstay headline of the tabloids—"Miracle Cure for Arthritis!" Arthritis is the kind of disease that's the perfect target for such scams. Arthritis is not well understood, so just about anything goes when it comes to proposed theories and treatments. And arthritis often strikes older people—favorite targets of charlatans.

If you suffer from arthritis, you know how desperate you can get for relief from the painful, crippling condition. You may feel you have nothing to lose by trying a reputed cure. After all, your own doctor may not be able to offer much relief, and what medications there are—primarily aspirin and steroids—have limited benefits and potential side effects.

Most important for scam artists, the disease is unpredictable, with natural flare-ups and remissions. This, of course, makes it nearly impossible to know for sure if a treatment is working or if the improvement is just a normal remission that would have occured with or without the treatment. Arthritis is a natural for the placebo effect, when the expectation that something will work can actually result in improvement.

The Un-disease

Arthritis isn't really a single disease. It's a term used to describe over 100 disorders that are collectively known as rheumatic diseases. And although the Greek word arthritis literally means "joint inflammation," even this hallmark is not present in all types.

Take osteoarthritis (OA), the most common form of arthritis, for instance. Often, it involves no inflammation. It's a degenerative joint disease; in other words, weight-bearing joints simply wear themselves out. This is a stereotypical condition of old age, but it's not uncommon in the younger crowd. It's particularly common among athletes (baseball players, golfers, tennis players), typists, pianists—anyone who pounds joints.

OA may start, for whatever reason (there may be a hereditary component), with the cartilage between joints thinning out and eventually being destroyed. This creates a painful bone-on-bone situation, resulting in wear and tear.

If you're overweight, you're more likely to develop OA, because there's more stress and strain on your joints, particularly the knees. Research shows that, conversely, if you lose excess weight—at least 11 pounds, according to a recent study of overweight middle-aged women—you can cut in half your risk of developing OA in your knee.

Rheumatoid arthritis (RA) is practically a different disease all together. It's characterized by the classic inflamed knuckles and joints and, often, misshapen hands. People who have RA and other forms of arthritis must endure endless episodes of swollen, red, painfully stiff joints.

RA, like the related disorder lupus, is an autoimmune disease, which means the body is literally fighting against itself. And the battle does not confine itself to the joints. It's a condition of the entire body, which can cause fatigue, loss of appetite, even fever.

The desperation that often stems from the mystery and misery of RA could explain the estimates that most sufferers have tried as many as 13 different arthritis remedies. Special diets and food cures seem to lead the pack.

Although the inventory of unfounded arthritis cures is long, there is a short list of hopeful diet connections. Most of the promising avenues of research in the food and nutrition arena involve RA. Here's what we know so far:

Fishy Ammunition

Hope has been raised most by fish oils, of all things. It's the omega-3 fatty acids in fish—the same stuff people were popping in the mid-80s to fend off heart disease—that may offer relief.

It's not such a fishy finding. Omega-3 fatty acids are known to exert anti-inflammatory action by causing the body to decrease inflammation. Several studies of RA sufferers have reported an easing of joint pain and less fatigue after taking fish oils; the discomfort and fatigue returned when the supplements were discontinued.

FISHING FOR OMEGA-3S

A 3.5 ounce serving of the following fish provides at least 700 milligrams (0.7 grams) of omega-3 fatty acids:

Anchovies *
Bass, striped
Bluefish
Herring *
Mackerel *
Sablefish *
Salmon
Sardines *
Shark
Trout, brook and lake (*lake only)
Tuna, white

* These contain double the omega-3s, or at least 1.4 grams. (In general, the darker the flesh, the fattier the fish, and the more omega-3s.)

But this connection is far from proven and certainly not a cure. Despite optimistic results from omega-3s, the disease remains active, the relief is modest, and it appears that the therapy may need to be continued on a long-term basis to be of any real help. Don't start popping fish-oil capsules without your doctor's OK, either. There can be serious side effects, including prolonged bleeding and an increased risk of stroke.

OMEGA-3S FOR LANDLUBBERS*

Beans, dry	Tofu
Canola oil	Walnut oil
Purslane	Walnuts
Seaweed	Wheat germ
Soybean sprouts	

*It's unclear whether omega-3s from nonfish sources are as potent or have the same effects as those from fish oils.

Then again, it certainly can't hurt to start eating more fish; it's part of a healthful diet anyway. Some reports say a half pound of fish a day may do the trick. If you can't manage to eat that much fish, try two or three servings a week. (See "Fishing for Omega-3s" to find out which fish provide the most omega-3s.) Omega-3 fatty acids are also found in some non-fish sources, such as canola oil, purslane, and walnut. Whether the omega-3s in these plant-based foods might have the same effects to the same degree as do omega-3s from fish sources, however, is as yet unclear. (See "Omega-3s for Landlubbers" for nonfish sources of these fatty acids.) Still, they can all be included in a healthy diet in moderation.

The Allergy Angle

Because RA symptoms come and go, it's tempting to blame food allergies. About a third of RA sufferers claim that certain foods trigger flare-ups of symptoms. The connection could just be coincidence. But if an allergic reaction can indeed provoke symptoms, it's likely to be very individual. There is no one food that can trigger arthritis symptoms in everyone. So there is no one food everyone can be told to avoid.

If you want to test yourself for food allergies, visit a registered dietitian so you can be monitored on a nutritionally

"IT WAS SOMETHING I ATE..."

There is one type of arthritis that actually can be predicted following outbreaks of food poisoning. It's a "reactive" arthritis, called Reiter's disease. It develops in two or three of every hundred people afflicted with diarrhea from intestinal bacteria. Because symptoms don't appear until weeks after the diarrhea subsides, most sufferers don't even connect the two. But, a few years back, health officials in Chicago predicted an outbreak of reactive arthritis following an outbreak of salmonella food poisoning. Their prediction was dead on.

What's the connection? It seems the diarrhea damages the intestine's protective barrier of mucosal cells, leaving them vulnerable to food allergens. These, in turn, cause Reiter's disease, which may seem like typical arthritis, with pain in weight-bearing joints. It may also be accompanied by eye and urinary-tract infections. The biggest difference between this and other types of arthritis is that although symptoms can last for weeks, months, or years, Reiter's is usually temporary.

sound elimination diet. Such a regimen starts with a simple diet that eliminates any possible allergy-producing foods, then adds them back one at a time, so that any consequences can be observed. A caution: Beware of any diet that eliminates entire food groups for a long period of time.

You should, at any rate, protect yourself from food-borne illnesses (see Good Food Gone Bad in Part III for advice on how to do that), because food poisoning can actually precipitate an allergic reaction that mimics arthritis (see "It Was Something I Ate...").

BIRTH DEFECTS

Pregnant women eating for two is an old joke. The new twist to that old wives' tale (but this time it's backed by solid scientific research) is that women should be eating for two before they become pregnant—at least in terms of the quality of their diet, if not in terms of the quanity of food they eat.

Women have always known that, ideally, they should build up their body's stores of nutrients—particularly iron and calcium—before they become pregnant. But, until recently, it wasn't appreciated just how much is at stake if a woman's nutritional well-being is not at its peak prior to pregnancy. There are several instances where nutrition before conception is most important—one of the most crucial is the link between the B vitamin, folic acid, and neural-tube birth defects. Being at an appropriate weight prior to pregnancy also appears to have a beneficial effect on pregnancy outcome.

Of course, a woman's nutritional and lifestyle habits during pregnancy can also greatly affect her chances of having a healthy baby. Adequate weight gain during pregnancy is important for reducing the risk of having a low-birth-weight infant, who may have resulting health problems. Avoidance of potentially harmful substances—such as alcohol, tobacco, marijuana and other illegal drugs, and even many legal medications—during pregnancy is also important for increasing the likelihood of having a healthy baby.

Folic Acid and Neural-Tube Defects

Most experts are now convinced that an adequate intake of folic acid during the first few weeks of pregnancy can help prevent a type of birth defect known collectively as neural-tube defects—or NTDs—in which the spinal column or brain does not develop properly. (The neural tube is the part of the embryo that gives rise to the brain and spinal cord.)

FOODS RICH IN FOLATE

Asparagus	Greens (mustard, turnip)
Bananas	Kale
Beans, dried (black, garbanzo, kidney, lima, pinto, white)	Lentils
	Lettuce (chicory, endive, escarole, romaine)
Beets	Liver (calf, chicken, pork, turkey)
Bread, whole wheat	
Brewer's yeast	Oranges, orange juice
Broccoli	Peas, dried
Carrots	Spinach
Cauliflower	Wheat germ
Cereal, ready to eat (enriched)	

In spina bifida, part of the spinal cord is exposed or defective; in anencephaly, there may be no brain at all. Spina bifida is currently the number-one disabling birth defect. The hope is that, now, with the knowledge of the folic-acid connection, many future tragedies of this type can be prevented.

NTDs are the only birth defects to be so directly linked to a pregnant woman's nutritional status. But, in an ironic twist, traditional prenatal care may not prevent NTDs; often, by the time a pregnant woman visits her physician and begins taking prenatal supplements that provide folic acid, it may already be too late to prevent an NTD.

That's because all NTDs occur in the first four weeks after conception. After that, neural-tube development is complete. But most women don't even know they're pregnant until at least three weeks after conception; many don't seek medical care until much later than that. So, it's clear: Any woman who might become pregnant should get plenty of folate in her diet (folate is the general term for folic acid and its relatives).

Researchers have suspected the link for years. It's long been known that women with one NTD baby who take multivitamin supplements before a subsequent pregnancy are less likely to give birth to a second NTD infant. But it took a long time to prove that folic acid made the difference, and that folic acid could also help women who had never given birth to a child with an NTD. Finally, a handful of large studies in the late 1980s and early 1990s firmly established the link.

The most recent study astounded researchers when it showed that women not taking folic acid (with or without other vitamins) were $3\frac{1}{2}$ times more likely to give birth to a baby with an NTD than the women who were taking supplemental folic acid (with or without other vitamins). The results were so dramatic that, for ethical reasons, the researchers halted the study early.

The U.S. Public Health Service now recommends that any woman capable of becoming pregnant consume 0.4 milligrams (400 micrograms) of folic acid a day prior to conception and throughout the first three months of pregnancy. Foods that are rich in folate include leafy green vegetables, legumes (dried beans and peas and lentils), and oranges. Even though folate is found in many foods, more than half of it can be destroyed during food processing, storage, and cooking. So, whenever possible, fresh sources, such as fruits and leafy green vegetables, should be chosen. Soon, on the recommendation of the Food and Drug Administration (FDA), manufacturers may begin fortifying foods with folate, as they do with other B vitamins and iron. Prenatal vitamins and multivitamin preparations containing folic acid are also widely available.

What About Caffeine?

Resisting the urge for that morning cup of "joe" has tormented pregnant women ever since 1980, when the Food and Drug Administration warned them to avoid caffeine. The FDA was being extra cautious after birth defects—cleft palate and malformed bones and extremities—showed up in rats given large quantities of caffeine.

Unfortunately, later press reports of caffeine's clean bill of health never made headlines, even though follow-up studies that contradicted earlier scare stories began appearing as early as 1982. Numerous studies were never able to uncover a danger to human fetuses.

We now know that rats only develop the birth defects when they are force-fed an unusually large amount of caffeine all at once, instead of over the course of a day, as people generally consume it. The human equivalent to the rats' intake would require you to drink 25 to 30 cups of coffee or over fifty 12-ounce colas within an hour—a feat not even the heaviest caffeine addicts could accomplish.

Just recently, the most definitive study ever conducted found caffeine not guilty of inflicting any harm whatsoever to a developing human fetus. It even convinced the FDA to do an about-face and recant its original warning. The study was more conclusive than others, because pregnancy was identified within three weeks of conception and caffeine intake was monitored throughout the nine months of pregnancy. No connection was found between the pregnant women's caffeine intake and birth defects, miscarriage, birth weight, or head circumference.

The FDA now agrees that caffeine in moderation is OK for pregnant women. But it won't rule out a danger from excessive doses, because the study only looked at caffeine up to 300 milligrams a day (about three 8-ounce cups of coffee, more than seven cups of tea, or five 12-ounce cans of cola)—a reasonable limit to set for a substance known to be a stimulant.

Artificial Worries from Artificial Sweeteners?

Anything that's not "natural" tends to make pregnant women nervous. After all, that's precious cargo they carry. The most commonly consumed of these are artificial sweeteners, dominated in the foods you eat by aspartame (NutraSweet Brand sweetener).

This low-cal sweetener isn't really artificial, it's just that its natural components aren't found linked up with each other in nature. Aspartame is actually two amino acids that just happen to taste sweet when stuck together. One of the amino acids is phenylalanine. Persons with the rare hereditary disorder called PKU—short for the tongue-twisting phenylketonuria—must avoid this amino acid because they lack the enzyme needed to process it.

Some consumer groups have questioned aspartame's use by a pregnant woman, because she might be a silent carrier of PKU. But studies show that these women process phenylalanine the same as anyone else, and it appears the fetus suffers no harm. All major health organizations, including the American Medical Association, the FDA, the World Health Organization, and the American Dietetic Association, agree that aspartame is safe for pregnant women.

CANCER

Cancer. The word itself is enough to make you shudder. Perhaps one of the most frightening aspects of the disease is that there is still so much that we don't know about it. But progress is being made in understanding the contributing factors and developing treatments. Heredity influences your risk of developing certain cancers, but factors in the environment—such as smoking and alcohol consumption—appear to play important roles. Another environmental influence that is garnering more and more attention is diet—both in terms of its role in triggering cancer and its potential role in helping to prevent it. Indeed, according to one estimate, an average of 35 percent of cancer deaths are attributable to diet. And, according to the American Institute for Cancer Research, cancer researchers have found that 40 to 60 percent of all cancers are in some way related to diet. And, unlike heredity, diet is one of the possible cancer contributors that we can change (along with smoking and drinking habits).

So what dietary choices can you make to help lessen your risk? That's the catch. We don't know all the answers yet, but we suspect we're close to quite a few. And some of those suspicions may be worth acting on now.

The Big Picture

Cancer, the number two killer in the United States, isn't a single disease. Cancer is an umbrella term for more than 200 different conditions, which all have in common the out-of-control growth of cells. Each type of cancer is unique, with its own set of triggers and treatments. Likewise, protecting yourself against cancers is specific as well.

Still, there appear to be some common diet themes across the different cancers. Vegetables and fruits seem almost universally beneficial, as does the fiber they contain. And fat has been indicted, but not convicted. The more you look at it, the more you realize that a diet that may help protect against cancer is very similar to a heart-healthy diet and a weight-conscious diet. And the main components of all three are neatly summarized in the Food Guide Pyramid (see Variety, Balance, and Moderation in Part III for a discussion of this dietary guide). Could it be that eating right is the common theme?

Diet as Hero, Not Villain

Proving a dietary link to cancer is not easy. Although the connection to some types of cancer seems more solid, some suspected ties are merely guesses based on statistics that compare diseases in different cultures—a branch of science called epidemiology. Actual clinical trials that put theories to the ultimate test are expensive and cannot provide valid results for decades, because cancer takes that long to develop.

Best for Beta-carotene

For cancer protection, eat one or two servings a day of foods rich in beta-carotene, such as:

Apricots, fresh or dried; apricot nectar
Broccoli
Cantaloupe
Carrots, carrot juice
Grapefruit, red or pink
Greens, collard or mustard
Kale
Mango
Pepper, sweet red
Pumpkin
Spinach
Sweet potatoes
Swiss chard
Winter squash

For years, scientists focused on specific substances in foods that might cause cancer. At first, suspicions centered around man-made creations, such as additives, artificial sweeteners, and pesticides. Then researchers refocused their attention on the many natural toxins in foods that were potentially cancerous, such as aflatoxins in peanuts and solanine in potatoes.

Now, we've progressed even further. Where it's at today is prevention. Food doesn't have to be the enemy; it can be your ally, along with other healthy lifestyle choices such as avoiding tobacco and limiting alcohol consumption. It's more realistic to focus on what you can eat, not what you can't. So the goal of many new studies and programs at the National Cancer Institute (NCI) is to identify foods that can block or delay cancer. This may be the most promising route of all.

Here is an overview of what we know, what we suspect, and what we know we don't know about foods that may help protect against cancer and foods that may promote it.

Potential Cancer Protectors
Beta-carotene Hits the Big Time

Vitamin manufacturers are falling all over themselves to replace the vitamin A in their pills with beta-carotene—not just because it's a safer form of the nutrient, but because it's an antioxidant (see "Antioxidants—What's all the Fuss?" under Vitamins in Part I). One of the strongest diet/cancer connections is the protective power that beta-carotene appears to have against lung cancer. It has been estimated that having a low level of beta-carotene in your blood may quadruple your risk for lung cancer. There's also some evidence that beta-carotene protects against oral cancers and tumors of the stomach, cervix, uterus, prostate, and colon.

The newest beta-carotene link came in mid-1993, when the Nurses' Health Study in Boston found that women who averaged one to two daily servings of foods rich in vitamin A enjoyed 20 percent less risk of breast cancer than those who averaged less than a serving a day. Because vitamin A can be toxic in large doses, the emphasis is on getting it from fruits and vegetables, where it is primarily in the form of beta-carotene, and not from supplements of vitamin A. Other carotenoids, especially lutein and lycopene, may be protective as well, but they have not been studied as much, and information on their content in foods is limited.

Most people get about 1.5 milligrams of beta-carotene a day from the foods they eat. The NCI and the U.S. Department of Agriculture recommend a diet that includes about four times that much, or one to two servings of foods rich in beta-carotene each day. Smokers may want to get even more, but an increased beta-carotene intake is no substitute for quitting smoking altogether.

BEYOND CITRUS FOR C

For cancer protection, select four to five servings a day of vitamin C-rich foods, such as:

Broccoli
Brussels sprouts
Cabbage
Cantaloupe
Cauliflower
Greens, collard, mustard, or turnip
Kale
Kiwifruit
Mango
Pepper, sweet, green or red
Potatoes, white or sweet
Strawberries
Tomatoes, tomato juice

Vitamin C Does More Than Prevent Scurvy

Researchers are still arguing over vitamin C and colds. But vitamin C may offer protection against lots of other conditions, including cancer. Eating a diet high in vitamin C has been strongly linked to a lower risk of cancers of the mouth, throat, stomach, and pancreas. Weaker data exists for cancers of the breast, cervix, and rectum. However, it's hard to separate an effect of vitamin C from that of beta-carotene, because many fruits and vegetables are rich in both.

Of course, it may be the combination of the two that's important. Recent research supports that theory. A reanalysis of 24 years of data showed that, of the more than 1,800 middle-aged men studied, those who consumed the most vitamin C plus the most beta-carotene were the least likely to die of cancer, particularly lung cancer. In fact, their death rate over the

24 years from any cause was 30 percent lower than the group consuming the least vitamin C and beta-carotene. The difference in vitamin C and beta-carotene intakes between the two groups is the amount found in just two oranges and two carrots a day.

Vitamin C has long been known to protect against substances called N-nitroso compounds, or nitrosamines. These are stomach carcinogens that form from nitrates (found naturally in food, water, and saliva) and nitrites (added to hot dogs, bacon, and other cured foods to enhance color and prevent food poisoning). The vitamin C must be present in the stomach at the same time as the nitrates/nitrites to have that effect. So there's yet another reason to make vitamin C-rich foods a regular part of your diet.

Vitamin E Expectations

Research appears to support vitamin E's contribution to cutting the risk of cancers of the stomach and lung and possibly bladder, colon, and rectum. At least one study has calculated that low blood levels of vitamin E more than double a person's risk for lung cancer.

But vitamin E is unique. While its merit as an antioxidant is accepted by many scientists, it only appears to be of value when consumed in amounts far greater than what you can get from foods. Because vitamin E is fat soluble, the foods richest in it tend to be high in fat—such as vegetable oils, sunflower seeds, nuts, wheat germ—so it's not a very practical nutrient to seek out in large amounts in the diet. Otherwise, you may find yourself overloading on calories.

What to do? As a start, be sure to eat lots of whole grains, fortified cereals, leafy greens, and fish to obtain a baseline level of E. To get your intake into the potentially cancer-fighting range—about 100 International Units (IU)—without overdosing on fat, however, would require a supplement. (Although many studies are conducted using 800 IU, there's evidence to show you don't need this much to gain benefits.) Still, while many experts are optimistic about vitamin E's possibilities, they have stopped short of recommending such a supplement until further research is done. Certainly, at this point, if you are considering a vitamin E supplement, you should discuss it with your doctor first.

ANTICANCER CRUSADERS: FRUITS AND VEGETABLES

Confused as to how to cram all those important cancer conquerors into your diet? Just think fruits and vegetables. Study after study has linked a low incidence of cancer with eating lots of fruits and veggies.

Fruits and vegetables pack in both types of fiber—soluble and insoluble. They are virtually devoid of fat, as long as you can resist adding butter, margarine, cheese, or high-fat sauces and can stick to nonfat salad dressing. Yes, fresh produce is your best bet for getting plenty of vitamin C and beta-carotene—two famed antioxidant nutrients. And, lastly, fruits and vegetables boast a wide array of mysterious and promising phytochemicals, like sulforaphane in broccoli, indoles in cabbage, and liminoids in citrus fruits.

Selenium's Tightrope Act

This mineral is not actually an antioxidant. Rather, it is part of the enzyme glutathione peroxidase, which is part of the body's antioxidant defense system, helping to protect against free radicals. You don't hear as much about selenium, however, because we still don't know that much about it.

Getting the right amount is a balancing act that Mother Nature handles fairly well. Selenium is widely available in such foods as grains, lean meat, poultry, and fish. If you eat all the complex carbohydrates recommended in the Food Guide Pyramid, you should get enough selenium in your diet. Selenium, however, can be toxic in amounts not all that much greater than recommended amounts. So supplements are a distinctly bad idea.

The Calcium Connection

This newcomer to the cancer-prevention scene is a bit more controversial. The link is based largely on research at the University of California at San Diego that suggests calcium plays a role in blocking colon and breast cancer, perhaps by thwarting the ability of cancerous cells to gain a foothold in the lining of the intestines, or by binding with them, rendering them benign.

Many Americans get only about half the RDA for calcium, which is 1,200 milligrams for teens and young adults and 800 milligrams for adults age 25 and older. Amounts of 1,200 to 1,500 milligrams have been linked to an anticancer effect. In order to use the calcium, however, the body must also get an ample amount of vitamin D. Because vitamin D is toxic at fairly low levels, it's safest to meet your needs by consuming foods fortified with vitamin D, such as skim milk (see Vitamin D in Part I for additional food sources of vitamin D). Another option is to spend a mere ten minutes in the sun each day (face and arms is enough); your body does the rest. Calcium sources include skim or 1% milk, low-fat yogurt, low-fat cheese (all except cottage cheese), ice milk, bok choy, broccoli, kale, and sardines and salmon with the bones.

Fiber Fallout

The research on fiber in the prevention of colon cancer is pretty positive, even if the link has not been proven beyond a shadow of a doubt. That may be partly because many past studies failed to separate out the effects of soluble versus insoluble fibers. It's the insoluble type—as in wheat bran—that probably provides the most protection. But fiber's effect may also depend on whether your diet is high in fat.

Then there are the variety of ways fiber may protect: by diluting toxins in the digestive tract, by altering the conditions within the bowel, and by literally getting carcinogens out of the way faster (see Fiber in Part I). The numerous variables are what confuse the issue.

But don't mistake the forest for the trees. Because fiber is clearly beneficial to many other conditions, it's wise to make sure you are consuming adequate amounts. Experts advise aiming for 20 to 35 total grams of fiber each day. Most Americans, however, eat an average of only about 11 grams. If your diet is low in fiber, try opting for foods made with whole grains rather than refined grains and eat at least five servings of fruits and vegetables a day. (Again, see Fiber in Part I for good sources.) Following the Food Guide Pyramid, discussed in Variety, Balance, and Moderation in Part III, can help you ensure adequate fiber intake.

Cancer Promoters
Fat Is Where It's At

Fat has been found guilty in contributing to the development of a number of diseases, and cancer is no exception. There's strong evidence linking a high-fat diet to colon cancer. Until recently, the breast-cancer link was just as strong; however, the prestigious Nurses' Health Study at Harvard found no difference in cancer risk between those eating 50 percent of their calories from fat and those consuming less than 30 percent. This has definitely muddied the waters. However, the simplest explanation may be that the fat level in the nurses' diets wasn't low enough to make a difference—maybe below 25 percent would make a difference, or below 20 percent. We just don't know yet.

Few scientists, however, believe that fat is completely unrelated to breast cancer. It's more likely that this latest study has introduced yet another variable to consider. Perhaps it matters *when* a woman's diet is high in fat; it might be worse if it's

MAKING COOKING SAFER

• Choose lean cuts of meat. Trim all exterior fat and remove the skin from poultry before grilling.

• Parboil or partially microwave foods before grilling; it will reduce the fat content and limit the time the meat is exposed to flame and smoke.

• Avoid letting the flame come into direct contact with the grilling meat. Keep smoke away from food by wrapping it in foil or by venting the smoke.

• Cook meat until done (juices run clear, not pink), but avoid charring. Do not eat blackened surfaces.

• Avoid fried foods that are cooked very well-done.

high in fat when she's young. Or maybe the mix of saturated fats versus unsaturated fats influences fat's role.

In keeping with saturated fat's villainous reputation in heart disease, some evidence points to saturated fat as a possible contributor to both colon and breast cancer (heredity is also an important component). But other research fingers polyunsaturates as promoting breast tumors. Where's a confused shopper to turn? You might want to try substituting monounsaturated fats, such as olive and canola oil, for some of the saturated and polyunsaturated fats in your diet.

Even when fat does affect cancer risk, it's not as a cause, but rather as a promoter of the disease. That means it enhances the action of true carcinogens, such as tobacco smoke. Experts generally echo the advice given to prevent other chronic diseases—cut fat intake to less than 30 percent of calories—even though we aren't yet sure this is low enough. Since it's unclear which type of fat may have a greater influence, you might try limiting saturated fats to less than ten percent of calories and polyunsaturates to no more than ten percent of calories, filling the remaining ten percent or so of fat calories with monoun-

COMMONSENSE HABITS TO COMBAT CANCER

1. Maintain your optimal weight.
2. Cut down on the fat you eat—to 30 percent or less of calories.
3. Get 20 to 35 grams of fiber a day.
4. Eat five to nine servings of fruits and vegetables a day. Be sure to include those that are rich in beta-carotene and vitamin C.
5. Eat cruciferous vegetables a few times a week. They include: broccoli, brussels sprouts, cabbage, cauliflower, and kohlrabi.
6. Limit how much you eat of foods that are salt-cured, nitrite-cured (hot dogs, luncheon meats, bacon, sausage, and ham), pickled, or smoked. If you eat them, do so along with a food rich in vitamin C.
7. If you drink alcohol, do so only in moderation.

saturates, such as olive and canola oils (this is the breakdown of fat intake recommended to decrease risk of high blood cholesterol and heart disease, as well).

The Calorie Conundrum

It may sound a bit absurd to say calories can cause cancer. After all, you can't stop eating. But research does suggest that an excess of calories is cancer-promoting, while being slightly underweight affords protection. This may even be a crucial part of the fat connection, considering that fat is higher in calories than are protein or carbohydrate.

The cancer/calorie connection that appears most solid is for cancer of the endometrium—the lining of the uterus. It is much more common in women who are overweight. Other possible calorie links are to cancers of the cervix, colon, breast, gallbladder, kidney, prostate, and thyroid.

Alcohol Advice

There's no doubt that alcohol contributes to esophageal and other oral-cavity cancers. Add cigarette smoke, and the risk skyrockets. But is there danger only for alcoholics, or should social drinkers also abstain? There have been conflicting data on moderate drinking and breast-cancer risk. It's probably best to follow the advice given for other chronic diseases: If you drink, do so only in moderation.

Nitrate/Nitrite Alert

As already discussed, natural nitrates and manmade nitrites can be converted to carcinogenic nitrosamines in your body. Getting plenty of vitamin-C containing foods can help counteract their effect. Still, it may be best to limit your intake of these substances.

Although some vegetables naturally contain nitrates, they often also have the built-in protection of vitamin C. Not so for your local water supply. Nitrate contamination from fertilizers can be a problem. Check your local water department or health department to find out about nitrate levels. If they're high, you might look into bottled water.

The Japanese suffer a risk of stomach cancer much greater than that of other cultures. Part of the reason is thought to be their consumption of dried salted fish, smoked fish, and pickled vegetables, which contain high concentrations of salt, nitrates, and nitrites. Salt-curing and salt-pickling provide excessive salt, which may be corrosive to the lining of the stomach. One theory suggests that this irritation may make the stomach lining more susceptible to cancerous changes, such as those brought on by nitrosamines. So your best bet may be to consume these foods only in moderation, if at all.

Unwelcome Mutagens

Mutagens are substances that set off sudden changes in a cell's genetic makeup, creating potentially cancerous compounds. Whenever you brown food, mutagens form. The more well-done you cook meat, the more mutagens you serve up with it.

Research has identified as many as eight different mutagens that form in cooked hamburger, two of which have tested as carcinogenic in animals. Beef seems to be most susceptible, but pork may be as risky; poultry and fish perhaps less so.

Because these mutagens don't form until meat is at 300 degrees Fahrenheit for a significant time, rare and medium-rare meat is not affected (but be sure to cook meat enough to kill microorganisms). Fried and broiled meats are riskiest, because they involve the highest temperatures. Grilling is safer. Microwaving, boiling, and baking are safest.

Grilling, however, carries its own risks. Other carcinogens form on the surface of meats, in direct proportion to the amount of fat in the meat. The carcinogens form when the fat drips onto the coals, tiles, or rocks. The rising smoke then coats the meat with the toxins.

CATARACTS

Cartoon characters see spots or stars before their eyes, and everyone laughs. But there's nothing funny about it when you see the telltale spots that signal cataracts. A cataract interferes with your vision, and you might need surgery to correct it. It's also a hallmark of aging, not something about which many of us like to be reminded.

What Is a Cataract?

The reality is sobering. If you live long enough, chances are you'll get cataracts. As the population ages, the numbers creep ever upward—each year, more than a million people are diagnosed with cataracts severe enough to require surgery. Almost two-thirds of all 60-year-olds have them.

A cataract starts off as a cloudy spot on the clear lens of your eye (behind your colored iris), almost as if you smeared grease on it. Some cataracts develop so slowly, you aren't even aware of them. If the cataract is near the edge of the lens, it may not interfere with vision. But, often, the cataract gets worse, or you get more of them.

You may begin to notice double or blurred vision, sensitivity to light—glare may be especially troublesome—and changes in color perception. The upshot will be progressively more-frequent changes in your eyeglass prescription, until the glasses no longer seem to help the problem. The pupil of your eye—the black part—may even do a chameleon imitation, actually changing color to a yellowish or white hue.

HOW TO COUNTERACT CATARACTS

• Limit your sun exposure between the hours of 10 A.M. and 4 P.M., when sunlight is most intense.

• Wear a wide-brimmed hat when in the sun.

• Choose sunglasses with UVA and UVB protection (they are labeled voluntarily by the manufacturer) and wear them.

• Protect your children's eyes. Hats may be more practical for them; start when they are young, so they develop the habit and don't resist. If they wear sunglasses, choose high-impact-resistant lenses.

• Stop smoking. Smoking increases the amount of oxidative damage inflicted on your eyes.

• If you have diabetes, keep your blood-sugar levels under control. High blood-sugar levels can damage the lens of the eye.

• Eat a diet rich in fruits and vegetables. Aim for five to nine servings a day. Include those rich in vitamin C and beta-carotene. (See Vitamins in Part I for sources.)

Your eye doctor will probably detect your cataract, and, if it gets severe enough, suggest the latest in eye surgery. Until the late 1970s, cataract surgery was a pretty big deal—certainly no picnic. It never really restored vision, and you had to wear thick glasses, declaring to the world your advancing age.

Now, cataract surgery is a mere hour-long affair performed on an outpatient basis. The cloudy lens is removed and replaced with a plastic intraocular lens. Success—and a 20th century miracle.

But wait just a minute. Wouldn't preventing cataracts in the first place be even better? Tell those doctors to hang on to their scalpels and lasers, because cataracts may not be the inevitable consequence of aging we've come to expect.

Move Over, Surgeons

In the late 1980s, a study was published that revolutionized cataract thinking. Researchers studied over 800 professional fishermen in Maryland and proved a direct association between exposure to ultraviolet (UV) radiation—sunlight—and cataracts. The more UV exposure, the more cataracts—up to three times the risk.

Where there's UV exposure, there's oxidation going on. And wherever there's oxidation, there's the potential for antioxidant nutrients to prevent it. At last, researchers no longer laughed at suggestions that antioxidants might help prevent cataracts. And it makes sense.

The eye is constantly exposed to light and air—no doubt polluted air—and that's just the recipe for oxidation. Remember free radicals? When cells are oxidized, they set off chain reactions that can destroy whatever is in their path. (See Vitamins in Part I for a detailed explanation of oxidation.)

Suddenly, a dietary connection to cataracts no longer seems absurd. There actually is a Laboratory for Nutrition and Vision Research at Tufts University. Research from there and elsewhere has supported the idea that antioxidants may help delay or even prevent cataract formation.

In one study, people who took supplements of vitamin C were four times less likely to develop cataracts. In another, people with higher blood levels of the antioxidant vitamins C and E and beta-carotene were the least likely to get cataracts.

In one of the most practical findings to date, a recent study showed that women who eat lots of fruits and vegetables have a whopping 39 percent lower risk of developing severe cataracts (the kind that require surgery) than those who don't eat much produce. Among the strongest protectors were spinach, sweet potatoes, and winter squash, all high in carotene content. But it didn't seem to be the beta-carotene that was key, because carrots were not particularly effective. Perhaps other members of the carotene family are the heroes here.

Admittedly, we are still in the infancy of learning about the antioxidant/cataract connection. Not all results have been promising. But one estimate suggests that antioxidants could prevent half of all cataract surgeries. That would indeed be something to see.

So How Come Everyone Doesn't Benefit?

To be honest, we're not sure yet. But researchers are working on it. Even the National Eye Institute of the prestigious National Institutes of Health has begun long-term research.

It could be that the people in these studies who had high blood levels of antioxidants but still developed cataracts simply had too much UV exposure when young. It may have overwhelmed the body's ability to counteract with antioxidants—in other words, a case of too little, too late.

The lesson may be to start young. Avoid exposing your eyes to sunlight in the same way you avoid exposing your skin. Wear a hat and sunglasses. And eat your fruits and vegetables.

CONSTIPATION

Commercials promise lifelong regularity. But you would give anything if you could just go *now*. Laxative ads like these may elicit a snicker or two, but constipation is no laughing matter, as anyone who has experienced its bloating, straining, pressure, and all-around discomfort will tell you. The desperation of people suffering from constipation is evidenced by the estimated $450 million per year spent on laxatives, which ironically may actually perpetuate and aggravate the problem.

Most doctors define constipation quite simply as infrequent and difficult bowel movements. Constipation is probably the only self-diagnosis that physicians commonly accept without question from a patient. However, it's easy to confuse constipation with a condition called dyschesia—difficulty in having bowel movements due to weakened muscles. Constipation is merely the delayed movement, for whatever reason, of waste through the intestines. Many factors contribute to this often misunderstood and incorrectly treated condition.

Is It Constipation?

The only thing people have in common about bowel movements is that they have them. There is no "normal" definition

---

TURNING TO TEAS?

You may have seen a tea that boasts to make your next bowel movement a smooth one. But wait before you try sipping your laxative at high tea.

Most of these new-wave teas contain senna, a powerful mover and shaker of the digestive tract. While senna is safe when doses are standardized (they are in over-the-counter laxative products), uncontrolled consumption of senna in teas is definitely not what the doctor ordered.

---

of regularity. What's normal for you may be abnormal for someone else. "Normal" can be anywhere from three times a day to three times a week. But, generally, if you go three consecutive days without a bowel movement, stools tend to harden in the intestinal tract, making them difficult to pass. Misunderstanding the wide range that is considered normal is probably the most frequent reason for laxative abuse. Overuse leads to dependence, increased dosages, and ultimately, failure of the intestine to function properly on its own.

Causes of Constipation

Common contributors to constipation include a poor diet, inadequate fluid intake, lack of exercise, and overuse of laxatives. Moreover, medications such as antidepressants, antacids, antihistamines, diuretics, tranquilizers, iron supplements, anticonvulsants used for epilepsy, and anti-Parkinson drugs can cause constipation or make it worse. In older people, a poor diet may be made worse by a decreased interest in food, slower metabolism, and difficulties in chewing due to dentures.

Constipation can be a common symptom of pregnancy—an especially bad time to resort to laxatives. It's the result of changes in hormones and unfamiliar pressure on the bowel from the developing fetus.

Coping with Constipation

Diet and exercise are your best lines of defense for both preventing and treating constipation. A diet low in fiber and an inactive lifestyle are open invitations to sluggish bowels. Try including exercise, even something as mild as a walk every day, in your routine. And try boosting your fiber intake.

When to Be Concerned

Constipation can be an extremely troublesome, if harmless, condition. However, it can also be a signal that there is a more serious, underlying condition at work. Some common causes of constipation include ignoring the urge, hemorrhoids, lupus, Parkinson's disease, stroke, and neurological and muscular diseases, such as multiple sclerosis.

Any significant change in frequency that does not respond to an increase in fiber may signal potential problems that range from colon polyps to a malignancy. Likewise, if you notice spots of blood or have to strain uncomfortably with each bowel movement, and you go less than two times per week, see your doctor.

Start slowly, adding fresh produce first, then unprocessed bran. Trial and error will help you find the foods that work best for you. Just as regularity varies from person to person, so does the road to relief.

Here are some specific steps you can take to fight constipation:

• Consume 20 to 35 grams of fiber a day, especially fresh produce, bran, and whole-grain breads.

• Drink plenty of fluids—at least six to eight glasses of fluids a day.

• Exercise regularly, for 20 to 30 minutes, three to five times a week, for optimal results.

• Don't ignore the urge to go.

• Eat more prunes and figs and drink more prune juice. They all contain the natural laxative isatin. It works for some people. It may work for you.

• Try a cup of coffee. A strong cup of coffee is sometimes just what the doctor ordered to end constipation. It does not work for everyone, but if it does work for you, you'll get relief fast—in less than five minutes.

• If constipation lasts more than three weeks, seek the advice of a doctor.

• As a last resort, use laxatives, but only under the supervision of a doctor.

DENTAL DISEASE

Even Shakespeare in his time knew enough to say, "Bid them wash their faces, and keep their teeth clean." Perhaps he knew old age and dentures don't have to go together, nor do little kids and cavities.

Dental decay is not inevitable. It may have been around since prehistoric times, but we know enough now to prevent it. Yet, amazingly, only two percent of the population can boast of having no cavities or gum disease.

Starting Out Right

No one is sure why some people don't get cavities as easily as others. Most of it is brushing, flossing, a good diet, and fluoride. Part of it might be heredity; if you're lucky, you may have inherited naturally strong teeth. Some of it might even be how well your mom ate during your fetal development.

During pregnancy, it's important for a mom-to-be to get enough calcium and protein, as well as vitamins A, C, and D and assorted minerals to ensure strong, healthy teeth in the newborn. And diet is especially crucial in a child's developing years.

What Goes Wrong

You know sugar is bad for your teeth. But why? The plaque that forms in your mouth—and that your dental hygienist works so hard to remove—accumulates bacteria. Anything that ferments in your mouth is fodder for the bacteria. The soup du jour is sugar, but these bacteria aren't picky eaters; just about any carbohydrate will do.

As bacteria feast on sugars and starches, they form acids that eat away at the enamel protecting your teeth. This leaves your pearly whites wide open for decay. Eventually, cavities, or holes, develop.

Keeping that Smile Healthy

• Eat sweets with meals rather than as snacks.

• Limit your consumption of sugars and starches as snacks. Stick to cheese, nuts, yogurt, plain popcorn, and fruit. Especially try to limit sticky foods such as raisins and other dried fruits, crackers, and cookies as snacks.

• If you do eat sweets or starches by themselves, brush afterwards, or wash them down with a glass of milk.

• If you can't brush after a meal or snack, chew sugarless gum for ten minutes or nibble on a piece of aged cheese.

• Eat foods rich in vitamin C.

• Get enough calcium. It is important for developing teeth and in later years to maintain bone health. Loss of bone in your jaw can cause tooth loss and lead to poorly fitting dentures.

It Doesn't Stop at Sugar

Back up a minute. Yes, you read it right, almost any carbohydrate can be bad—sugars and starches. But it's only carbohydrates left on the teeth that invite trouble.

Which are the worst offenders? Those that stick to your teeth, like the notorious raisin. Even seemingly innocuous foods like crackers, cookies, and white bread are trouble, say researchers, because they have a knack for sticking in the cracks and crevices of your teeth.

The Good Guys

It turns out some foods long thought to cause cavities really aren't so bad. Milk chocolate and liquids like sugared soft drinks are not a big problem, because they wash over the teeth, with little lingering effect (unless you drink them constantly). Even kids' sugary cereals aren't so bad if they're eaten with milk, which helps wash away the sugar. And the calcium and phosphorus in the milk help neutralize the acids.

Researchers have identified seven cheeses, so far, that actually help protect teeth when eaten after carbohydrate-containing foods. They are: blue, Brie, aged cheddar, Gouda, Monterey Jack, mozzarella, and Swiss. Aged cheeses have the edge, researchers think, because their sharp taste promotes the flow of saliva. Other protein foods, like meats and nuts, have anti-cavity effects, too.

When Desserts Are Better Than Snacks

Most important, it's not how much sugar you eat that most affects your dental health, but how often you eat it, and what you eat it with. If your child has a stash of Halloween candy, it's better to eat it all at once (assuming he or she doesn't get a stomachache, of course), rather than spread it out, eating one piece now and one piece later.

Even better, eat sweets with meals, instead of as snacks. Chewing other foods helps wash sugar away and stimulates production of saliva—natural protection from acids. Crunchy, high-fiber foods, such as raw carrots and apples, can also help clean tooth surfaces of sticky foods.

Anything that promotes saliva production helps prevent decay. That includes chewing gum. Researchers have identified a protein in saliva, called sialin, that counteracts the acids produced by bacteria.

Nix the Nighttime Bottle

It's an awful sight—a toddler with decayed bottom front teeth. More awful because it doesn't have to happen. It's the telltale sign of nursing bottle syndrome—when a baby goes to sleep with a bottle in his or her mouth (or sucks on a bottle all day). Almost anything (except water) in the bottle does damage, even milk, because it contains the sugar lactose. As your child dozes off to sleep, whatever liquid is in the bottle pools around the bottom front teeth. Bacteria in the mouth then convert the sugar in the juice or milk into acids that eat away at the teeth. Because saliva flow is reduced during sleep, it can't protect against the acids. What to do at nod-off time? Feed a bottle in your arms. If your baby still needs to suck on something, try a pacifier or bottle of water.

The Facts on Fluoride

Getting enough fluoride—in the water supply or in a supplement—is most protective during the first eight years of life. Experts recommend a fluoride supplement for an infant if Mom is using ready-to-feed formula, is mixing formula with unfluoridated water, or is breast-feeding. (Even when a mother's drinking water is fluoridated, very little passes into her breast milk.) Otherwise, a supplement is in order only if your water is not fluoridated.

RECOMMENDED DOSAGES:

Birth to 2 years	0.25 mg a day
2 to 3 years	0.50 mg a day
3 to 12 years	1.00 mg a day

X MARKS XYLITOL

Chewing gum isn't just kid stuff. It helps promote saliva production, which counteracts the acids that cause cavities. Xylitol is a slowly absorbed type of sugar called a polyol. Unlike other sugars, it cannot be fermented by bacteria in the mouth, making it the perfect sweetener for gum. Research has shown xylitol the hands-down winner in tests on prevention of dental decay. But finding xylitol gum in the United States may be hard. It's a best-seller in Europe but has yet to make a big splash here.

How much is too much? Infants and toddlers should not exceed 1.5 milligrams a day; otherwise, a white mottling will appear on the teeth. More than 3.0 milligrams, at any age, results in brown staining of the teeth.

Don't Forget Gum Disease

With all the talk of cavities, it's often overlooked that gum disease, not cavities, is the number one dental problem. It's only given second-banana status here because what you eat isn't quite as directly influential with gum disease as it is with cavities. After religious flossing—probably your best ammunition—it's simply good basic nutrition that's needed to combat gum disease.

Vitamin C is essential for healthy gums. One of the first signs of scurvy is bleeding gums (although gums bleed for lots of other reasons, too, like not flossing). It doesn't take much vitamin C to be protective. A glass of orange juice every day will do the trick. Include fruits and vegetables to promote chewing and saliva production.

<u>DIABETES</u>

It's not likely to be the focus of a disease-of-the-week TV movie. Maybe that's because diabetes does not tend to generate the same sympathy or sense of urgency as cancer or heart disease. Instead, it's an insidious disease. Over 14 million Americans suffer silently with diabetes and almost 50,000 of them die each year from its complications.

Almost everyone knows someone with diabetes mellitus (the full medical term). But misinformation about diabetes is common. First, let's defuse the misconception you hear most often: Diabetes is not caused by eating too much sugar. But it's no coincidence that over three-quarters of diabetics are overweight.

Wayward Insulin

Diabetes strikes when insulin, for whatever reason, can't do its job right. Insulin is a hormone, a chemical messenger, whose duty it is to pass the word to your body's cells that food is coming. "Food," in this case, means glucose—the sugar that circulates in the blood after food is digested.

Insulin is the doorkeeper; without it, cell doors won't open and the cells won't get nourishment from the glucose waiting to enter. So what happens to the glucose piling up at the cells' doorsteps? It keeps circulating in the blood. That's why diabetics have high blood-sugar levels.

If you are diabetic, the irony is that even though there's too much sugar in your blood, your cells are literally starving. So they start breaking down fat for energy and, in the process, give off byproducts of metabolism called ketone bodies, or simply ketones.

Having too many ketones in your blood is called ketosis. The excess ketones are flushed out in your urine, which is why diabetics must test their urine for acetone, a ketone. If it's high, they need more insulin. In ketoacidosis, the blood is too acidic from the buildup of ketones, a dangerous situation that can lead to coma.

The One-Two Punch

There are two major types of diabetes. They differ based on what's gone awry with the body's ability to respond to insulin.

Type I, or insulin-dependent diabetes mellitus (previously called *juvenile diabetes*), typically appears in childhood or young adulthood. If you have type I diabetes, you may be genetically prone to the disease. But the diabetes may have been triggered by a virus or injury.

The problem with insulin in this case is there's just not enough of it to go around. So food sits outside cell "doors" because there's no insulin on duty to let it in. So, type I diabetics must give themselves daily injections of insulin for the rest of their lives. To be most effective, injections must be carefully timed with meals and snacks.

Type II, or non-insulin-dependent diabetes mellitus (also called *adult-onset diabetes*), strikes in middle age or later. It is by far the most common type in Western, technologically advanced nations. Your genes determine whether or not you are prone to this type of diabetes.

With type II, there's plenty of insulin to go around, but for some reason the cells don't recognize it as the doorkeeper. The insulin may knock, but the door may not open. The effect is the same as with type I; little glucose enters the cells, so they starve, while the sugar piles up in the bloodstream. We call this not being "sensitive" to insulin. A mild form of type II diabetes is a prediabetic condition called insulin insensitivity, or impaired glucose tolerance.

Your family tree will provide clues to whether you are likely to develop insulin insensitivity. But just because it runs in your family doesn't mean it's inevitable that you will develop diabetes. You may be able to prevent, or at least delay, the development of full-blown diabetes by losing excess weight. Being overweight doesn't cause diabetes, but if you have an inherited

---

WARNING SIGNS OF DIABETES

Excessive urination *
Insatiable thirst *
Constant hunger *
Weight loss *
Dry, itchy skin *
Fatigue, weakness
Blurry eyesight
Skin sores/infections
Numbness in fingers or toes

*More typical in type I diabetes.

KNOW THE DIFFERENCE

Ketoacidosis (diabetic coma): Nausea and vomiting, rapid breathing, sweet-smelling breath, dry mouth and skin (from dehydration), fixed and dilated pupils, coma. Immediate medical assistance is required.

Insulin reaction (insulin shock): Excessive sweating, rapid heartbeat, hunger, abdominal pain, weakness, fainting, clammy skin, paleness, tingling sensation in mouth and fingers, irritability, blurred vision, drowsiness, headache. You need sugar fast—without delay. Drink a cup of orange juice or a regular soft drink or eat raisins or a sugar cube. Do not rely on a chocolate candy bar to do the trick; the fat in it slows the sugar's absorption.

---

tendency for diabetes, your extra weight may overtax your body's weakened sensitivity to insulin, pushing you over the edge into the diabetic range.

Just how important can weight loss be? Very. And you don't have to be svelte to benefit. A recent study showed that if you are overweight, losing only five to ten percent of your weight—about 10 to 20 pounds, on average—can significantly lessen the likelihood that you'll develop diabetes (and high blood pressure and heart disease, for that matter). For those who are severely obese, losing just half their massive excess weight can prevent diabetes. For someone who's already diabetic, a weight loss of only 10 to 20 pounds can mean improved blood-sugar levels, lower blood pressure, and reduced cholesterol.

In susceptible women, being pregnant can trigger a form of the disease called gestational diabetes. The diabetes may disappear after the baby is born—although the tendency to redevelop diabetes will not—or it may stay with you forever after.

The Telltale Signs

How do you know if you have diabetes? The classic signs are an insatiable thirst and excessive urination (to the point where the need to urinate may wake you several times during the night). These two symptoms—caused by the need to get rid of excess sugar—are more noticeable with type I diabetes than with type II. Other signals are fatigue, sores on your hands and feet that won't heal (caused by poor blood flow), urinary tract infections, and blurry vision.

If you have type I diabetes, you may lose weight, because the glucose can't reach your cells. This doesn't usually happen with type II diabetes, because there's always some insulin that works; it just isn't 100 percent effective. That's why the symptoms for type II diabetes are often less dramatic and more easily ignored. In fact, there may be no noticeable symptoms in type II diabetes at all.

Three-Pronged Approach

Type I diabetes must be treated with insulin injections, along with a proper diet and exercise program. Type II diabetics may need medication called oral hypoglycemics and may even occasionally need insulin, but the ultimate goal is to control blood sugars well enough with diet and exercise to avoid all that.

Exercise acts a little like insulin—that is, it opens cell doors to glucose. So when you exercise, you need less insulin, which is good. But it also means you must carefully watch your blood-sugar levels and adjust your insulin dosages, medication, or diet accordingly, so you don't experience an insulin reaction.

An *insulin reaction,* or *insulin shock,* happens when your body has too much insulin—from injecting too much insulin, from eating too little food, or from exercising too much without eating. It's not to be confused with *diabetic coma,* or *ketoacidosis,* which is what happens if your blood-sugar levels go sky high, eventually resulting in a buildup of ketones, a problem more likely to happen in type I diabetics.

Because the symptoms of these two life-threatening situations are easily confused, familiarize yourself and your family and friends with the differences (see "Know the Difference"). Wearing a medic-alert bracelet or other identification can be a lifesaver. It's not unusual for bystanders to think someone having a diabetic reaction is simply drunk or on drugs.

If you exercise, have a longer-acting snack with protein before you start, like half a sandwich, yogurt, cheese, or milk. Be sure also to keep a quick-acting snack with you to counteract the low blood sugar you may have after (see "Quick-Acting Snacks"). If you exercise regularly, build these snacks into your daily diet plan.

QUICK-ACTING SNACKS

(For exercise or insulin reaction)
Banana
Glucose tablets
Honey
Orange juice
Raisins
Regular soft drink
Sugar cube

Timing Is Everything

In the past, treating diabetes was a constant balancing act between too much insulin in the blood versus too much sugar in the blood. Like Goldilocks in the Three Bears' house, it was always too this or too that, never just right.

The trend in treatment today is to aim for "tight control"—keeping blood-sugar levels as close to normal as much of the time as possible. What you want to avoid are dramatic "peaks" and "valleys"—when blood sugar is especially high or has sunk too low. This blood-sugar roller coaster may be what damages major arteries and smaller blood vessels, leading to the complications of diabetes that can kill and debilitate, such as heart disease, kidney failure, blindness, nerve damage, and poor circulation.

WHAT ABOUT SUGAR SUBSTITUTES?

Go ahead and enjoy foods sweetened with noncaloric sweeteners, such as the popular aspartame (NutraSweet), that old standby saccharin, and the newer acesulfame-K (Sunette). Prominent organizations, including the American Diabetes Association, the American Dietetic Association, and the American Medical Association, say these are safe.

But bear in mind that "sugar free" does not mean carbohydrate-free or calorie-free. Many artificially sweetened foods may contain just as many calories as their sugar-filled counterparts. To be sure, check food labels.

For that matter, few people realize that tabletop sweeteners like Equal (aspartame), Sweet 'n' Low (saccharin), SugarTwin (saccharin), and Sweet One (acesulfame-K) have calories. Ironically, that's because the sweeteners themselves are so sweet very little is needed, so manufacturers add a "carrier" to create enough bulk to be easily sprinkled. What do they use? Dextrose, otherwise known as glucose.

In one packet of any of the four sweeteners, there's one gram of sugar and four calories (equivalent in sweetness to two teaspoons of sugar at 32 calories). That's not a lot, but if you're diabetic, it could total up over the course of a day, so it needs to be considered in your diet plan.

Likewise, fructose and "polyol" sweeteners like sorbitol and xylitol, all of which are carbohydrates, contribute calories and must be taken into account when planning your diet.

A recently completed ten-year study of type I diabetics has provided dramatic proof that tight control of blood sugars to near-normal levels helps keep at bay the chronic conditions that result from damage to blood vessels. Intensive therapy to the 1,441 diabetics in the study resulted in a striking 50 percent drop in the risk of blindness, kidney disease, and nerve damage. It also resulted in fewer diabetics with high blood-cholesterol levels. The evidence was so overwhelming, the study was halted a year early so everyone could benefit. Although not included in the study, type II diabetics may benefit from this approach as well.

For diabetics whose blood-sugar level is particularly pesky, maintaining tight control may mean multiple injections of insulin or multiple doses of medication throughout the day. But for many type II diabetics, simply losing some weight and manipulating diet may be all that's needed to control blood sugar without the need for insulin or medicine.

So what diet changes are in store? It's really nothing new—pretty much the same heart-healthy, anticancer diet recommendations being made for everyone, as you'll see in "What to Expect." So it's not so much the foods you eat, it's when you eat them. What you can't afford to do as a diabetic is skip meals. You must keep to a regular schedule of eating. Some research shows that eating smaller meals more often can keep your blood sugar closer to the normal range.

What's to Eat?

The recommended diet for diabetics has done an about-face in the past two decades. Experts used to think if you restricted carbohydrates, you wouldn't overtax your insulin any more than necessary. But a diet low in carbohydrates dictated a higher fat content, and that contributed to higher-than-average rates of heart disease among diabetics. At the same time, researchers were discovering the benefits of soluble fiber for diabetics.

Why is soluble fiber so good for diabetics? The gums and gels that soluble fiber forms in your intestines slow down the absorption of glucose into cells, lowering what would otherwise be peaks in your blood-sugar level. Research shows that a diet that is high in soluble fiber can stabilize blood-sugar lev-

---

AN ALTERNATIVE APPROACH

A controversy of sorts is brewing in the diabetes world. Diabetics typically have high blood levels of unwanted triglycerides (the storage form of fat) and low blood levels of "good" HDL-cholesterol. But the now-traditional high-carbohydrate diet sometimes raises triglycerides even more and lowers HDLs further, neither of which is desirable, because it may increase your risk of heart disease. So some researchers are suggesting a compromise diet that cuts back on carbohydrates and ups the fat, on the condition that the increase in fat comes from monounsaturated fats, like olive and canola oils and peanut butter. The best advice for now is to be sure your doctor monitors your blood-lipid levels if you are following a high-carbohydrate diet, paying particular attention to triglycerides and HDLs. That way, if they move in the wrong direction, you and your doctor can decide whether it's appropriate for you to cut back on carbohydrates and up your intake of monounsaturated fats.

---

els to the point where medication sometimes can be reduced or even stopped in adult diabetics. The same soluble fiber also helps to lower blood cholesterol. And, a high-fiber diet can help you lose weight. It provides bulk that fills your stomach, staving off hunger and taking the place of fattier foods. (For soluble fiber sources, see Fiber in Part I.) So, a low-fat diet that is high in complex carbohydrates has been adopted as best, with an emphasis on soluble fiber, the kind found in legumes, oats, barley, fruits, and some vegetables.

But, if you're looking for a diet plan, you won't find it here. You can't hand someone a preprinted diet for diabetes; it doesn't exist. Well, it probably does, but it shouldn't. That's because there are no pat answers that work for everyone. Each and every diabetic needs individual diet counseling. That way, a diet plan is personalized to your calorie needs, taking into account how your blood sugar reacts, how much and when you exercise, when you snack, and what your food preferences and habits are. We'll give you the rationale for dietary treatment, but you must visit your doctor and a registered dietitian for your individual diet plan.

What to Expect

Since maintaining a healthy weight is paramount to preventing and controlling diabetes, a registered dietitian will work with you to develop a meal plan suited to your needs, whether it's weight loss or maintenance. Such a plan is likely to follow these American Diabetes Association guidelines—almost the same as what's recommended for the general public:

Carbohydrate: This should make up the bulk of your daily calories—50 to 60 percent. Go for unrefined carbohydrates, such as whole-wheat bread, whole-grain cereals, brown rice, and whole-wheat pasta. Don't forget other complex carbohydrates, such as fruit, vegetables, and legumes. Go easy on refined carbohydrates, such as sugar, white bread, and baked goods. Sugar is not taboo; it's allowed in small amounts, as long as your weight is in an acceptable range and your blood sugar is under control. It's best tolerated when eaten along with other foods.

Protein: This recommendation is no different for diabetics than for anyone else—about 15 to 20 percent of total calories. That amounts to about 45 to 50 grams a day for a typical woman weighing between 125 and 140 pounds and about 60 to 65 grams a day for a typical man weighing between 165 and 180 pounds.

Fat: Keep your intake at 30 percent or less of daily calories. It's most important to limit saturated fats; emphasize monounsaturated or polyunsaturated fats instead. (See Fat in Part I for fat sources.)

Cholesterol: Limit your dietary intake to 300 milligrams a day. That means you can still enjoy about four eggs a week.

Fiber: Make an effort to get about 40 grams of fiber a day. Concentrate on soluble-fiber sources, such as dried beans and peas, lentils, oats, barley, and fruit. (See Fiber in Part I for more sources.)

DIVERTICULAR DISEASE

Anyone who has it will tell you the pain and discomfort sometimes seem unbearable, but the condition is seldom serious. Diverticulosis and diverticulitis are different stages of the condition known as diverticular disease. In diverticulosis, small pouches develop in the wall of the large intestine. These pouches can become irritated and infected. When they do, the condition becomes diverticulitis and can trigger constipation or diarrhea, gas, abdominal pain, fever, and mucus and blood in the stools.

Symptoms vary from person to person. In fact, many people don't even know they have diverticulosis because they have no symptoms.

No one knows how many people have diverticular disease. One estimate puts it at 30 percent of adults aged 50 and older and 50 percent of adults over age 80. Though younger people are not immune to it, it becomes more common with age.

For years, diverticular disease was considered a normal part of aging. But that view is seldom held anymore. The disease is virtually unknown in primitive cultures. It is strictly a disease of Western civilization and the eating habits that go with it.

A diet low in simple carbohydrates, but rich in complex carbohydrates and fiber is your best preventative.

A Diverticular Diet

Ironically, in years past, the diet recommended for diverticulosis sufferers was a low-fiber diet. It was thought that "roughage" might irritate the diverticular pouches and trigger inflammation. Today, however, we know how wrong we were. People who eat a low-fiber diet with few whole grains, fruits, and vegetables are actually more likely to develop diverticular disease and have a tougher time of it than those who eat a high-fiber diet.

Experts believe that pockets form as a result of the increased pressure needed to eliminate the small, hard stools characteristic of a low-fiber diet. The idea that diverticular disease is the result of a lack of dietary fiber is supported by animal studies. In addition, if fiber intake in several countries is compared with the incidence of diverticular disease, it seems clear that a low-fiber diet increases the risk of developing the condition. Several human studies have found that eating bran and other high-fiber foods clearly decreases pain, constipation, and other symptoms.

There is no correct dose of fiber to add to your diet to help prevent diverticular disease. But do start off slowly. If you get overzealous, you could make matters worse. Employ trial and error to find an amount that relieves your symptoms. But give it time—at least three months.

Another age-old no-no for people with diverticulosis was eating nuts, seeds, and hulls. Foods like pecans, tomatoes, and blueberries were off-limits. The rationale was that seeds and the like might lodge in diverticular pouches, triggering a bout with diverticulitis. But experts now say not to worry.

EATING DISORDERS

They are dramatized in made-for-TV movies and featured on the covers of national magazines. But, despite their notoriety, eating disorders are anything but glamorous.

The debilitating and destructive disorders *anorexia nervosa* and *bulimia nervosa* affect mostly women. Men make up only about five to ten percent of all cases. Anorexia and bulimia combined strike up to 15 percent of all adolescent girls and teenagers. Among college-age women, the incidence may be as high as 19 percent.

It's believed that anorexia and bulimia are triggered by a combination of psychological and environmental factors such as extreme social pressure to be thin; an abnormal or over-protective family environment; and yet-to-be identified physiological factors such as imbalances in brain chemicals.

One study suggests that women who develop bulimia have low serotonin levels in the brain, which trigger binge eating, possibly by affecting the appetite. Serotonin is a chemical produced in the brain that is known to have a relaxing effect.

Some researchers believe there is a connection between depression and bulimia. In one study, 70 percent of bulimics treated with antidepressants were able to reduce the number of episodes of binge eating. Despite ongoing research, none of these contributing factors is completely understood.

Eating disorders usually begin innocently enough with a desire by young girls to lose weight or prevent weight gain. Symptoms common to anorexia and bulimia include a fear of obesity, erratic eating patterns, severe body-image disturbance (sufferers see themselves as too fat even when emaciated), and purging (self-induced vomiting or heavy use of laxatives or diuretics).

Defining the Disorders
Anorexia Nervosa

Eating disorders afflict middle- or upper-middle-class adolescent girls or young women most often. Only a small percentage of those with either disorder—less than ten percent—are boys. Three symptoms are necessary for a definitive diagnosis of anorexia nervosa: fear of weight gain and/or obesity; food aversion; and distorted body image. Other red flags for the condition are continued efforts to lose weight despite a drastic drop in weight, food and weight phobias, and obsessive exercising.

Anorexia may be triggered by a single attempt to diet or begin gradually and then worsen over a period of years. A young woman suffering anorexia may well lose more than 25 percent of her original body weight. An anorexic may get down to 60 or 70 pounds, and still look in the mirror and see a fat body. Despite the fatigue that results from virtual starvation, anorexics often are quite dedicated to rigorous exercise programs in order to burn what few calories they take in.

Not to place the blame on parents, but the "typical" anorexic comes from a family that places a premium on appearance and academic achievement. It's been suggested that teenage girls view eating, either consciously or unconsciously, as the single aspect of their lives over which their parents have no say and they alone have complete control. Whatever its causes, anorexia kills. The death rate is estimated to be from 2 to 19 percent. Anorexics who do not receive treatment eventually die from starvation or from illnesses related to malnutrition, such as heart or kidney failure or hypothermia.

Bulimia Nervosa

Combine excessive food binges with purging (self-induced vomiting or excessive use of laxatives or diuretics) and you have the eating disorder bulimia nervosa. Bulimia is a disease by itself, but it also occurs in about one-half of all anorexia sufferers. The most common profile includes: obsession with body weight; binge eating; and purging (by self-induced vomiting and the use of over-the-counter laxatives and/or diuretics). Though the methods differ, like anorexia, the driving force behind bulimia is an exaggerated fear of weight gain and an almost phobic fear of loss of control. Unlike anorexics, bulimics are usually of normal weight. So a bulimic is able to remain "in the closet" for longer than an anorexic, whose major symptom—extreme weight loss—is there for everyone to see.

Research indicates that on average, a bulimic binges for about an hour and 15 minutes, and is likely to take in on average more than 3,000 calories in that time—more than most of us eat in three complete meals. In extreme cases, it has been reported that a binge can last as long as eight hours, with as many as 20,000 calories consumed—the amount most of us would consume in about ten days. Favorite foods for bingeing are "forbidden" foods such as cakes, cookies, ice cream, pastries, and candy.

Some binges are planned while others are spur-of-the-moment, triggered by negative feelings of stress, loneliness, or boredom. Some bulimics purge only after eating high-calorie foods. Others will binge 14 times a week or more, regardless of what they eat.

In addition to vomiting, some bulimics resort to regular use of over-the-counter laxatives to purge their bodies of the enormous quantities of food they eat.

For sufferers, bingeing and purging become a vicious out-of-control cycle of eating to soothe bad feelings, followed by guilt over the bingeing and shame over the possibility of being found out. The natural result of guilt and shame is stress, which leads to yet another binge followed by another episode of purging.

Identifying an Eating Disorder

People who suffer from an eating disorder leave telltale signs that loved ones can look for as clues to their affliction.

You just need to know what to look for. Someone with an eating disorder will go to great lengths to cover up their secret life, but friends and family may eventually notice changes taking place. Look for physical changes. With anorexia, these include unexplained weight loss, chronic fatigue, and light-headedness. With bulimia, there are likely to be dental problems from purging, facial puffiness from dehydration, and rebound fluid retention. (When bulimics purge, dehydration results; then, when they eat or drink, the body overcompensates by retaining fluid.) The following list can help you identify signs and symptoms of an eating disorder:

- Severe weight loss, continued efforts at losing weight
- Food phobias
- Intense fear of becoming obese, which does not diminish as weight loss progresses
- Severe body image disturbance (Sufferers perceive their body weight, size, or shape irrationally, claiming to "feel fat" even when emaciated.)
- Refusal to maintain even minimal normal body weight (15 percent below normal weight)
- In adolescents, failure to gain weight as expected, leading to body weight 15 percent below expected norm
- In women, absence of at least three consecutive menstrual cycles; in young adolescent girls, failure to begin first menstruation
- Antisocial eating patterns
- Chronic fatigue
- In anorexics, eating only a few bites of food at mealtime, insisting they are full
- In anorexics, development of unusual rituals at mealtime, such as repeatedly pushing their food around the plate, to cover the fact that they are not eating
- With anorexics, unexplained disappearance of large quantities of food from the kitchen

• In anorexics, possible swelling of joints due to loss of the fat that usually cushions them

• Obsession with food-related activities, like collecting grocery coupons, recipes, and cookbooks

• Compulsive exercising (for both anorexics and bulimics), often to the point of physical exhaustion

• In bulimics, possibly spending as much as $50 a day to support their "habit;" may consequently resort to shoplifting in supermarkets or stealing money

• Recurrent episodes of binge eating (rapid consumption of a large amount of food, usually in less than two hours); a minimum average of two binge eating episodes per week for at least three months

• Regularly engaging in self-induced vomiting, use of laxatives, or rigorous dieting or fasting to counteract the effects of binge eating

• Dental problems from repeated purging, and facial puffiness from dehydration

Seeking Help

Much like someone with alcoholism, a person who's had an eating disorder once in life will always be vulnerable to a relapse. Although people with eating disorders cannot be cured, they can be helped to keep it under control and to recover.

Those least likely to recover are those whose illness has gone untreated for a long period of time, those who developed the eating disorder at an older age, those who lost a tremendous amount of weight, and those who suffer from a combination of anorexia and bulimia (bulimarexia).

About one-half of anorexics who survive and undergo treatment return to their normal body weight. But the other half continue to battle the disease for years, if not for life.

Effective programs combine psychological, family, and biological components. No specific regimen can guarantee complete recovery for any one person, but early identification and therapy (medication, psychotherapy, family counseling) increase the chances of a lasting recovery and can prevent the most drastic consequence—death.

FIBROCYSTIC BREAST DISEASE

For some women, it just goes with the territory. Each month, swollen breasts, pain, and tenderness arrive with an irritating predictability. And just as predictably, they disappear with the start of each menstrual period. The lumps that come and go each month are what your doctor would call "fibrocystic breast disease." Most women just refer to it as lumpy breasts.

Not every woman's pain comes and goes with their menstrual cycle. In some women, lumpy breasts do little more than cause occasional discomfort. For others, the pain and tenderness are chronic and severe. It's not unusual for the pain and tenderness to spread to the armpit, where lymph glands can swell and become uncomfortable.

Indeed, most women—as many as 80 percent—experience lumpy breasts at least occasionally. Some experts insist it's a normal phenomenon of a woman's breast tissue during her childbearing years. But others say that's not so and warn that the potential complications are too serious to ignore.

What's the Cause?

Lumps that come and go with each menstrual cycle are the result of the ups and downs in the levels of the hormones ⁺rogen and progesterone. Some doctors have suggested that an imbalance of these hormones is actually to blame. Fibrocystic breast disease is most common in women 30 and over, and symptoms generally become more severe as a woman approaches menopause. But it can affect women in their twenties as well. Women who suffer from premenstrual syndrome are more likely to develop fibrocystic breast disease. That's not surprising, since both conditions are directly influenced by hormones. Other risk factors include early onset of menstruation, no pregnancies, and a history of miscarriage.

The Cancer Connection

The answer to the $64,000 question of whether women with lumpy breasts are at a greater risk for breast cancer is still uncertain. Though fibrocystic breast lumps are not cancerous, some research does suggest that women who have fibrocystic breast disease may be at higher risk for developing breast cancer later on.

But it may be that there are several different types of fibrocystic tissue, and that only a few types actually increase a woman's risk of developing breast cancer. In fact, researchers have identified 13 different kinds of fibrocystic tissue, but only atypical forms appear to be at increased risk; common forms of fibrocystic lumps do not become cancerous. Only a biopsy of your breast tissue can tell if you have the type considered to be high risk. For women with the high-risk type of tissue and for women who don't know if they're at high risk for breast cancer, some doctors recommend breast exams twice a year.

Is Caffeine a Culprit?

Whether caffeine increases or aggravates fibrocystic breast disease is uncertain. Some research has linked the consumption of coffee, tea, and chocolate to lumpy breasts; some studies have found no connection. Each of these foods contains caffeine or related compounds called methylxanthines, which are suspect in causing the condition.

In a nutshell, some studies have shown that cutting back or cutting out caffeine improves symptoms, while others have not. The first report that suggested a connection between caffeine consumption and fibrocystic breast disease was published in 1979. Several studies since then have found the same connection. In one study, women who drank four or five cups of coffee a day were at more than double the risk for lumpy breasts, regardless of their age. But the researchers found no connection between breast lumps and the amount of cola or chocolate the women consumed, which would seem to absolve caffeine and point to something else in coffee.

SOME COMMON CAFFEINE SOURCES

Food or Beverage	Amount	Caffeine (milligrams)
Coffee, roasted, ground, perked	5 oz.	79
Coffee, instant	5 oz.	64
Coffee, roasted, ground, drip	5 oz.	112
ground, decaffeinated	5 oz.	2
Coffee, instant, decaffeinated	5 oz.	3
Tea, bagged	5 oz.	42
Tea, instant, iced	12 oz.	70
Tea, leaf	5 oz.	41
Cocoa beverage	5 oz.	5
Milk chocolate	1 oz.	11
Chocolate milk	8 oz.	5
Baking chocolate	1 oz.	35
Soft drinks		
Colas, regular	6 oz.	15–23
Colas, decaffeinated	6 oz.	trace
Colas, diet	6 oz.	1–29

Bolstering that idea is a large study of more than 3,300 women with fibrocystic breast disease conducted several years ago by the National Cancer Institute. The researchers found no relationship between caffeine consumption and fibrocystic breast disease.

Despite the lack of scientific evidence, many women say their symptoms improve when they cut back on caffeine. Many practitioners seem to believe in cutting back as well. One of the first questions your doctor is likely to ask is, "How much coffee do you drink?" Since there's no "down" side to cutting back on caffeine—except that you may have a little more trouble geting going in the morning—you might want to give it a try.

Does "E" Spell Relief?

Supplements of vitamin E have come in and out of favor over the years as a treatment for fibrocystic breast discomfort. One small study several years ago found that when women took 600 IUs of vitamin E a day, 85 percent of them experienced improvement in their symptoms. But other larger and more well-controlled studies found no benefit from taking vitamin E supplements.

A Lumpy Goodbye

The only sure-fire way to rid yourself of fibrocystic breast disease is to experience menopause. Some three to five years after menopause, when your ovaries stop secreting female hormones, you're unlikely to suffer the problems you did while you were menstruating.

Estrogen replacement therapy (ERT) may, of course, prolong your discomfort from fibrocystic breast disease. If the hormones are there, whether from your ovaries or from a pill, your breasts will react in the same way. Therefore, you will need to discuss the pros and cons with your doctor.

FLATULENCE

Everyone has it at some time. It's universally embarrassing (except, perhaps, for small children), but no one dare speak its name. It's gas, or flatulence. Experts say it's not unusual for a person to pass gas anywhere from 14 to 23 times a day. The buildup of intestinal gas is rarely serious, but it can be embarrassing and at times uncomfortable or even painful.

What Causes Gas?

Barring a serious medical condition, food is the major reason why gas builds up. In fact, intestinal gas is a normal by-product of your body as it handles the food you eat. When undigested carbohydrates migrate from the stomach to the lower intestine, they encounter bacteria that feed on the undigested matter, releasing gas in the process.

Certain foods are just natural gas producers. Fruits, vegetables, beans, and most dairy products fall into this category. Carbohydrate-rich plant foods and milk offer intestinal bacteria a virtual feast.

Gas is also associated with high-fiber diets, but you can get gas even if you eat a low-fiber diet. In fact, eating refined wheat products like bagels, pasta, and pretzels can increase flatulence. Dried beans and peas tend to produce the most gas, with wheat, oats, corn, and potatoes not far behind. Beans are particularly high in nonabsorbable carbohydrates.

Of the carbohydrate-rich foods, rice is least likely to trigger gas production. Animal foods and oils, which contain few or no carbohydrates, are also unlikely to set off rumbling.

The sweetener sorbitol is a gas producer and causes diarrhea as well. In fact, sorbitol's value as a sweetener is due to the body's inability to digest it as completely as sugar. Fewer calories are absorbed, and the gas it produces is simply proof that it is not being readily digested.

Occasionally, gas is more than just a normal reaction to eating. It can be a symptom of an underlying disorder. If gas is particularly troublesome to you, don't automatically dismiss it. For people who suffer from excess gas production, the most common problem is lactose intolerance, a condition in which the body is unable to handle lactose, the sugar found in milk (see Lactose Intolerance).

Less common causes of excessive gassiness are malabsorption syndromes such as celiac disease. In this condition, the body cannot handle gluten, a protein in wheat products.

Bloating, or the sensation of gas, may be a sign of a sluggish digestive tract or of an irritated intestine. If the bloating and discomfort persist, you should see a doctor. But in general, there's no reason to be alarmed by occasional gassiness; it's a normal side effect of eating.

FOODS THAT TRIGGER GAS

Low Octane	High Octane
Eggs	Broccoli
Fish	Brussels sprouts
Meat	Cabbage
Oils	Cauliflower
Poultry	Dried beans and peas
Rice	Milk and milk products (for the lactose intolerant)
Regular	
Apples	Onions
Bananas	Rutabagas
Bread products	Soybeans
Carrots	Turnips
Celery	
Eggplant	

Why Me?

It's not only what you eat that affects gas production. How your body reacts to the foods you eat is just as important. A bowl of bran may make your abdomen blow up like a balloon but may leave someone else unaffected. The particular collection of bacteria in your intestines may explain why. Some bacteria produce gas, others actually consume it. The bacterial balance varies from person to person.

The best approach for pinpointing the foods that give you gas is with trial-and-error dieting. However, the problem with trying to control gas with diet is that some of the gassiest foods are also among the healthiest. Dried beans and cruciferous vegetables (the cabbage family), which are notorious gas producers, are also high in fiber and low in fat and may help reduce the risk of cancer.

Stopping Gas

It's impossible to get rid of gas completely, but you can reduce it. Here are a few tactics.

• Eat and drink slowly. Don't gulp; chew thoroughly.

• Avoid sugar-free gums and sugar-free candies that contain sorbitol or xylitol, both sweeteners that are poorly digested.

• Don't make sudden changes in your fiber intake. If your diet is low in fiber, increase it gradually over weeks or months. If, for instance, your diet now provides ten grams or less of fiber and you suddenly increase to 30 or 35 grams, you are likely to experience bloating and gas.

• The "explosiveness" of beans can be subdued to some extent by soaking the beans overnight, then draining, rinsing, and cooking them thoroughly. The process makes the carbohydrates in beans more digestible. Also, start by choosing more easily digestible types (lentils, limas, split peas) and then gradually trying other types. Or try canned beans instead of dried; they're usually well cooked and are therefore less likely to cause as much gassiness.

• Soybeans are one of the worst gas offenders. Tofu or soybean curd is less likely to be a problem; most of the indigestible sugars are washed out with the whey when fermented soybean products are made.

• Eat only small amounts of gas-causing vegetables at a sitting. If possible, try not to mix two in the same meal or recipe.

• Consider trying Beano, over-the-counter drops you add to food just prior to eating. Beano contains an enzyme that breaks down indigestible carbohydrates in food.

If none of these tips works for you, ask your pharmacist to recommend an over-the-counter antiflatulent product, or see your doctor.

FOOD ALLERGIES AND INTOLERANCES

Can you spot who has a food allergy? Here are three people who think they do:

Henry, a healthy 55-year-old accountant, develops a nasty rash each time he eats shellfish.

Ethan, a 30-year-old self-confessed hypochondriac, breaks out in hives at the mere smell of chocolate.

Allison, an active 25-year-old graduate student, gets horrible gas each time she drinks milk.

All of these people are convinced they have a food allergy. Not so. Henry is the only one of the group with a real allergy to a food, in this case, shellfish. Ethan has been tested often and allergists can find no physical cause for his reaction. But hives can be brought on by emotions. His belief that he is allergic to chocolate could be enough to trigger the hives.

Allison has lactose intolerance, not an allergy to milk. She simply lacks the enzyme needed to digest lactose, the sugar in milk (see Lactose Intolerance).

It's estimated that true food allergy affects less than two percent of the population. About five percent of young children are believed to have food allergies, most of which show up in the first years of life. But most affected children outgrow their allergies.

As many as 80 percent of people who believe they have food allergies don't actually have them. The mistaken 80 percent actually have what some experts have dubbed "pseudo food allergies." Though the symptoms, such as headaches and hives, are quite real, the cause may be a simple intolerance, for instance, or be psychological—believing you're allergic to a food may be enough to trigger symptoms.

Misunderstanding food allergies is common, and people like Ethan and Allison sometimes unnecessarily restrict what they eat because of fear of a life-threatening reaction. Here are the real food-allergy facts.

Anatomy of a Food Allergy

Anyone can develop a food allergy. But your tendency to become allergic is often inherited from your parents. A child with one allergic parent is twice as likely to develop a food allergy than a child whose parents are not allergic. If both parents have allergies, the child's risk doubles again and the child is about four times more likely to be affected. The substances to which a child is allergic, however, may well differ from what the parents are allergic to.

A food allergy is any adverse reaction by your immune system to a normally harmless food or food ingredient. If the immune system is not involved, it is not a food allergy, but a food intolerance. A single food can contain many food allergens, or allergy "triggers." Most food-allergy triggers are proteins rather than carbohydrates or fats. In allergies, something goes awry and the body treats a protein as if it were an invading bacteria, setting off a complex chain of reactions.

If you have inherited the tendency to develop allergies, your body makes greater-than-normal amounts of immunoglobulin E, or IgE—a type of antibody in the immune system—when you eat certain foods. As millions of IgE antibodies circulate in your blood, they activate specialized immune cells, called basophils and mast cells. These immune cells release histamine and other substances that produce allergy symptoms. You've heard of antihistamines? They are medications designed to combat the histamine released when you have an allergic reaction.

Although allergic reactions to almost any food can occur, most reactions are caused by a small number of foods: milk, eggs, fish, shellfish, soy, wheat, peanuts, and tree nuts such as walnuts.

People who are allergic to plant foods, however, may experience cross-allergies. For example, if you're allergic to peanuts, you may also be allergic to other legumes, including green peas, soybeans, and lentils. Or if you're allergic to cantaloupe, you may have a reaction to cucumber or pumpkin. Allergic to shrimp? You may also have an allergy to crab.

Allergic reactions usually begin within minutes to a few hours after eating the offending food. But in very sensitive people, simply touching or smelling the food can trigger an allergic response. The most common type of food allergy is immediate—within two hours of eating the offending food. But symptoms can begin within seconds of eating or perhaps simply smelling or touching the food.

Delayed allergic reactions can appear from a few hours to 48 hours after you eat the food. Generally, symptoms from a delayed allergic reaction are less severe than those from an immediate response. Symptoms of delayed food-allergy reactions include eczema, hives, and asthma. By virtue of their nature, delayed food reactions are more difficult to identify. They are also much less common. Keeping an accurate, detailed food diary for at least a week may help in fingering the offending food.

Among the most common food-allergy symptoms are swelling or itching of the lips, mouth, and/or throat. Once the offending food enters your digestive system, nausea, vomiting, cramping, and diarrhea may begin. Itching, hives, eczema, and redness of the skin are also common. But you might experience symptoms that resemble an allergy to ragweed or pollen—sneezing, a runny nose, or shortness of breath. This is called allergic rhinitis.

When Allergies Are Life-or-Death Conditions

Thankfully, most cases of allergic reaction are relatively mild. But a small percentage of people with food allergies experience reactions severe enough to be life-threatening. Anaphylaxis is the rare but potentially fatal condition in which several parts of the body experience allergic reactions simultaneously. Symptoms can progress rapidly and include severe itching, hives, sweating, swelling of the throat, breathing difficulties, lowered blood pressure, unconsciousness, and, if left untreated, even death.

In one study of fatal allergic reactions to foods, deaths occurred away from home when people had accidentally eaten a food to which they knew they were severely allergic. If you know you are severely allergic, be extremely cautious when eating out. Some allergenic ingredients are well hidden.

You're at higher risk of dying from an allergic reaction if you have asthma or if you don't have a dose of epinephrine (adrenaline) on hand to administer quickly after your reaction begins. Sold only by prescription, epinephrine is usually packaged as a bee-sting kit for those who react severely to insect bites. Talk to your doctor about it.

People with severe reactions should be instructed on when and how to give themselves a shot of epinephrine in the event of a severe reaction. Oral antihistamines may be helpful in treating mild reactions, but the early administration of epinephrine can be a lifesaver.

A small segment of the population is highly allergic to sulfites, a chemical used to preserve the color of foods such as dried fruits and vegetables. If you are allergic, you may develop shortness of breath or fatal shock shortly after eating a sulfite-treated food. Sulfites can also trigger severe asthma attacks in sulfite-sensitive asthmatics. For that reason, in 1986, the FDA banned the use of sulfites on fresh fruits and vegetables (except potatoes) that are sold or served raw to consumers, like what you might find at a salad bar. If sulfites are added to packaged and processed foods, it must be listed on the ingredient label. Sulfites are sometimes added to red wines, but all wines have some sulfites present that are produced naturally.

Tartrazine, or FD&C Yellow (dye) #5, may induce asthma attacks in a very small minority of asthmatics. According to a report from the National Asthma Education Program of the National Institutes of Health, this type of reaction is probably limited to those rare individuals who appear to have an immunologically mediated sensitivity to the dye. Nonetheless, manufacturers of foods containing this dye are now required to include it in the list of ingredients.

Diagnosing Food Allergies

You should consult an allergist or other qualified health professional to determine whether your symptoms really are being caused by a food allergy or if you have some other problem. Because food allergies can affect many different organs and systems in your body, they have become a popular dumping ground for a host of unexplained medical problems. Misconceptions about food allergies are sometimes reinforced by some practitioners, who blame almost every unexplainable ache or pain on food allergies.

A growing number of self-proclaimed specialists calling themselves "clinical ecologists" would have you believe that food allergies affect millions of people, causing conditions that range from obesity and fatigue to hyperactivity and insomnia. In addition, some well-meaning qualified allergists overdiagnose food allergies because they use inappropriate diagnostic tests. Consulting a board-certified allergist is your best bet for an accurate diagnosis.

The diagnosis of your food allergy should start with a thorough medical history, followed by: questions about the amount of food you have to eat to trigger a reaction; how long it takes to develop symptoms; and how often you have an allergic reaction. A complete physical examination and laboratory tests should be given to rule out other medical conditions.

Elimination diets are often helpful both in the diagnosis and treatment of food allergies. Here's what generally happens on an elimination diet: For several weeks, you completely eliminate or restrict foods you suspect you are allergic to and stick with foods least likely to cause allergic reactions. Foods that rarely cause allergies include apples, artichokes, carrots, gelatin, lamb, lettuce, peaches, pears, and rice.

If your symptoms improve on the restricted diet, then you can introduce the suspect foods one at a time and see if the symptoms return. If they do, you should continue to avoid that food. One caveat: You should try elimination diets only with your doctor's OK and only under the supervision of a registered dietitian. Never eliminate entire groups of food for weeks at a time.

Several tests are available to determine if your immune system overreacts to certain foods. In skin-prick testing, a diluted extract of the food is placed on your skin, and the skin is scratched or punctured. If no reaction occurs at the site, then the skin test is negative. If a bump surrounded by redness (it will look like a mosquito bite) forms within 15 minutes, then the skin test is positive and you may be allergic to the food being tested. But skin testing is not the most reliable indicator of food allergies. It tends to give false positives—that is, it indicates a sensitivity that is not really there or that triggers no symptoms. False negatives can also occur (in other words, no reaction to the test occurs, but the individual is still allergic to the food).

Blood tests known as the radioallergosorbent test (RAST) or the enzyme-linked immunosorbent assay (ELISA) are also used to test for allergies. These test for antibodies in your body. Though the tests are more reliable than the skin prick, they, too, can give false positives.

If your medical history, physical examination, or skin and laboratory tests suggest a food allergy, and if your reactions to the food are not severe, then your doctor may conduct a food challenge to find out just how much you can tolerate. In a food challenge, you are given increasing doses of the suspected food until you develop symptoms.

Two controversial methods advertised to diagnose food allergy are cytotoxic testing and symptom-provocation testing, in which a dose of the food extract is placed under your tongue or injected. But according to the American Academy of Allergy and Immunology, these methods are expensive and unreliable for detecting food allergies.

After the Diagnosis

Once you've been diagnosed with a food allergy or allergies, the only effective treatment is to avoid the offender(s). An eating plan that eliminates the offending food(s) should be developed carefully. Your diet should take into account your ability to tolerate certain amounts of the food, the need to eat a balanced diet, and an understanding of how difficult it is to follow the diet.

To successfully follow an allergy diet, you must become adept at reading food labels. All food products are required by law to provide a list of ingredients. But be sure to recheck labels periodically, as product formulations frequently change. You can also get very specific information about food ingredients by contacting the consumer affairs departments of food companies.

In some cases, strictly avoiding an allergenic food seems to help people outgrow food allergies. One study found that after rigorously following allergen-free diets for one to two years, about one-third of older children and adults were no longer sensitive to the offending foods. However, allergies to peanuts, nuts, fish, and shellfish may last a lifetime.

Food Intolerance

Often confused with food allergies, a food intolerance is the inability to consume normal amounts of a food for reasons unrelated to the immune system. Lactose intolerance, for instance, falls into this category (see Lactose Intolerance).

Certain food additives can cause intolerances. A small number of people may experience mild and short-lived reactions after eating monosodium glutamate (MSG), a flavor enhancer used in processed foods. The intolerance is also known as "Chinese Restaurant Syndrome." The manufacturers of MSG say no such reaction exists. But many who have experienced it beg to differ.

In certain sensitive individuals, the amino acid tyramine may promote headaches (see Headaches).

GALLBLADDER PROBLEMS

Fat, female, forty, and fertile is the not-so-flattering profile often used to describe someone who is most at risk for developing gallbladder disease. No one seems to know exactly what causes gallbladder disease. But it's doubtful that any one factor is to blame. It is probably due to several factors including heredity, diet, hormones, and infections. But the four F's noted above do offer clues.

The medical terms for gallbladder disease are almost unpronounceable. Cholelithiasis (ko-le-li-THY-a-sis) refers to gallstones, and cholecystitis (ko-le-sis-TY-tis) refers to an inflamed gallbladder.

What Does the Gallbladder Do?

The gallbladder is a small, muscular, pear-shaped sac that resides just under the right side of your liver. It has the capacity to hold about a quarter cup of bile, a yellowish-green material produced by the liver. Bile is made up of water, bile salts and acids, cholesterol, and phospholipids (compounds that help dissolve fats). Bile's main function is to help break up large globs of fat into smaller globs, which is the first step in digesting fat.

A healthy gallbladder keeps bile moving, making stone formation unlikely. However, if something goes awry, the sludgelike contents of the gallbladder can crystalize, creating a gallstone. The most common type of gallstone forms when bile becomes supersaturated and cholesterol crystals form. Stones can grow to be quite large, and your gallbladder may contain hundreds of them. They can be detected through a special X ray called a cholecystogram.

Secret Stones

About half of the people who have gallstones don't even know it. Over 60 percent of the people with gallstones will experience symptoms only once. These symptomless stones probably float freely in the gallbladder. But watch out—if a stone settles in the duct that leads to the small intestine, it will surely let its presence be known. If the stone is large enough to block the flow of bile out of the duct, it will trigger severe pain and nausea, maybe even vomiting, fever, bloating, belching, and jaundice.

The most serious scenario is when pressure builds in the gallbladder to the point where it bursts. Left untreated, this could lead to peritonitis, a severe infection of the abdominal cavity. A blocked gallbladder duct can also damage your pancreas and your liver. Fortunately, all of this is unlikely to happen. If you see a doctor when you have symptoms, the gallbladder will probably be removed before your condition reaches this critical point.

Who Gets Gallstones?

Gallstones are quite common in the United States. Approximately 20 million people have them. If you think that's high, consider Sweden, where 44 percent of the population is affected. Or consider the Pima Indians of southern Arizona; more than three-quarters of them develop gallstones by the age of 35.

Getting older carries with it a risk of gallbladder disease. But age isn't the only risk-raising factor. Other high-risk groups include overweight women, American Indians from the southwestern United States (such as the Pima), and diabetics.

The Diet Connection

Experts say that some—though not all—gallbladder disease can be prevented. And it looks as if diet plays a crucial role. The composition of your bile strongly affects your chances of developing gallstones. And what you eat influences bile composition.

High-fiber diets seem to offer some protection against gallstones. And a small protective effect has been seen in women who eat a lot of vegetables.

The strongest diet connection relates to eating too much. Research has found, at least in women, that the heavier you are, the higher your risk of developing gallstones. Even being moderately overweight almost doubles your risk. That risk increases sixfold if you're very overweight. By age 60, almost one-third of obese women can expect to develop gallbladder disease.

If you are overweight, you need to lose weight. But take it slowly. Ironically, rapid weight loss is a suspect in gallstone formation.

Super-low-fat diets—less than ten grams of fat a day—are also risky. Without enough fat to stimulate it, the gallbladder becomes inactive, allowing stones to form. For years, patients suffering from gallbladder disease were instructed to eat low-fat diets because it was thought that by reducing dietary fat, the gallbladder would be used less and this would provide relief from symptoms. However, there is little evidence that restricting fat helps much. On the other hand, some people with gallstones do experience discomfort when they eat certain spicy, greasy foods. You should be the judge of what triggers your symptoms and simply stay away from foods that seem to produce problems for you.

Though cholesterol is a major component of gallstones, the amount of cholesterol in your diet probably has little, if any, effect on whether or not you develop them.

When Diet Isn't Enough

Doctors use a variety of treatments to provide some degree of relief. But the standard treatment for chronic gallbladder disease is simply to remove the organ. After surgery, you can gradually return to a normal diet. If some foods still bother you, cross them off your menu. But generally, the liver manufactures enough bile to handle a normal diet.

Though surgery may sound like drastic treatment, some doctors actually consider it a preventive measure. For example, diabetics who have symptomless gallstones are candidates for preventive surgery, to ensure that gallstones don't make trouble in the future.

Having your gallbladder removed is considered major surgery. It takes about a month to recover. However, a simpler surgical technique called laparoscopic laser cholecystectomy, in which the gallbladder is removed through a tiny incision, is coming into vogue. This latest "Band Aid" surgery (so-called because it requires a tiny incision) eventually may replace traditional gallbladder surgery. Most people can return to normal activities within a week of having this type of surgery.

Drugs are used to dissolve small gallstones in people who aren't strong enough to undergo surgery. But the medications do have drawbacks. Diarrhea is a common side effect. And one-half of patients develop new stones within five years of stopping drug treatment.

HEADACHES

It's back. That pounding in your head that just won't go away. You would do anything just to feel like you again. Millions of Americans suffer from headaches, whether sinus, tension, stress, or the granddaddy of headaches—migraine. A headache can be simply annoying or it can be debilitating, interfering with your ability to function normally. Getting rid of a headache once you have one can be difficult. Your best strategy is to stop it before it ever gets started. One of the most common headache triggers, over which you have complete control, is food.

Though all kinds of headaches have other influencing factors besides diet, food can sometimes be the straw that breaks the camel's back. Certain substances in foods, for example, may trigger some migraines in sensitive individuals. Migraines occur when blood vessels in the scalp contract and expand, producing throbbing pain usually on one side of the head. Seventy percent of migraine sufferers are women.

Some headache specialists agree that there is a strong connection between diet and headaches. However, others believe that diet management in the treatment of headaches is a gimmick for some headache clinics to make money.

Tyramine

Eating foods rich in tyramine, a substance related to amino acids, may cause migraine attacks if you're sensitive to it. Tyramine appears to prompt attacks by causing blood vessels in the skull to constrict and dilate. It's been estimated that people who suffer migraines may have a metabolic defect that prevents them from breaking down tyramine. The result is a buildup of tyramine in the blood and, ultimately, a migraine. Migraines triggered by tyramine are most common in people taking monoamine oxidase (MAO) inhibitors, used to treat depression.

Tyramine is found in aged and fermented foods, such as Chianti wine, overripe bananas, avocados, peanuts, chicken liver, and aged cheeses. If aged cheeses are a headache trigger for you, be aware that some cheeses are blends that contain aged cheeses as an ingredient. Check labels.

Alcohol

Any alcoholic beverage can provoke headaches. Alcohol not only dilates blood vessels, but by-products of the fermentation process, called congeners, can provoke headaches. The greatest amount of congeners are found in cognac and Scotch whiskey.

Chocolate

Chocolate is double trouble. It contains phenylethylamine—a naturally occurring substance that affects blood vessels in the same way as tyramine—and a small amount of caf-

FOODS THAT CAN BRING ON THE PAIN

Cheeses—American, blue, Bourseault, brick, Brie, Camembert, cheddar, Emmentaler, Gruyère, mozzarella, Roquefort

Beverages—Beer, Chianti, coffee, cognac, colas, scotch, tea, any red wine

Other Foods—Avocados, bananas, chicken livers, chocolate, fava beans, nuts, peanut butter, peanuts, pepperoni, pickled herring, sausages, sour cream, soy sauce, freshly baked yeast products

Food Additives—aspartame, monosodium glutamate (MSG), nitrates (sodium nitrite), hydrolyzed vegetable protein

feine. Migraine sufferers should moderate their caffeine intake because a headache can be set off when an excessive intake of caffeine is suddenly stopped (see "When Cutting Back on Caffeine Makes You Sick"). For example, many people suffer "caffeine withdrawal" on weekends.

Food Additives

Some food additives such as sodium nitrites—used in smoked ham, bacon, hot dogs, pepperoni, sausages, and cold cuts as a preservative and coloring agent—dilate blood vessels and can be headache triggers. Monosodium glutamate (MSG), a flavor enhancer found in over 2,500 food products, has also been suggested as a possible cause of migraines.

Timing of Meals

Just as eating the wrong foods can trigger migraine headaches, skipping meals can have the same effect. Prolonged

WHEN CUTTING BACK ON CAFFEINE MAKES YOU SICK

If you're a coffee drinker, a recent study published in *The New England Journal of Medicine* probably came as no surprise. It found that people who suddenly stop consuming caffeine are likely to experience a long list of unpleasant side effects, including drowsiness, depression, anxiety, fatigue, and headaches—even nausea and vomiting. In the study, more than one-half of those who stopped caffeine reported moderate to severe headaches. The average coffee intake was about 1½ cups per day.

So, big deal, you say? Well, this study was important because it was the first to clearly show that caffeine withdrawal occurs even in people who are low to moderate coffee drinkers. Earlier studies focused on people who drank at least three cups a day. Moreover, withdrawal symptoms were more prevalent in this study than in earlier ones.

If you are trying to cut back, keep in mind that coffee isn't the only source of caffeine. It's also found in some over-the-counter medications, colas, teas, and chocolate. (See "Some Common Caffeine Sources" in Fibrocystic Breast Disease.)

The number one rule: Cut back gradually, or you may suffer the consequences. Try halving your caffeinated coffee, tea, or cola intake during week one (mix half your regular brew with decaf), then halve it again the second and third weeks, until you're drinking straight decaf.

fasting can make blood-sugar levels drop and bring on headaches. The problem is compounded if you consume large amounts of caffeine-containing beverages to keep hunger at bay. The result can be a whopper of a headache. Eating regular meals can stave off this migraine trigger.

Food Allergies

There are some researchers who say headaches can result from food allergies or intolerances. The theory is that the body's immune system identifies some foods as allergic compounds and sets off vascular changes, leading to headaches. Whether or not you react, they say, depends on your own level of sensitivity. But most experts insist that the immune system is not involved in triggering headaches.

HEARTBURN

That fire you feel at the base of your breastbone after you overindulge is the result of acid indigestion, also known as heartburn. Almost half of all adults suffer from it regularly. Women are more likely to experience it during pregnancy. And the burning sensation can be severe enough that it sometimes does a great imitation of a heart attack.

Heartburn is a common symptom of what doctors call gastroesophageal reflux. Simply stated, the acidic contents of the stomach back up into the esophagus—the tube in your throat that connects your mouth to your stomach. Normally, a muscle at the base of the esophagus, called the lower esophageal sphincter, prevents what's in the stomach from sloshing back up through the esophagus. But some people have a weakened esophageal sphincter—so weak, that coughing or straining may be enough to bring on a bout of heartburn. Why isn't known. But it is more common once you pass age 50.

When it happens, you may have a burning chest pain lasting up to two hours, an acid or bitter taste in your mouth, stomach pain, nausea, and even breathing difficulty.

Heartburn Triggers

Though food is most often the prime suspect as the cause of heartburn, other factors in your life may bring it on. Most common: stress, medications, excitement, and depression. Smokers are likely candidates for heartburn. Smoke weakens the contractions of the lower esophageal sphincter muscle.

Common Food Offenders

Some people, just by their nature, may be more vulnerable to heartburn. But it's still what, when, and how much you eat that are the most common culprits. Mexican food has been cited as most likely to cause heartburn, followed by Italian food, pizza, and hamburgers served at fast-food restaurants. Other food triggers include coffee, tea, colas (substituting decaf doesn't help), any spicy or high-fat food, tomato products, citrus fruits and juices, and alcoholic beverages.

A food seldom thought of as a heartburn trigger is chocolate, but it, too, can start the fire. An after-dinner peppermint or spearmint, sometimes used to relieve heartburn, can actually make it worse.

While you may need to avoid or limit all of these foods, keep in mind that everyone has their own unique trigger foods. Note which foods you are most sensitive to and avoid them. It's really just a matter of common sense.

Late-night eating may be an invitation to heartburn. Give yourself some time to digest your food before you go horizontal. And sleep on an angle (elevating the head of your bed six inches). Doctors say this is the single most important self-help measure. Changing your diet may be enough if you suffer only mild symptoms, but persistent heartburn may be a red flag for more serious conditions.

Reflux Complications

Heartburn is generally more of an annoyance than a danger. But remember, it is a symptom of gastroesophageal reflux. While many people with reflux never experience anything worse than an occasional bout with heartburn, be aware that untreated reflux can have serious consequences.

For example, over a period of time, if the esophagus is repeatedly irritated by acid reflux, complications may result: anemia, caused by blood loss from a damaged esophagus, or permanent scarring of the lower esophagus that can interfere with swallowing.

TYPICAL HEARTBURN PRODUCERS

Alcohol	Garlic
Allspice	Ginger
Carbonated beverages	Hot peppers
Chili powder	Milk
Chocolate	Milk shakes
Chocolate milk	Nutmeg
Cinnamon	Onions
Citrus fruits and fruit juices	Pastries
Coffee	Peppermint
Cumin	Pepperoni
Deep-fried foods	Spearmint
	Tomato products

Acid reflux that occurs while you sleep can seep into the lungs and cause coughing and inflammation of the bronchial tubes. You may become hoarse if gastric reflux burns your vocal chords.

No need to worry if you experience heartburn only occasionally—say once or twice a week. But if your heartburn is chronic or if sleeping becomes a sort of "Mission Impossible," it's time to see a doctor. Your doctor may do nothing more than recommend antacids (they seem to help most heartburn sufferers, at least temporarily). But you may have to take them as often as every hour until your symptoms subside.

There are also prescription medications that may help. For chronic, severe heartburn, the doctor may order an "upper GI series," a series of X rays of the esophagus, stomach, and small intestines that enables the doctor to take a closer look and see if any damage has been done.

As yet, no one knows why some people have weak esophageal sphincters. And there's no cure for gastro-esophageal reflux. But there are steps you can take to lessen the likelihood that your symptoms will become worse:

• Avoid eating large meals.

• Don't eat within three to four hours of going to sleep or even lying down on the couch in front of the television.

• If overweight, lose weight. Being overweight increases the chance that you will suffer from heartburn.

• Wait a couple of hours after you eat to exercise.

• Don't bend over shortly after you eat.

• Stop smoking.

• Elevate the head of your bed six inches from the floor by placing blocks or books under the legs; gravity helps clear the esophagus of acid reflux. But don't extra use pillows under your head. This position could actually make your heartburn worse, by altering the angle of your neck and throat.

• Stimulate your production of saliva by chewing gum, antacids, lozenges, or hard candy; just thinking about biting into a sour lemon can also increase salivation. Saliva is naturally alkaline, and extra production may help to neutralize the acid in your esophagus. But avoid peppermint-flavored candies. Peppermint tends to aggravate heartburn.

• See your doctor if you are taking antacids three or more times a week.

HEART DISEASE

A lot of ingredients go into the "recipe" for a heart attack. Some are handed to you when you're born. Some you acquire as you age. Fortunately, some of them you can change. If you do, you may be able to modify that recipe enough to avoid cooking your own goose.

It's likely that your first encounter with "risk factors"—ingredients for disease—is when you find out your blood cholesterol level.

Making Sense of Alphabet Soup

Don't feel bad if you're confused by all those acronyms your doctor, the media, and even this book throw out at you—LDLs, HDLs, and the like. (You may want to refresh your memory about fat and cholesterol by referring back to Fat in Part I.) For our purposes here, just remember that HDLs are the "good" kind of cholesterol that gets carried away from your heart and arteries, and LDLs are the "bad" cholesterol that causes cholesterol buildup around your heart and arteries.

The cholesterol in your blood is always a combination of HDLs and LDLs (plus a few VLDLs, very low-density lipoproteins, and chylomicrons, but we won't concern ourselves with those here). Your blood cholesterol is usually about one-third HDLs and two-thirds LDLs, but some people have more HDLs and fewer LDLs than others. Some of this is luck—your family tree might favor HDLs—but some of it depends on your diet and how much you exercise.

Your age and sex also influence your blood cholesterol level. In childhood, females tend to have higher total cholesterol values. Males actually show a significant decline during adolescence, when testosterone starts flooding their bodies. Adult males over the age of 20, however, generally have higher levels of cholesterol than females do. Once women reach menopause, though, they tend to have higher cholesterol levels than their male counterparts.

What's Your Cholesterol?

When you get your cholesterol tested at a health fair or at the mall or if you test yourself at home with a home cholesterol kit, the number you get is your total cholesterol. Total cholesterol is easier to measure than the individual lipoproteins, because it can be done from a fingerstick and doesn't require you to fast beforehand. (However, this type of quick cholesterol test may not be as accurate and reliable as a cholesterol test done on blood that is drawn and sent to a laboratory for analysis.)

For years, it's been known that the higher your total cholesterol, the greater your chances of suffering a heart attack. In general, you want your total cholesterol to be below 200. Above 240 is entering the danger zone. But, experts concede that knowing your total cholesterol is not a foolproof warning system.

A total cholesterol reading tells you the sum total of HDLs, LDLs, and VLDLs you have in your blood, but it doesn't tell you how much you have of each. Because it's good news to have a lot of HDLs in your blood, but bad news to have a lot of LDLs and VLDLs, this is important information you're missing. So, while total cholesterol is useful, it isn't the whole story.

The latest thinking is that your blood level of HDLs is a better indicator of your heart-attack risk. In mid-1993, the National Cholesterol Education Program (NCEP) added a recommendation that initial testing of cholesterol include an HDL measurement. A blood level below 35 increases your risk of heart attack, while an HDL above 60 is protective.

Best of all for predicting heart attacks might be what's known as your ratio of total cholesterol to HDL (TC:HDL). Some experts, including William Castelli, M.D., director of the famed Framingham Heart Study, have relied on this indicator for years. By some accounts, you're at low risk for heart trouble if your TC:HDL ratio is less than 4.5 (men) or 4.0 (women). Anyone with a ratio above these cutoffs is at higher risk and should act to lower total cholesterol, raise HDLs, or both. Regular exercise is a way to boost your HDLs, as is stopping smoking and losing excess weight. But it may be easier to lower your LDLs, which will automatically lower your total cholesterol and your TC:HDL ratio.

CHECK OUT YOUR RISK

Total Cholesterol:	Less than 200 = Desirable
	200-239 = Borderline-high
	240 and above = High
LDL Cholesterol:	Less than 130 = Desirable
	130-159 = Borderline-high
	160 or above = High
HDL Cholesterol:	Less than 35 = Increased risk
	35 or above = Acceptable
	Above 60 = Decreased risk
Triglycerides:	Less than 200 = Normal
	200-400 = Borderline-high
	401-1000 = High
	Above 1000 = Very high

What about triglycerides, the storage form of the fat that you eat and the fat that you make from carbohydrates and protein? That's a toughie. Researchers have waxed and waned on the importance of a high triglyceride level. A high triglyceride level increases your risk for heart disease, but maybe only because it's usually accompanied by high LDLs, low HDLs, or high blood sugar.

To worry over triglycerides or not? That is the debate. While there's no clear answer as to whether high triglycerides alone raise your risk of heart disease, a new 12-year study from the University of California at San Diego identifies who should pay most attention: those with high triglycerides who are younger than 70 or who have low HDLs (below 35 in men; below 45 in women) or low LDLs (below 160).

If your triglycerides are high (see sidebar, "Check Out Your Risk"), the new NCEP guidelines recommend you lose weight (if you are overweight), avoid alcohol, and increase your physical activity. Limiting refined carbohydrates—like sugar, honey, corn syrup, molasses—may be wise as well.

The Dreaded Heart Attack: How It Starts

No, we don't mean when you feel the crushing weight in your chest and the pain radiating down your left arm. We mean when it really begins, years before. Trouble starts when LDL cholesterol finds "nicks" in the vessel walls—places to grab onto. The LDLs cling to these weaknesses in artery walls, attracting other substances like minerals and cell debris, to form a substance called plaque.

Plaque is what hardens along the inside of your vessel walls, narrowing the diameter through which blood can flow. The more LDLs you have floating around, the more there are to initiate the plaque process.

Experts think this process starts in the teenage years or young adulthood, as something they call fatty streaks. Over the years, the plaque grows larger. It becomes fibrous and calcifies, almost like scar tissue, literally "hardening" your arteries. Eventually, it can completely block an artery, preventing blood flow and the passage of oxygen to the heart. If this happens in a small artery or if the blockage in a major artery is incomplete, you may notice only chest pain, called angina. But if complete blockage occurs in a major artery, you'll have a full-blown heart attack, what doctors call a myocardial infarction, or MI, for short. This is what you want to prevent.

Prevention Is the Name of the Game

It makes sense that if heart disease starts early, that's when prevention should start, too. Don't wait until it's too late. You may not get an early warning. For one of every four persons who suffer a heart attack, sudden death is their first sign of the underlying damage.

Does that mean it's a lost cause to try to mend your ways later in life? The good news is, no! If you've been lucky enough to survive a heart attack, or even if you have no symptoms, changing your lifestyle still can halt and maybe even reverse clogged arteries; it's just more difficult to do than when you are young. But, at any age, the steps you can take to prevent heart disease remain the same.

And there's lots you can do. True, you can't change the genes you were born with. Some people are just more prone to heart disease than others. But if you know heart disease runs in your family, you have the advantage of knowing about your inherited tendency, plus a strong incentive to fight it.

What else can't you change? Time marches forward for all of us, so the added risk as we age is a given. If you're a man, however, you're more vulnerable to heart disease at an earlier age. That doesn't mean women should feel they're immune to this disease. After menopause, the rate of heart disease quickly evens out. And women at this stage in life are actually more likely to die if they suffer a heart attack.

What can you change? We won't dwell on the nondiet-related things you can do, but they include probably the most important changes, like stopping smoking, treating high blood pressure, and being more physically active. Then there are the various dietary changes that may make a difference.

The Semantics of Cholesterol and Diet

You often hear people say they're on a "low-cholesterol" diet. While that may be true, it's more important to be following a "cholesterol-lowering" diet. What's the difference? More than se-

WHAT PUTS YOU AT RISK FOR A HEART ATTACK?

• Being a male age 45 years or older
• Being a woman age 55 years or older (or experiencing early menopause and not taking estrogen replacement therapy)
  • Family history of premature heart disease
  • Smoking
  • High blood pressure
  • Diabetes
  • LDL-cholesterol level of 240 or above
  • HDL-cholesterol level less than 35

[Note: Obesity and physical inactivity are not direct risk factors, but both contribute to many of the above conditions, and attempts to correct them should be part of a treatment plan.]

mantics. A diet that's low in cholesterol limits the amount of dietary cholesterol you eat. But that's just one small part of a cholesterol-lowering diet, which lowers the level of cholesterol in your blood.

The most important part of a cholesterol-lowering diet is limiting the amount of saturated fat and total fat in your diet. Saturated fat increases your blood cholesterol levels even more than the cholesterol you eat does. (Remember that while animal fats tend to be high in saturated fats and plant foods tend to have more unsaturated fats, there are exceptions. The tropical oils—coconut oil, palm oil, and palm kernel oil—are high in saturated fats.) Limiting total fat not only lowers total blood cholesterol, it helps to keep you at a healthy weight, or helps you get to a healthy weight if you are carrying excess pounds.

Polyunsaturated fats are OK, but no longer revered, because besides lowering "bad" LDL cholesterol, they also lower "good" HDL cholesterol. Monounsaturates lower LDLs without lowering HDLs, so they are preferred as replacements for

THE STEPS TO A HEALTHY HEART

Diet is the first line of defense against cholesterol levels that are too high. First up, a Step I cholesterol-lowering diet. If that doesn't bring your levels down far enough in a month or so, a Step II diet is in order. (For tips on how to cut the fat in your diet, see "Cutting Saturated Fat and Cholesterol" on the following page and Fat in Part I.)

Step I Diet
Total fat: Less than 30% of total calories
Saturated fat: Less than 10% of total calories
Polyunsaturated fat: Up to 10% of total calories
Monounsaturated fat: 10-15% of total calories
Carbohydrates: 50-60% of total calories
Protein: 10-20% of total calories
Cholesterol: Less than 300 milligrams/day
Calories: To achieve and maintain desirable weight

Step II Diet
Same as for Step I, except:
Saturated fat: Less than 7% of total calories
Cholesterol: Less than 200 milligrams/day

some of the saturated fat in your diet. Olive and canola oils are rich in monounsaturates. Peanut oil is, too, but it contains more saturated fats than the other two.

It's important to remember, however, that polyunsaturated and monounsaturated fats that have been hydrogenated—forming *trans* fatty acids—are bad news when it comes to blood cholesterol levels. As mentioned in the Fat chapter of Part I, *trans* fatty acids can raise blood cholesterol, possibly as much as saturated fats can.

Cutting Saturated Fat and Cholesterol

• Make complex carbohydrates the centerpiece of your meals. Add meats as a condiment, only two or three ounces per serving, on the side or mixed in with rice, potatoes, pasta, or couscous, for example.

• Choose meats graded "select;" there's less marbled or "invisible" fat that you can't cut out. Trim all visible fat, then broil or grill the meat, so fat drips away.

• Choose lean cuts of meat. For beef: anything with "round" or "loin" in its name, such as bottom round, top round, eye of round, top loin, sirloin, and tenderloin. For pork: center or tenderloin cuts. For ground meat, ask for ground round, or rinse ground meat in warm water first (to cut the fat content).

• Remove the skin from poultry; that's where most of the fat hangs out. You can keep it on during cooking, to hold in juices, but remove it before eating.

• Drink skim or 1% milk. Switching from whole to skim milk saves over 60 calories and almost eight grams of fat for every cup you drink. Don't try it cold turkey, though. First switch to 2%, then to 1%, then to skim. Give yourself time to get used to each lower fat level, even mixing 2% and 1% for a while if necessary. Choose low-fat or nonfat versions of other dairy products like yogurt, cottage cheese, American and hard cheeses, and buttermilk.

• Switch from butter to a liquid margarine or a tub margarine with liquid oil listed as the first ingredient. But go easy—it still has calories and fat.

• When making eggs, throw away every other yolk, using just the white. In recipes, substitute two egg whites for every whole egg called for.

• Read labels so you can avoid highly saturated coconut and palm kernel oils used in processed foods. Beware of foods listing partially hydrogenated oil as the first or second ingredient.

How Low Should You Go?

Talk about a hot topic. This one has researchers in heated debate. The question is: Is it dangerous for your cholesterol level to go very low? Some studies have uncovered a higher death rate—from all causes, not just heart disease—in people with very low total cholesterol levels—generally below 140. But such a low cholesterol level might be the result of undiagnosed disease, including cancer, making it more a symptom of possible trouble than a cause.

Scientists also discovered an odder link: People with a total cholesterol below 189 are more likely to die from accidents or suicides. A theory has sprung up suggesting that a low cholesterol level could trigger a drop in serotonin levels, a brain chemical that normally inhibits harmful behavior impulses. But a recent analysis of statistics from a study of men found that healthy men with low cholesterol levels did not die any sooner. Those who died early were either heavy smokers or heavy drinkers, were found to have liver disease, or had had a portion of their intestines removed.

• If you make soup or gravy, leave enough time to chill it, so you can skim off the fat that congeals on top. Then heat.

• When eating out, ask for meats and fish to be broiled or grilled; avoid sauteed. Order sauces and dressings on the side and use them sparingly. Select sorbet or fruit for dessert.

• On menus, watch out for key words that spell trouble: Alfredo, au gratin, béarnaise, béchamel, beurre blanc, escalloped, hollandaise, and parmigiana.

• Try cutting the oil in recipes by one-half; often it won't make a difference in how the dish turns out.

Get Rid of that Excess Baggage

If you're overweight, losing some of those excess pounds can help lower your blood cholesterol. Experts now consider

FAT'S FATAL FACTOR

Here's still another reason to watch your fat intake. A British researcher has pointed a finger at fat as the reason for high levels of a dangerous blood-clotting protein called factor VII. Having factor VII around raises your risk that an artery-blocking blood clot will form, leading to a heart attack. Eating a lot of fat apparently revs the blood-clotting system into high gear, triggering increased production of factor VII. Presumably, low-fat meals offer protection against this fatal factor.

weight loss (for anyone who's overweight) and physical activity just as important as a cholesterol-lowering diet if you're trying to prevent or treat heart disease. You'll get better results from following a cholesterol-lowering diet if you also lose excess weight and exercise.

But be careful how you lose that weight. Crash diets are not the answer; slow and steady is your best bet (see Overweight/Obesity). Why? You're more likely to keep it off that way. And research shows that extreme fluctuations in weight may increase your risk of heart attack even more.

Pump Up the Volume

Regular aerobic activity that gets the heart pumping does not need to be at Olympic-caliber level. Even walking three or four times a week is beneficial. Besides exercising your heart—which, after all, is a muscle—physical activity helps keep your blood pressure and weight down. Aim for 70 to 85 percent of your maximum heart rate (see "Target Heart Rate"). You can calculate your target rate for your exact age by subtracting your age from 220 (that gives you your maximum heart rate), then multiplying by 0.70 (for a novice target rate) or by 0.85 (for an experienced target rate). If you already have heart disease, however, be sure to talk with your doctor before beginning any exercise program.

TARGET HEART RATE

Age	Maximum Heart Rate	Target Range
20	200	140-170
30	190	133-161
40	180	126-153
50	170	119-144
60	160	112-136
70	150	105-127

Oat Bran and Beyond

You may have thought oat bran died a much-deserved death at the end of the 80s. But as with Mark Twain, reports of its death were greatly exaggerated. Oat bran has repeatedly been shown to help lower cholesterol levels because of its soluble-fiber content.

There are a few caveats, however. It's most helpful to people whose cholesterol levels are in the danger range above 240. And you need to eat quite a bit to notice a difference. A recent study found that three grams of soluble fiber a day—a large bowl of oat bran cereal or three packets of instant oatmeal—reduced high blood-cholesterol levels by five or six points beyond what a low-fat, low-cholesterol diet could do.

Increasing fiber by any amount provides benefits, simply because it takes the place of more-refined foods high in fat and calories. But a new study now reports that soluble fiber can reduce cholesterol levels another five percent in people who already have lowered their cholesterol on a low-fat, low-cholesterol diet. And it doesn't have to be oat bran, either. Fruits are generally high in soluble fiber, as are some vegetables, but legumes are king of the soluble fiber hit parade. (See Fiber in Part I for specific foods high in soluble fiber.)

Antioxidants to the Rescue!

You remember antioxidants—those nutrients that fend off dangerous free radicals that form whenever oxidation occurs? Researchers are finding them to be important in preventing heart disease. That's because they've discovered things are even more complicated than we thought. Just when we've all gotten straight in our minds the difference between LDLs and HDLs, along comes the news that there are "good" LDLs and "bad" LDLs. The bad ones are oxidized LDLs, or just ox-LDL for short. It seems LDLs are not particularly harmful until they become ox-LDLs. So, if you can prevent their oxidation, it might not matter so much how many LDLs you have.

You may see lots of supplements boasting they contain antioxidants. To get enough vitamin E so it will act as an antioxidant, you probably need a supplement. But you can get plenty of vitamin C, beta-carotene, and other substances with antioxidant properties from foods, by eating a wide variety of fruits and vegetables. (See Vitamins in Part I for good sources).

Fishing Around for Answers

Fish oils made big news a few years back, then quietly faded away. But the evidence that they help prevent heart disease has

---

GARLIC WARDS OFF MORE THAN VAMPIRES

The link between garlic and prevention of heart disease is legendary. Now, researchers have discovered a chemical in garlic that's thought to thin the blood so it's less likely to clot into dangerous plaques. It may also lower LDLs and even raise HDLs. (Check out Garlic in Part IV for more information on this aromatic vegetable.)

not gone away. What has been tempered is the enthusiasm for fish-oil supplements. No one is really sure how much helps, and too much can cause bleeding problems. So, the emphasis these days is on fish itself. You can't overdose on fish, and some studies suggest as little as one to two servings of fish a week may be protective.

Just what do fish oils do? The oils in fish are known as omega-3 fatty acids. The first inkling that they may be of value emerged in studies of Eskimos, who eat lots of omega-3s because they eat so much fish. They also rarely suffer heart attacks. Since then, researchers have discovered that omega-3s prolong blood clotting time, making plaque less likely to congeal on the inside of blood vessels. They may also lower blood-triglyceride levels and blood pressure.

Fish aren't the only sources of omega-3s. Fish get the fatty acids from plankton they eat, which is why seaweed is also a rich source. (See Arthritis for other sources of omega-3 fatty acids.)

Coffee Confusion

Does it or doesn't it? Researchers have gone 'round and 'round debating whether coffee contributes to heart disease. Different studies have arrived at exact opposite conclusions. Part of the problem is that people who smoke and people who drink alcohol (both known risk factors for heart disease) are more likely to be heavy coffee drinkers, often biasing study results.

There is some evidence that coffee can raise LDL-cholesterol levels. But scientists now think it all depends on how you brew the coffee. Only boiled coffee—the kind that's popular in Scandinavia, but not here in the United States—seems to increase the risk for heart disease. Filtered coffee appears to be safer. Although more than four cups a day may raise your cholesterol slightly, both LDLs and HDLs are increased, canceling out the effect. Caffeine is not thought to be the problem, so

BEEF, BUTTER, AND CHOCOLATE VINDICATED?

Not exactly. What you may have heard bandied about on the nightly news and in comedy routines is media hype. Here's the real scoop on all three.

Researchers have found that one type of saturated fat, called stearic acid, doesn't raise cholesterol levels like other saturated fats do. It just so happens to be one of the main saturated fats in beef and chocolate. But—and here's the catch—it's not the only one. So, while beef and chocolate might not be as artery-clogging as we once thought, they are still high in other cholesterol-raising saturated fats. Lean cuts of beef, and chocolates once in a while, are fine.

Butter is not better, as headlines might have you thinking. It's just that margarine is not as good as we once thought. It seems the hydrogenated fats in margarine contain *trans* fatty acids, which raise LDLs and lower HDLS—just the opposite of why you're eating margarine in the first place. But that doesn't mean it's worse for your heart than butter, which, after all, is full of saturated fat. It means you should choose a liquid or soft tub margarine, which are lower in *trans* fats than stick margarine, and use very small amounts of it, just as you should for butter.

decaf is not necessarily off the hook. The bottom line? Moderate consumption of coffee—less than four cups a day—is probably safe.

HEMORRHOIDS

What product advertises on television that it can relieve the "...awful itching and burning..." of hemorrhoids? Hint: It's a "preparation." But nothing can prepare you for the pain no one likes to talk about.

You may think hemorrhoids are a problem of the modern world, born of our refined diet and sedentary ways. But, while our "civilized" lifestyle certainly contributes to the condition, people have been suffering from hemorrhoids for centuries.

Years ago, hemorrhoids were known as "piles." Then as now, they're caused by stress on the veins in the rectum. Today, hemorrhoids are one of the most common problems doctors encounter in patients.

What Causes Hemorrhoids?

In a word, pressure. But it's more than just the stress of standing upright. There's the pressure caused by pregnancy, constipation, diarrhea, "straining" to go, sitting too long, obesity, and even prolonged coughing and sneezing.

Too much pressure can cause veins in the rectum and anus to swell and stretch out of shape. Internal hemorrhoids form just under the tissue that lines the inside of the rectum. They are not visible unless they become so big they "prolapse," or protrude through the anus. External hemorrhoids form outside the rectum, in the veins surrounding the anus.

Either type of hemorrhoid can bleed, although external ones are more prone to bleeding, because they're easily irritated. But the infamous itching, burning, and pain typically results from external hemorrhoids. If an internal hemorrhoid develops a "fissure"—a tear or ulcer in the anal canal—or forms a blood clot, it can cause severe pain. But normally, internal hemorrhoids don't burn or itch, because there are no nerve endings inside the rectum. That's why the Food and Drug Administration, in 1991, banned 30 over-the-counter hemorrhoid preparations from the market as unsafe or ineffective. Now, products must be labeled "for external use only."

Almost all rectal bleeding is due to hemorrhoids, but because such bleeding can, in rare instances, be a signal of other serious disease, notably colon cancer, you should always consult a doctor if you spot blood in the toilet or on the toilet tissue after you wipe yourself if that bleeding lasts more than a day. External hemorrhoids are easily diagnosed, but to detect internal hemorrhoids, a doctor may need to use a special instrument called a proctoscope to look inside.

How to Prevent Them

Hemorrhoids aren't dangerous; they don't lead to cancer or other serious conditions. They rarely bleed enough to cause anemia. In fact, they often cause no symptoms. Still, they can be extremely uncomfortable, and most people would just as soon not have them.

Prevention is the best course. One of the best ways to prevent hemorrhoids is to develop good bowel, exercise, and dietary habits when you're young. But it's never too late.

Good bowel habits mean going when you have the urge, not necessarily every morning, and not holding it in until a more convenient time. There are limits to this, of course, but in general, try to go when nature calls. This develops what doctors call good bowel "tone." A sure way to ruin good tone is to rely on laxatives. Overuse makes your intestinal muscles eventually "forget" how to work. The result is increasing difficulty passing a stool, which in turn requires more straining. Remember, everyone's body has a different rhythm; some people may go twice a day, but it's perfectly normal if you only have bowel movements every three days. Avoid labeling yourself as constipated unless you have bothersome symptoms.

Try to avoid sitting too much—especially on the toilet. This position relaxes your rectal muscles, allowing blood to fill your veins and creating pressure. Physical activity, on the other hand, stimulates all your muscles, including those in the rectum, helping prevent constipation.

RX: Fiber + Fluids

Constipation is the classic cause of hemorrhoids, but diarrhea can create similar pressure-filled situations. Both consti-

HEMORRHOID PREVENTION

• Eat a high-fiber diet, with an emphasis on wheat bran. Include five servings a day of fruits and vegetables, switch over to whole grains, and make beans, not meat, a major part of your meals. If necessary, use a bulk softener, but not a laxative.

• Drink lots of fluids. Six to eight glasses a day is not too much.

• Listen to your body; answer nature's call without delay whenever possible.

• Avoid straining when you're on the toilet. Wait for the "urge."

• Avoid sitting for long periods of time. Break it up with walks.

• Include regular physical activity in your daily plan.

• Practice good hygiene. Wipe off well, but not excessively. Use water if necessary. Warm-water soaks can help relieve discomfort.

pation and diarrhea, fortunately, can be treated with a high-fiber diet. Bran, specifically wheat bran, is the time-honored cure-all, because it creates a bulky stool. But also look to other whole grains, fresh fruits and vegetables, and legumes. (See Constipation for good sources of fiber and bran.) If necessary, you can use an over-the-counter bulk-forming laxative such as psyllium (Perdiem Fiber, Metamucil), but stay away from other types of laxatives. Keep in mind that it's better to get your fiber from foods.

Drinking adequate fluids is essential for keeping your bowel working well. You should drink several glasses a day—up to eight—of water or any fluid. This is especially important if you're eating more bran. Too much bran can actually cause constipation if you're not also drinking adequate fluids.

When All Else Fails

Your doctor may recommend some over-the-counter medications, but they do nothing to heal hemorrhoids; they merely ease the pain and itching. Other than the measures above, your doctor will probably hesitate to do more, since hemorrhoids are a relatively harmless condition.

If you truly are in pain, however, your doctor may recommend surgical treatment. There are many options: rubber-band ligation, infrared photocoagulation, laser coagulation, sclerotherapy, and traditional surgery with a knife. But what you should know about any surgery, besides the complications that can arise—infection, incontinence—is that it is not a cure. It's only temporary. Hemorrhoids are likely to return, especially if you have not changed to a high-fiber diet, with adequate fluids and daily exercise. So surgery should only be considered as a last resort.

HIGH BLOOD PRESSURE

If you knew there was a silent killer lurking, just waiting to strike its next victim, and that there was a one in four chance it might be you, would you be worried? Would you do everything you could do to avoid this killer? Of course. Well, it's all true, and the silent killer is high blood pressure.

How silly, you're probably thinking; I'll know when my blood pressure is high. No, you won't, at least not until it's too late. That's why it's called the silent killer. Apparently, the message is getting across. Until recently, only half of the 60 million Americans with high blood pressure knew they had it. But now, only 16 percent are in the dark. And that's a dangerous place to be.

The statistics are sobering. More than 30,000 Americans will die this year from high blood pressure. That doesn't even include the thousands more that die from heart attacks and strokes that are related to high blood pressure. According to one estimate, if you have high blood pressure, you are seven times more likely to suffer a stroke than if your blood pressure is normal.

At younger ages, more men are afflicted, but after age 65, more women suffer. And women account for more deaths. In fact, more than one-quarter of adult women have high blood pressure; after age 55, it's up to more than half of American women, with the percentages rising every year after that.

Scarier still are the stats for minorities. Blacks are twice as likely to have high blood pressure, and they're four times more likely to die from it. Puerto Ricans, Cuban-Americans, and Mexican-Americans are at greater risk, as well.

The Enigma Called Hypertension

If you have high blood pressure, odds are 90 to 95 percent that you have what's known as essential hypertension. That simply means doctors have no idea what caused it, although heredity and age play large roles. A small minority of people have secondary hypertension, meaning high blood pressure is a symptom of an underlying problem, which if corrected may correct the high blood pressure. But essential hypertension has no cure. You must treat it for life, whether that's with lifestyle changes or drugs or both.

Although the technical term for true high blood pressure is hypertension, it's not a fitting label. The disease is not caused by tension, nor does it make you "hyper." But maybe because that misconception abounds, most people don't realize that hypertension usually has no symptoms. So we'll stick with the more descriptive high blood pressure for most of our discussion, as an interchangeable term for hypertension.

If there are no symptoms, how do you know you have it? Good question. Here's where the first preventive step comes into play. You must have your blood pressure checked regularly. Be sure to ask what your reading is every time. Don't just take the nurse's or doctor's word that it's "within the normal range." You should know what your numbers are, so you'll know if you're straying from your norm.

It's normal for blood pressure to vary throughout the day, depending on your emotions, activity, and even eating. Often, just being in a doctor's office is enough to raise your blood pressure slightly. That's why it's so important to check it regularly. But one abnormal reading is nothing to get excited about; high blood pressure is never diagnosed from one reading alone.

What the Numbers Mean

Most of us are familiar enough with blood pressure readings to know that there are two numbers, the higher one is given first "over" the lower number, like a fraction. But do you know what the numbers refer to?

Briefly, blood pressure is a measure of the force that your blood exerts against your blood-vessel walls. The higher number is called the systolic pressure—the pressure of the blood when the heart pumps. The lower number is the diastolic pressure—the pressure of the blood between heartbeats, when it's at rest.

The more resistance there is to a smooth blood flow, the higher the numbers. If your arteries are clogged, your heart has to work harder than it should to pump blood throughout your body; there will be more resistance to flow, hence a higher pressure. And that's not good. It can lead to a dangerously enlarged heart. The extra pressure on blood vessels can weaken them, making them susceptible to hardening. Blood flow to the body's organs may be slowed, leading to kidney disease, stroke, or heart attack.

So what should your numbers be to avoid all that? In general, it's best if your systolic is below 120 and diastolic is below 80. There's a grey area of uncertain risk, but scientists have

TRANSLATING YOUR BLOOD PRESSURE

Here's how adult blood pressure (BP) readings are classified by the NHLBI, and what action you should take. You fall into the higher risk category even if just one of the two numbers fits the higher range.

Blood Pressure Systolic	Diastolic	Hypertension Classification	Recommendation for Action
< 120	or < 80	Optimal	Have BP checked again within two years.
< 130	or < 85	Normal	
130-139	or 85-89	High Normal	Have BP checked again within one year, and make lifestyle changes.
140-159	or 90-99	Stage 1 (Mild)	Have BP checked again within two months, and make lifestyle changes.
160-179	or 100-109	Stage 2 (Moderate)	Have a complete medical evaluation within one month.
180-209	or 110-119	Stage 3 (Severe)	Have a complete medical evaluation within one week.
≥ 210	≥ 120	Stage 4	Have a complete medical evaluation done immediately.

Key

< = less than   ≥ = equal to or greater than

agreed on certain cut-off points above which definite danger lurks. This new way to classify high blood pressure was announced by the National Heart, Lung, and Blood Institute (NHLBI) in 1993 (see "Translating Your Blood Pressure").

Previously, doctors paid more attention to diastolic pressure readings as being more indicative of trouble. Now, the recommendation is to give equal concern to both numbers; the systolic number is actually thought to better predict the complications that arise from high blood pressure. For those individuals who are diagnosed with hypertension, the aim is to reduce blood pressure down to at least 140/90, perhaps even to 130/85.

Your Secret Weapon: Lifestyle Changes

If you can prevent or lower high blood pressure, then you immediately and dramatically improve your chances for living free of heart disease, stroke, and kidney disease. It's that simple, and that important. And, after quitting smoking, what's the number one way to prevent and treat high blood pressure? No, it's not cutting out salt. The best and surest way for everyone to reduce their blood pressure—even if it's not particularly high to begin with—is to lose excess weight.

Here's the lowdown on weight loss and other "lifestyle changes" experts urge you to make to prevent high blood pressure from becoming serious.

Lose excess weight. This is the most effective diet-related change you can make. The largest hypertension prevention study ever conducted recently concluded that weight loss was by far the most effective of all the lifestyle changes made, including sodium restriction, nutritional supplements, and stress management. And it's likely, say the researchers, that the higher your blood pressure or the more overweight you are to begin with, the more dramatic the effect losing weight will have on your blood pressure.

Study results recently released from the University of Texas in Houston reveal that for overweight, but not obese, people with mild hypertension, losing just 6 to 12 pounds of excess weight helped them lower their blood pressure and keep it in the normal range. Similar weight loss in people taking blood-pressure medication helped them keep their blood pressure under control without having to increase their dosages of medication.

The moral of the story? You may do better to focus on just a small weight loss at first. You'll be far more successful than if you try to get rid of all your excess weight at once (see Overweight for more information). Also, with your doctor's permission, include regular exercise as part of your daily routine. It needn't be a vigorous workout to get results. Even a simple daily walk will help keep excess pounds at bay and blood pressure down. For the ideal cardiovascular workout, check out "Target Heart Rate" in Heart Disease.

Cut back on salt. Actually, this is not the cut-and-dried advice you probably think it is. Salt—and the sodium in salt—has gotten more than its fair share of bad press. Studies of different populations around the world paint a fairly convincing picture of sodium as a culprit in causing high blood pressure. Hence, the admonition to avoid it. But what's good for a population as a whole is not necessarily helpful to you as an individual.

In truth, restricting sodium intake may, at best, be helpful to only one-third to one-half of people with high blood pressure, which translates to barely 10 to 15 percent of all Americans. Then why is everyone encouraged to cut back? For the simple reason that we don't know who it will help and who it won't. So we're all told to make the sacrifice, perhaps unnecessarily so.

If you benefit from a sodium restriction, you are what's called sodium-sensitive. That means you have a tendency to retain fluid when you take in too much salt, probably because of a defect in your kidneys' ability to get rid of the sodium. Your body then tries to dilute the concentration of sodium in the blood by conserving fluids. This forces your blood vessels to work extra hard to circulate the additional blood volume. The nerves on the blood vessels become overstimulated and start signaling the vessels to constrict, or get smaller. This only makes it harder for the heart to pump, eventually causing your blood pressure to rise.

Researchers are hard at work trying to find a way to identify just who is sodium-sensitive. If they succeed, one day we'll be able to predict just who will benefit from a sodium restriction.

Even the time-honored thinking that it's only the sodium in salt (which is 40 percent sodium and 60 percent chloride) that's the guilty party has been challenged. Researchers have suggested it is sodium chloride—a.k.a. table salt—that is the problem. Sodium in other forms—like sodium bicarbonate and monosodium glutamate—doesn't seem to cause so much trouble; besides, it contributes less than ten percent of our sodium anyway. So we'll stick to talking salt here.

Perhaps the who-is-sodium-sensitive question is moot, because there's little argument that Americans eat far more salt than they need. If you're typical, you probably eat anywhere from 6 to 20 grams of salt (that's about 2½ to 8 grams of sodium) a day. As much as 75 percent of the salt in our diets comes from processed foods. Only ten percent of what we eat is there naturally, and 15 percent comes from what's added at cooking and at the table.

Fortunately, since the taste for salt is learned—it's not an innate desire like the taste for sugar is—cutting back is possible and probably desirable. The NHLBI recommends trying to cut down to just over 6 grams of salt (2½ grams of sodium), or about one teaspoon, a day. Don't even try to cut out salt entirely. First of all, your body needs some sodium to function; it's an essential nutrient (though ⅕ of a gram is all you need).

Second, you couldn't eliminate sodium even if you tried; it's found naturally in nearly all foods. And third, you still need a practical and palatable diet, which is certainly doable with less salt, but may become less than pleasurable if you have to resort to sodium-free foods.

It makes more sense to cut back on salt where you can, without becoming paranoid about it. That's not so hard to do if you make the right choices in the supermarket and learn to rely on spices and herbs. Heating up your palate helps; heap on some hot peppers or hot sauce and you won't miss the salt. Most important, start eating more whole foods—like the ones discussed in Part IV—and fewer packaged, processed foods; by doing so, you can cut your salt intake in half. Then, just learn to live without the salt shaker, and you're set. (See "Shake the Salt Habit.")

Rack up the potassium. Some people who are hypertensive take potassium-losing thiazide diuretics (Diuril, for example) and are told to eat a banana a day to replace the potassium. But researchers now think extra potassium may be a good idea for everyone. Not only do we eat too much sodium, we take in too little potassium. It's the balance between sodium and potassium that is thought to be important to blood pressure.

But we don't want you running out for potassium supplements. That could be dangerous. Both too much potassium and too little potassium can trigger a heart attack. Stick to foods high in potassium to be safe. But rest assured, bananas are not your only choice. (See Minerals in Part I for good sources of potassium.)

A caveat if you already have high blood pressure and are taking a potassium-sparing diuretic (such as Aldactone) or if you have kidney disease: Discuss with your doctor first whether extra potassium is a good idea for you. If it's not, be aware that many salt substitutes contain potassium chloride.

SHAKE THE SALT HABIT

• Limit your intake of highly processed foods, like frozen dinners, packaged mixes, or prepared sauces used to "extend" meats. They may not always taste salty, but they are, often more than foods that look and taste saltier.

• Buy soups that are sodium-reduced. You'll save sodium but still get flavor, as opposed to truly bland-tasting sodium-free soups. Better yet, make your own low-sodium soups in bulk on the weekends, then freeze individual portions.

• Go easy on the condiments. Ketchup, mustard, mayonnaise, and dressings are loaded with salt; you just don't taste it.

• When eating out, ask for sauces, dressings, and gravies on the side. You'll cut the salt, fat, and calories all in one fell swoop.

• Don't salt your food before tasting it, either. However, you're better off cooking your foods from scratch and salting your own portion lightly than relying on heavily salted processed foods.

• Limit your intake of exceptionally high-sodium foods, like soy sauce, bouillon, olives, pickles, salad dressings, ketchup, smoked and cured meats, tomato and vegetable juices, instant hot cereals, sauerkraut, canned meats and fish, sausage, bologna, and hot dogs.

• Experiment with herbs and spices to find ones that can take the place of salt. Make your own spice combo to put in your salt shaker and use as a salt substitute. Start with the three "P's"—paprika, parsley, and pepper.

• Beware hidden sources of sodium, like "lemon pepper" and "garlic pepper," which both contain salt as an ingredient. Read labels!

• Try squirting lemon or lime juice on vegetables, or steam them with garlic.

Count on calcium. This may be news to you, but calcium is critical to how your heart maintains its rhythm and to how your kidneys regulate sodium and water balance in the body. And, indeed, research has shown that people with high blood pressure generally don't get enough calcium in their diets.

Other studies show that getting extra calcium can actually lower blood pressure. But that may not be true for everyone. As with sodium, only some people may be calcium-sensitive, and they may even be the same people who are sodium-sensitive.

It doesn't appear that amounts greater than the adult RDA of 800 milligrams are helpful, however, so supplements are not the answer. Rely, instead, on foods rich in calcium (see Osteoporosis for calcium sources.)

Increase fiber—decrease fat. Some research shows that eating more fiber can lower blood pressure. A Harvard Medical School study found that people eating less than 12 grams of fiber a day were 60 percent more likely to develop high blood pressure than those who ate more than 24 grams a day. The fiber in fruits was found to provide the most protection from high blood pressure. Meanwhile, studies from Finland show that replacing saturated fat with polyunsaturated fat can lower blood pressure. Does all this sound familiar? It should. We're talking a heart-healthy diet here, so there's every reason to try it.

Don't forget the fish. Here's yet another case where fish may prove fantastic because of their omega-3 fatty-acid content. Researchers gave supplements of omega-3s to people with high blood pressure and were able to lower their blood pressure up to ten points. How? Omega-3s are thought to increase production of a certain type of prostaglandin; these prostaglandins serve as vasodilators, which simply means they make blood vessels expand, thus easing the pressure of blood on the vessel walls.

The amount of fish oil given in studies, however, is equal to what you'd find in a pound of fish a day. That's a lot. So we wouldn't recommend relying solely on fish to keep your blood pressure under control, but it may prove to be one of many positive steps you can take.

Go for the garlic. Numerous researchers have pointed to garlic's ability to lower blood pressure. It also has obvious potential as a flavor replacement for salt. So if you enjoy its flavor, go ahead and indulge. (See Garlic in Part IV.)

Let fruits and vegetables reign. Vegetarians, not surprisingly, have much less incidence of high blood pressure. You, too, can benefit from this approach, even without becoming a vegetarian per se. Just start eating more fruits and vegetables and less animal protein. You'll be eating less fat and more fiber, less salt and more potassium, and you'll very likely lose weight. All this will help your blood pressure.

Curb the nasty habits. Not surprisingly, both smoking and alcohol are strongly associated with high blood pressure. Heavy drinkers probably double their risk of high blood pressure. The NHLBI recommends no more than one ounce of alcohol a day—the amount found in two ounces of 100-proof liquor, eight ounces of wine, or 24 ounces of beer.

It may be a surprise to learn that caffeine does not appear to be particularly risky for blood pressure. While it can raise your pressure temporarily, if you routinely drink a certain amount of coffee, tea, or cola every day, your body adapts to the caffeine level, and your blood pressure is no longer affected.

Adding Medication

The many medications available for treating high blood pressure are beyond the scope of this book, and besides, most experts still consider lifestyle changes to be the first line of defense for treating mild hypertension. But medications are playing an increasingly more important role. Most people are familiar with diuretics, drugs that rid your body of excess fluid. But other drugs may now be taking their place, such as beta-blockers, calcium-channel blockers, and ACE inhibitors. A new study of people with mild hypertension shows that prescribing medication on top of lifestyle changes (diet and exercise) is often more effective than either alone in preventing future heart attacks and strokes. And physicians are finding that if they prescribe lifestyle changes along with medication for people with more severe hypertension, they can use smaller doses of the drugs, cutting both cost and the chance of side effects.

KIDNEY STONES

There's no romancing these stones. But with good nutrition, you may be able to prevent kidney stones from inflicting their pain upon you.

Here's how stones are created: Substances that you get from your diet and that your body produces, including calcium and oxalate, dissolve in urine as it passes through the kidneys. If the urine becomes "supersaturated" with them and is unable to dissolve anymore, the crystals settle out and collect into clumps that accumulate into hard stones.

About ten percent of us will develop kidney stones at some time. You're most likely to suffer from stones if you are male, age 40 or over, have gout, have a family history of kidney stones, or drink heavily. But even if all of these conditions apply, drinking plenty of water may be enough to keep stones at bay.

Kidney stones don't always cause problems. But when they grow large enough to block the flow of urine through the ureter, the pain can be excruciating. You're likely to first feel pain in the lower back, but it can spread to the thighs and groin. Other symptoms of the nasty infection a stone can cause: nausea and vomiting, fever and chills, blood in the urine, and abdominal bloating.

Sound Waves of Relief

Getting rid of kidney stones used to be a much-dreaded surgical procedure followed by weeks of slow recovery. Today, thanks to lithotripsy, a high-tech procedure, invisible sound waves are passed through the body to pulverize stones to the consistency of sand. Prior to the FDA's approval of lithotripsy in 1984, kidney stones could only be removed one of three ways: surgically, with drugs that dissolved the stone, or by "passing" the stone in the urine—an extremely painful experience. Today, lithotripsy is quite common. No anesthesia is required and you can go home the same day.

The Return of the Stone

Just because you made it through one bout with kidney stones doesn't mean you're home free. Your chance of having a repeat performance is great—as much as 80 percent over the next several years. That's why prevention, as always, is the best medicine. Estimates suggest that the right diet can prevent up to 50 percent of kidney stone recurrences. But experts butt heads over what that "right diet" is.

Ironic Prevention

Most kidney stones—about 90 percent—are made of calcium and oxalate, a chemical found in some plants. So, the standard advice doctors gave for years seemed reasonable: If you're a stone former or at risk for stones, cut back on foods rich in calcium and oxalate.

That conventional wisdom was recently turned on its ear when someone decided to test the time-honored advice. New research discovered that a diet low in calcium actually in-

---

Possible Stone Formers

Oddly enough, it's not always the foods that are highest in oxalate that trigger the highest oxalate levels in the urine. Recent research identified the following eight foods as the ones most likely to increase oxalate excretion. Some are high in oxalates, others are not. Avoid them if you know you have a tendency to form kidney stones.

Beets	Spinach
Chocolate	Strawberries
Nuts	Tea
Rhubarb	Wheat bran

---

creased the risk of forming kidney stones. Imagine that. Logic does not always prevail. In a study of 50,000 middle-aged men, those who ate diets rich in calcium were about one-third less likely to develop calcium-containing kidney stones than the men on low-calcium diets. Not only was there no benefit from cutting back on calcium, but a calcium-rich diet appeared to protect against kidney-stone formation. Why? It seems the extra calcium may help carry oxalates out of the body, leaving less of either for stone formation. The study also confirmed what doctors already knew: A high-protein diet contributes to stone formation, while potassium and fluid intake protect against it.

What an eye-opener this study has been. Now, experts think that restricting calcium actually results in more oxalate being absorbed and more stones being formed. Getting plenty of calcium, on the other hand, keeps those oxalate trouble-makers too busy to form stones.

Your diet usually contributes only ten percent of the total oxalate in your body. The rest comes from the breakdown of the amino acid glycine and vitamin C (only megadoses of vitamin C are problematic, however).

So, what's the bottom line? If you're prone to kidney stones, whether you get them is most influenced by how much oxalate is present in your urinary tract, not by how much calcium is there. You can best prevent kidney stones by getting plenty of calcium in your diet; not overdoing the protein; boosting your intake of fruits and vegetables, which are rich in potassium; and, most importantly, drinking lots of fluids to dilute the concentration of minerals that can crystallize into stones and limit the time they hang around. Try to get about two 8-ounce glasses of water every four hours.

Singular Stones

Uric-acid stones are another, less common type of kidney stone. As you might have guessed, they contain uric acid. That's a substance that forms when purines in protein foods are broken down. When your urine is acidic, these stones are more likely to form. Acidic urine is a problem for people who suffer from gout. Not surprisingly, people with gout are more likely than other people to develop uric-acid kidney stones. If you suffer from these stones, you may need to cut back on protein, particularly foods high in purine. High-purine foods include anchovies, beer, brains, fish roe, heart, herring, kidney, liver, mackerel, mussels, sardines, shrimp, sweetbreads, and wine. Your doctor may also prescribe medications to reduce urine acidity.

LACTOSE INTOLERANCE

Milk is often called the "perfect food," but for about 70 to 80 percent of the world's population, drinking milk or eating any dairy product can trigger gas, bloating, and cramping. The cause? Lactose intolerance.

It's what happens when you don't have enough of an enzyme called lactase to break down lactose in your intestinal tract. You may be missing just a little or a lot. Depending on the degree of your enzyme deficiency, drinking milk or eating dairy products, such as ice cream or cottage cheese, can trigger bouts of diarrhea, cramping, and gas 30 minutes later.

The Lactose Lowdown

What's your nationality? It's a good clue to whether you are lactase deficient. The hereditary condition is common among Asians, with about 90 percent suffering from some degree of lactose intolerance. An estimated 70 percent of blacks and about 50 percent of Native Americans and Mexican Americans lack the enzyme. In fact, the only population left relatively unscathed are people of Northern European descent, in whom the incidence is only about 15 to 20 percent.

But lactose intolerance is not an all-or-nothing proposition. It's normal for the level of lactase in the intestinal tract to begin declining after the age of three. How steep that decline is varies greatly among individuals, accounting for a spectrum of symptoms ranging from none to a lot of diarrhea, cramping, and gas. The severity of symptoms depends on just how low your levels of the enzyme are. The gradual decline in your ability to digest lactose is believed to be genetically programmed. It's not affected by how much lactose you consume. So, the older you are, the more likely you are to be lactose intolerant.

There is, however, a rare inherited disorder called congenital lactase deficiency, in which the affected individual, from the time of birth, is either incapable of making lactase or can make only very limited amounts of it. The condition is life-threatening. As soon as an affected infant is given breast milk or a milk-based formula, symptoms such as gas, colic, diarrhea, and a failure to gain weight will appear. Special formulas that do not contain lactose are available. If your child has this disorder, discuss it thoroughly with your child's pediatrician.

Any illness that affects the lactase-producing cells of the small intestine, such as inflammatory bowel disease or even the flu, can trigger a temporary lactase deficiency. In these cases, the condition, referred to as secondary lactase deficiency, is usually temporary; once the illness is over and the damaged cells recover, they begin producing the enzyme again. However, if you have stomach or intestinal surgery, your inability to produce lactase can be permanent.

The variability of symptoms from person to person is so great that one person with lactose intolerance may be able to drink a glass of milk with no symptoms, while someone else with a more severe deficiency or a complete lack of the enzyme might not be able to tolerate even a spoonful of milk in coffee without feeling the effects. And the person who had no symptoms from a single glass of milk could invite trouble if they have ice cream for dessert, by exceeding their ability to handle lactose.

With time, each person learns their own tolerance and eats accordingly. Also, some over-the-counter products in tablet, caplet, or drop form can be taken or added to dairy products to predigest lactose. However, these preparations are not the answer for everyone.

Intolerance *vs.* Allergy

One of the most common misconceptions about lactose intolerance is that it is a milk allergy. Though the two are often confused, the difference is a critical one. The inability to completely digest lactose rarely translates into the need for a milk-free diet. But if you have a milk allergy, even minute amounts can trigger a life-threatening reaction. Symptoms of a true milk allergy include a runny nose, puffy eyes, skin rash, vomiting, tightness in the throat, and difficulty breathing. There is no connection between having a milk allergy, which is due to an immunological response to a protein, and having lactose intolerance, which is an enzyme deficiency.

Lactose intolerance is most common in adults, whereas milk allergies are seen mostly in children. Essentially all children who develop a milk allergy develop it in the first year or so of life. But true milk allergy is a rare occurrence compared to the incidence of lactose intolerance. Only about 2.5 percent of children under the age of three have milk allergies, and the vast majority will outgrow them. In the end, only about one-half of one percent of people carry milk allergies with them into late childhood and possibly into adulthood.

Testing Your Tolerance

Aside from the undeniable symptoms you experience each time you consume dairy products, there are two accurate ways to be sure you have lactose intolerance. One is an oral lactose tolerance test, and the other, more reliable method is a breath hydrogen test for lactose absorption. The level of hydrogen in your breath is measured after consuming lactose, as an indicator of the amount of lactose not being digested.

Living Without Lactose

Lactose is not lurking in milk just to cause you gastrointestinal upset. It serves a specific function. It appears to help your intestines absorb and hold on to calcium, a crucial nutrient for preventing osteoporosis (see Osteoporosis). So, when you cut back on foods high in lactose, you're not only cutting back on calcium, you also may be reducing the absorption of calcium you get from nondairy sources.

Fortunately, most people who are lactose deficient don't have to completely cut dairy foods from their diets. In fact, it's been estimated that about 80 percent of people with lactose intolerance are still able to drink enough milk for good nutrition. But to keep plenty of bone-building calcium in your diet, it's smart to try some of the lactose-reduced and lactose-free milks available. The milks are not bad, though they do taste sweeter than regular milk. Or you can add special enzyme drops to regular milk to predigest the lactose in the milk for you before you drink it. But you must add the drops about 24 hours in advance.

ADD TO YOUR GROCERY LIST:
FISH AND YOGURT

The omega-3 fatty acids in fish have made news in the fight against autoimmune diseases, such as some forms of arthritis. Apparently, they suppress the body's inflammatory response to fighting within the ranks. Some researchers believe they may also fight the spread of cancer cells.

Yogurt may finally be living up to its hype. Recent work at the University of California at Davis found that eating two 8 ounce cartons a day of yogurt with live cultures increased blood levels of a natural disease-fighter called interferon. But, more important, the people eating the yogurt suffered many fewer colds and allergy symptoms. There's also been a study linking the consumption of acidophilus-containing yogurt to prevention of vaginal yeast infections. Expect further research to shed more light on yogurt's potential.

You can also try one of the tablets designed for you to chew before you eat dairy products. Some experts say, however, that the chewable tablets don't digest lactose as efficiently as the drops you add to milk.

Just how diligent you must be in avoiding lactose depends entirely on how sensitive you are. But here are a few tips for avoiding problems.

• Give yogurt a try. Many people who suffer lactose intolerance are able to tolerate yogurt much better than they tolerate milk. And yogurt is an excellent calcium source. But not all yogurts are the same. Research has proved that different brands of yogurt may not be digested equally well. And you may tolerate plain yogurt better than flavored. Use trial and error to find the one that causes you the least distress. Also, be aware that if the yogurt is pasteurized, any benefit is destroyed with the heat process, and the lactose that is present is likely to cause you trouble.

• Drink chocolate milk. The calcium is thought to be just as well absorbed as that in regular milk and you may tolerate flavored milk better than plain. Cocoa may even stimulate lactase enzyme activity.

• You may tolerate aged cheeses like cheddar, Swiss, blue, mozzarella, parmesan, or Monterey Jack well. They contain little lactose compared to milk because the whey, which contains most of the lactose, separates from the cheese during processing.

• Drink milk with meals or pour milk over cereal and fruit. For people who are able to tolerate some lactose, taking in other food with lactose appears to make it go down easier and cause fewer symptoms.

• Drink smaller amounts of milk more often throughout the day. If you can't tolerate a cup of milk, you might do just fine with ½ cup taken at two different times of the day.

• Be aware that besides being present in dairy products, lactose is in about 21 percent of all prescription drugs and 6 percent of all over-the-counter drugs as an "inactive ingredient." Ask your pharmacist.

• Some nondairy foods that may contain lactose are breads, frozen vegetables, soups, salad dressings, cereals, cake mixes, and candies.

• Treat buttermilk and acidophilus milk the same as regular milk. They contain lactose and, contrary to what you may have heard before, they are no better tolerated than regular milk.

• Avoid skim milk. It may cause more problems than milk with a higher fat content. But you shouldn't drink whole milk because of its high fat content. Try 1% and 2% milk.

• Avoid high-lactose cheeses such as cottage cheese, ricotta, and sapsago.

• Try lactose-reduced and lactose-free dairy products like Dairy Ease lactose-reduced milk and Lactaid lactose-free and lactose-reduced milks and lactose-reduced cheeses. Both Dairy

Ease and Lactaid milks are available in whole, low-fat, and nonfat varieties. The Lactaid company makes chocolate and calcium-enriched varieties as well.

OSTEOPOROSIS

If ever there was a disease that fit the old saying, "An ounce of prevention is worth a pound of cure," it's osteoporosis. For years, it was thought that calcium was important only for kids. Once you were grown, your bones were built and that was that. Right? Wrong. That view was forever altered in 1984 when a National Institutes of Health (NIH) conference concluded that, to prevent osteoporosis, women needed more calcium than most of them were getting in their diets.

Osteoporosis is a condition of progressive bone loss that causes bones to become fragile and fracture easily. It is painful, disfiguring, and debilitating. It affects 25 million Americans—about two-thirds are women. For both men and women, age is the biggest risk factor. Osteoporosis usually becomes detectable once you reach your sixties and seventies. There's no cure, so the best line of defense is prevention. If you wait until menopause to worry about getting osteoporosis, it's too late to completely reverse the damage. The good news, however, is that there are steps that can be taken to prevent further bone loss.

The stereotypical "little old lady" image reflects the changes that can occur with osteoporosis: the loss of several inches in height due to the collapse of the spine as bone is lost. As a result, the woman develops a hump known as "dowager's hump" that causes frequent back pain. But that image isn't one that women are destined to live up to.

About 45 percent of your bone mass is laid down during your teen years. But, bone density begins to decrease by about age 35. In women, after menopause, the drop in bone mass is dramatic. By the age of 65, the average woman has only about 74 percent of her peak bone mass. A 65-year-old man, on the other hand, still has about 91 percent. Why do you often hear of older people who break their hips? It's a common clue to osteoporosis, just like the minor bone breaks in the spine that cause loss of height. More than a million people suffer bone fractures each year in the United States due to osteoporosis. Many of those with hip fractures die within a year. It's not uncommon for a person not to even know they have the disease until a bone fractures. As bones become thin and weaken, they are no longer able to withstand the physical stresses of everyday life. If bone loss is severe, something as simple as opening a window can cause bones to break.

How Much Calcium?

Not long after the NIH conference in 1984, calcium was heralded as the secret weapon against bone disease. Calcium was the star nutrient of the decade, and supplement sales soared. But, by the late 1980s, calcium's popularity faded, as studies began to suggest that estrogen and exercise were more important than calcium in preventing bone disease.

It's now pretty much agreed that there are three inseparable aspects of bone health: estrogen, exercise, and calcium. The interest in calcium has been revived by several recent studies that have clearly shown that extra calcium can help build more bone in young children and adolescents. But the biggest surprise came from research showing that postmenopausal women who get adequate calcium can cut bone loss more than 40 percent. And further research has shown that postmenopausal women can actually lay down new bone if they also take estrogen and exercise along with getting enough calcium.

The Recommended Dietary Allowance (RDA) for calcium for adults over age 24 is 800 milligrams per day, the amount found in about three 8-ounce glasses of milk. Some experts

COUNTING ON CALCIUM

	Serving	Calcium (milligrams)
Low-fat yogurt	8 oz.	300-400
Milk, goat's	8 oz.	326
Milk, skim	8 oz.	302
Milk, whole	8 oz.	302
Cheese, romano	1 oz.	302
Orange juice, calcium-fortified	8 oz.	300
Milk, 1%	8 oz.	300
Buttermilk, cultured	8 oz.	285
Cheese, cheddar	1 oz.	204
Salmon, canned with bones	3 oz.	181
Collard greens, chopped, boiled	1/2 cup	179
Cheese, mozzarella	1 oz.	147
Figs, dried	5 figs	99
Kale, boiled	1/2 cup	90
Almonds, dry roasted	1 oz.	80
Cheese, cottage	1/2 cup	68
Biscuit, from a mix	1 biscuit	58
Hamburger roll	1 roll	54
Broccoli, frozen spears	1/2 cup	47
Almond butter	1 tbsp.	43
Corn tortilla	1 tortilla	42
Cheese, goat, soft	1 oz.	40
Brussels sprouts	1/2 cup	28
Cheese, cream	1 oz.	23
Whole-wheat bread	1 slice	11
Soy milk	8 oz.	10

believe that to reduce the risk of osteoporosis, adults should consume closer to 1,000 milligrams a day. However, there is no general consensus on this. So your best bet at this point may be to make sure that you are meeting the RDA for calcium every day.

For women who do not like milk, are lactose intolerant, or are concerned about calories, fat, and cholesterol, there are calcium-rich nondairy foods and low-fat dairy products. Still, most women do not get enough calcium-rich foods to meet the RDA. For them, the only practical way to meet calcium needs may be a calcium supplement.

Seeking a Calcium Supplement

First, avoid supplements that contain bone meal or dolomite; they have sometimes been found to be contaminated with lead.

There's not a lot of evidence that one type of supplement offers more protection from osteoporosis than another. But, there are a few things you should know.

The number of tablets you need to take depends on the type of calcium your supplement contains. Calcium carbonate is the most widely used supplement because it contains the most calcium per tablet. Other calcium sources such as calcium lactate, calcium gluconate, or calcium citrate contain less per tablet, so you'll need to take several each day.

Check the label to find out how much calcium each tablet contains. With some brands, you'll have to take as many as 17 tablets a day to get 1,000 milligrams of calcium. That's a lot to swallow.

A relatively new alternative to calcium supplements is calcium-fortified juices and juice drinks, which provide between 150 to 300 milligrams per eight ounces.

How well you absorb calcium may depend on when you take it. Calcium is best absorbed when it's taken in divided doses rather than all at once. Also, if you're taking calcium carbonate supplements, take them with meals. The digestive juices secreted after a meal help absorb the calcium.

Not all calcium supplements are easily absorbed by the body. It has more to do with how the pill is made rather than what type of calcium is used. There's a simple home test you can perform on your calcium supplement to see just how available it is to your body. Take your calcium supplement and place it in several ounces of vinegar. It should disintegrate or break up within 30 minutes. If the tablet is still in one piece after 30 minutes, switch to another brand.

Antacids can be wonderfully inexpensive sources of supplemental calcium. Some antacids, such as Tums, provide about 200 to 300 milligrams of calcium per tablet; others contain aluminum, which actually robs your body of calcium. Check labels to be sure you're getting the right kind.

Other Bone Builders

Though calcium leads the pack of bone-building nutrients, there are other members of the group that play smaller, but equally critical roles in building and maintaining bone.

Magnesium. Though it is required for bone formation, magnesium's exact role isn't completely understood. About 60 percent of the human body's magnesium is found in bones. In animals, magnesium deficiency causes osteoporosis. Good food sources of magnesium include bananas, chocolate, nuts, seeds, soybeans, buckwheat, beans, and purslane.

Vitamin D. Without enough vitamin D, your body can't take full advantage of the calcium in your diet. Some calcium supplements come with vitamin D, but be careful not to overdose. Too much vitamin D can be toxic. Instead, you can get plenty of vitamin D from vitamin-D-fortified milk or by spending 5 to 15 minutes in the sun two or three times a week. Your skin can manufacture vitamin D when exposed to ultraviolet rays (unless they're blocked by sunscreen).

Manganese. Though the details of how it works aren't known, manganese appears to affect bone synthesis. Rich sources include pineapple, oatmeal, nuts, cereals, beans, whole wheat, spinach, and tea.

Boron. Boron is not yet recognized by the National Academy of Sciences (developers of the RDA) as an essential trace mineral, so there is no RDA for it. However, boron does appear to play a role in your body's ability to retain calcium. Fortunately, fruits and nuts provide boron, so as long as you're following the Food Guide Pyramid (see Variety, Balance, and Moderation in Part III), you're likely to get the boron you need. Foods richest in boron include apples, pears, grapes, dates, raisins, peaches, legumes, almonds, peanuts, and hazelnuts.

Bone Protectors

Besides making sure you get plenty of bone-building nutrients, there are several lifestyle changes you can make and medications you can take to ward off osteoporosis. You'll need to talk to your doctor about the medications. But you can take care of the lifestyle changes on your own. These are the factors that are protective:

Exercise. Regular weight-bearing exercise is crucial for the development and maintenance of healthy bone tissue. This is true for everyone, from young children to postmenopausal women. Walking is a good weight-bearing exercise, and one that most people can do.

Estrogen replacement therapy. After a woman experiences menopause, estrogen therapy can help forestall bone loss. The amount of estrogen required to both prevent bone loss and alleviate the symptoms of menopause is small, actually less than that in a typical birth control pill.

TIPS FOR BOOSTING YOUR CALCIUM INTAKE

• Use bone-in cuts of meat when making stew and soups. If you cook it slowly for a long time, some of the calcium in the bones will leach out into the broth.

• Sprinkle low-fat cheeses on vegetables and salads.

• When you make salads, use the deep-green lettuce leaves of romaine and kale. They are richer in calcium.

• Try adding some powdered nonfat dry milk to some of your foods, such as coffee, tea, soups, casseroles, and batters for bread, cake, cookies, or muffins. Try about ¼ cup per recipe; you'll never even know it's there.

• Make creamed soups with evaporated skim milk.

Overweight. This may be one of the few conditions where being overweight actually offers protection. It's not known exactly why. It could be because the extra weight strengthens bone or it could be that overweight women produce more estrogen than slender women.

Pregnancy. Your risk of developing osteoporosis is greater if you have never been pregnant. Though being pregnant lowers your risk, it's not known if multiple pregnancies lower your risk further or whether they might actually increase it.

The Calcium Robbers

Be aware that there are also bone destroyers:

Too much alcohol. It's been suggested that small amounts of alcohol, say three to six drinks a week, may actually help retain calcium and prevent osteoporosis by raising estrogen levels. But too much alcohol weakens bones and damages your overall health. The flip side to the estrogen coin, however, is that higher estrogen levels associated with moderate alcohol

WHO'S AT RISK?

Here's a checklist of osteoporosis risk factors.

Female. Women are several times more likely to develop osteoporosis than men.

Race. If you're white, you're at greater risk for developing osteoporosis sometime in your life than darker-skinned people are. Far fewer black women develop osteoporosis than do whites. People of Asian descent are also at higher risk for osteoporosis.

Bone structure. Petite women are at greater risk because of their small bones. If they experience the same rate of bone loss as a larger woman, they will develop osteoporosis sooner, because they have less bone to start with.

Early menopause. The earlier you experience menopause, the greater your risk of osteoporosis. Your risk also increases if you have a surgical menopause—a hysterectomy—at an early age and are not on hormone replacement therapy. If only the uterus is removed, but the ovaries are left intact, a woman will experience normal menopausal symptoms in her early 50s, on average.

Family history. Many women with osteoporosis have at least one family member who has the disease. Still, a lack of family history doesn't rule out the possibility that you will develop osteoporosis.

Long-term use of certain medications. People suffering from asthma or rheumatoid arthritis who take cortisone for long periods may diminish their bone strength.

intake may be linked to an increased risk for breast cancer, so go easy.

Too much caffeine. Drinking too much caffeine causes your body to flush out calcium, robbing your bones of the critical mineral. Though researchers haven't pinpointed the level of caffeine consumption that causes problems, it's probably a good idea to keep your daily caffeine intake to no more than about two or three cups of average brewed coffee or four or five cups of average brewed tea. Keep in mind that other food products, including caffeinated soft drinks, can add to your caffeine intake.

Inactivity. It's been proven that exercise is crucial to maintaining bone health throughout life. We're not talking killer aerobics. Simply taking a walk several times a week will do. But it must be weight-bearing exercise. Swimming is good for your heart, but it won't build stronger bones.

Excess protein. In the United States, we generally eat far more protein than we need. And it's believed that high-protein intake causes calcium to be excreted. Over time, this calcium loss, if not compensated for with dietary calcium, will come from the bones.

Smoking. Women who smoke tend to reach menopause earlier than nonsmokers, and this may be what increases their risk for osteoporosis. Or, smoking may encourage bone loss in other ways that haven't yet been identified.

OVERWEIGHT

The headlines about weight loss are positively dismal: "Experts Warn, Diets Don't Work," "Obesity Is Hazardous; So Is a

Failed Diet," "Fanatic Dieters May Shed Years Along with Pounds." Yet, the battle of the bulge is being fought by nearly 70 percent of American women and more than 50 percent of American men. So, what's the answer? The fact is, there is no one answer. How much you should lose, how you should lose it, and whether you should even try to lose it require highly individualized responses.

Why Me?

Though svelte bodies may be the ideal in this country, they are certainly not the norm. This is partly due to the fact that, generally, we eat too much and exercise too little. But it's also the result of genetics. You inherit the tendency to gain weight, just as you inherit blue eyes. And now, research has shown that the influence genetics has on weight and build is much greater than previously thought.

People who try to ignore the hereditary realities of their body size and shape are bound to be frustrated when endless diets and aerobics do not produce the body of their dreams. Genetically, only a tiny fraction of the population is destined to be model-thin. But losing weight depends on far more than mere willpower. If you try to fight your body's preferred weight, you have a lifelong uphill battle ahead of you. So, why do it at all? Because being obese carries with it enormous health risks.

The Price of Excess Pounds *vs.* Yo-Yo Dieting

The health risks of obesity are serious indeed. Stay overweight and you may be increasing your risk of heart disease, high blood pressure, colon cancer, breast cancer, gallbladder disease, osteoarthritis in the knees, diabetes, and back problems.

So, if you're overweight, you should lose weight, right? Well, experts aren't so sure anymore. It's been found that, for some people, losing weight may actually pose a greater health risk than staying overweight. Some research indicates that a drastic change in weight—up or down—may bring with it a significantly increased risk of dying from cardiovascular disease. It may sound weird that losing weight might increase your risk of dying. But that's only if you're a "yo-yo" dieter. "Yo-yo dieting" is when you repeatedly lose and regain weight. Maintaining a stable weight—even if not quite ideal—and avoiding major weight gain seem to be better moves.

The Creeping Pounds of Middle Age

A small percentage of people struggle with obesity from childhood and become obese adults. More common, however, are people who maintain a normal weight most of their lives but then gain 10, 20, or even 30 pounds in middle age and beyond. There are two major changes that take place with age that make it so easy to put on pounds. You tend to become less physically active, and so you lose muscle. That's not good, because muscle burns calories more rapidly than does fat tissue. The lack of activity and loss of muscle mass allow your weight to gradually drift upward as you age.

Though your weight is likely to rise steadily between the ages of 20 and 55, that may not necessarily be bad. In fact, some research suggests that the health risks of being moderately overweight lessen or perhaps disappear as you age. Some experts even suggest that being slightly overweight in your older years increases your longevity.

Am I Really Overweight?

The standards by which weight is measured have changed over the past several years. So has the terminology. "Ideal weight" is a thing of the past. In its place, nutritionists now speak of "desirable weight," "natural weight," and "reasonable weight." Instead of imposing an impossible ideal, the new view is that your goal should be a weight that will provide health benefits and be one that you can realistically reach without starving yourself.

Here's one method experts use for calculating "desirable" weight.

Calculating "desirable" weight:

Men: Allow 106 pounds for the first five feet of height, then add six pounds for every inch over that.

Women: Allow 100 pounds for the first five feet of height and add five pounds for every inch above, or subtract four pounds for every inch under five feet.

This formula gives desirable weights that are somewhat lower than the height and weight charts that are currently popular. Other charts take age into account, allowing for increasingly more weight as you get older.

You're considered "overweight" by the experts if you weigh ten percent over your desirable weight and "obese" if you're 20 percent above your desirable weight.

...Or Am I Overfat?

Aside from weight, researchers now say that the percentage of those pounds that are fat tissue and the way the fat is distributed on your body are better indicators of how much your excess weight is affecting your risk of health problems.

For example, many researchers now use the body mass index, or BMI, rather than weight alone to measure fatness. Both your height and weight are taken into consideration in the calculation. The formula may sound complicated, but it's easy if you use a calculator.

Calculating BMI

Multiply your weight in pounds by 700, divide by your height in inches, then divide by your height in inches again.

A BMI of 25 or less puts you at low risk for heart disease. Between 25 and 30, you're considered to be at low to moderate risk. If your BMI is 30 or more, you're at moderate to very high risk for heart disease.

Fat Distribution

In recent years, the distribution of excess fat on the body has become part of the "equation" for determining the degree of health risk associated with overweight. Some people, especially men, are shaped like apples—that is, their fat settles mostly around their waists and stomachs. Others, mainly women, tend to be more pear-shaped, with their fat mostly around the hips and thighs. Experts measure which tendency you have by calculating your waist-to-hip ratio. It's important because it turns out to be a good predictor of your heart-disease risk. The higher your waist-to-hip ratio—in other words, the more apple-shaped you are—the greater your risk for cardiovascular disease. Men should aim for a waist-to-hip ratio of less than 0.95; women less than 0.80.

Determining waist-to-hip ratio:

To find your waist-to-hip ratio, take a tape measure and measure the circumference of your waist at its narrowest point, when your stomach is relaxed. Then measure the circumference of your hips at their widest. Lastly, divide your waist measurement by your hip measurement. Remember, the lower the number, the lower your risk.

Diets Don't Work

The headlines have screamed this sound bite ever since a National Institutes of Health conference came to that conclusion in 1992. Actually, there are few scientific studies that have carefully evaluated the safety and effectiveness of the various weight-loss methods. But we don't need research to confirm the obvious: For most people, diets indeed do not work—at least not in the long run. Regardless of the type of diet people follow—very-low-calorie, fasting, behavior modification,

DIETING DISASTERS

If you decide to go the commercial-diet-plan route or to follow the plan in a magazine or book, keep in mind that inappropriate, overpriced, and sometimes dangerous diet plans abound. Here are a few things to look out for:

• Avoid diet plans that focus on a particular food.

• Avoid diet plans that completely omit one food, food group, or nutrient.

• Steer clear of plans that offer bizarre, but often appealing, theories as to why their unique system of food combining or timing of meals will make the pounds melt away. It's usually nonsense.

• Don't follow a diet that recommends less than 1,200 calories a day, unless you're under the care of a doctor.

• Forget about diets that recommend megadoses of special "fat-burning" vitamins, minerals, and herbs.

prepackaged meals—and regardless of how much weight they lose—10, 20, even 100 pounds—the weight usually returns when they stop "dieting" and start eating in the real world.

Still, Americans spend an estimated $30 billion a year on weight-loss efforts. Few of the weight-loss programs you see advertised on television or in the newspaper have been studied to find out the proportion of people who complete the program, how much weight they lose, or their success in maintaining the weight loss. Without these statistics, testimonials are meaningless. Just about anyone can lose weight, but who can actually keep the weight off?

When You Plateau

If you've tried to lose weight before, you know the feeling. Despite adhering to your low-fat diet plan and exercising regularly, you've reached a point where the pounds refuse to budge. It's commonly referred to as a dieting plateau. While no one argues that plateaus occur, experts disagree as to what causes them. Here are a few theories:

• Yo-yo dieters are more likely to experience plateaus than first-timers. Some researchers say that's because each weight loss and regain may permanently lower a person's metabolic rate, which translates into fewer calories burned and lower calorie needs.

• If you lose weight too fast, you'll lose muscle along with the fat. Because muscle requires more calories than fat to maintain itself, your calorie requirements will drop.

• Research suggests that once you've lost a lot of weight, your body becomes incredibly efficient, getting the most out of each calorie. In other words, once you've lost weight, it takes fewer calories to do the same job it did before you dieted.

• In many cases, simply cutting back on calories can slow your metabolic rate by about ten percent.

So, What Does Work?

Despite the overall bad news about dieting, there are a few weight-loss techniques that seem to offer the greatest chance for success.

Personalizing Your Plan

One recent study found that women who design their own programs for diet and exercise are the most successful at maintaining lost weight. In other words, to achieve long-term weight-loss success, a prepackaged strategy from a class, a diet book, or a counselor cannot be expected to work for everyone. You need to personalize your eating plan to your habits, food likes and dislikes, schedule, and lifestyle. If you don't, you won't stick with it.

Keeping a Food Diary

Some experts say that keeping a food diary is one of the best things you can do to get a handle on your eating habits and to identify your diet downfalls. You may think you know how much you're putting in your mouth, but you can't be sure unless you carefully weigh and measure your food, at least for a while. One study exposed a huge gap that exists between the amount of food people perceive they eat and what they actually eat. Among severely obese people, the gap can be as large as 1,000 calories a day.

Your diary can be as simple as writing down the date, the time, and what you ate, or it can be more detailed, including your feelings when you ate, how the food was prepared, who you ate with and where.

Exercising

The same study that discovered the success of personalized weight-loss plans also found that the women who exercised regularly had better track records for keeping weight off than nonexercisers.

Exercise alone is not enough to pare off all of your excess pounds, but it certainly can help you lose weight quicker and keep it off longer—if you make exercise a regular part of your life in addition to a healthy diet.

For weight loss, exercise doesn't have to be a "marathon" affair. Walking, taking the stairs, or vigorously scrubbing the tub add to your fitness total. In one study, such "mild" exercise cut the death rate of a group of men by almost 60 percent compared to a similar group of inactive men.

Eating More

That's right, eating more, not less, can actually make it easier for you to take weight off and keep it off, but only if you eat the right foods. Cut back on calories too much, say by 60 percent a day, and your body slows down its metabolism to conserve energy and ultimately slows weight loss. A modest cut in calories, however, say by only 30 percent a day, and your body is more likely to continue metabolizing food at its usual rate.

The result? A higher metabolic rate and more calories burned over the long haul.

It's even been suggested that cutting back too much can by itself trigger binge eating, causing dieters to regain all the weight they have lost, and sometimes even more.

Eating a Low-Fat Diet

For years, nutritionists insisted that a calorie was a calorie. Whether your calories came from carbohydrates, proteins, or fats was thought to matter little. It was the total number of calories that was considered the key to weight control. Well, that's changed. Research now strongly suggests that calorie for calorie, excess fat calories are more fattening than excess calories from carbohydrates or protein. In other words, 100 calories of mayonnaise is more likely to be deposited on your hips, thighs, and belly than 100 calories of sugar.

In fact, some research has found that the number of calories from fat in your diet may be the single strongest predictor of weight gain, much stronger than the total number of calories you take in.

Official recommendations for healthy eating that come from the government and from organizations like the National Cancer Institute and the American Heart Association recommend that we keep fat intake to 30 percent or less of calories. However, proponents of the fat-is-more-fattening theory say that 20 percent of calories from fat is better, while ten percent is ideal.

But a diet so low in fat is not for everyone. It takes determination and commitment to a totally new way of eating. The best advice: Cut back on fat wherever you can. One study found that the simplest and most effective ways to cut back on your fat intake are to replace high-fat foods with lower-fat alternatives. Try skinless chicken instead of fatty beef, fruit instead of fatty desserts, cereal instead of eggs for breakfast, jam instead of margarine on toast and bagels; eat vegetarian-style a

---

PRACTICING PORTION CONTROL

The key to knocking off extra pounds while following a balanced diet may be to become well acquainted with portion sizes. Most of us are pretty poor estimators of the portions of foods we eat. In fact, most of the time it's hard to even remember what you had to eat yesterday.

So, for the first few weeks of your new weight-loss plan, it's a good idea to keep a precise diary of everything you eat and drink. Don't be tempted to leave out toppings, gravies, garnishes, or nibbles you take here and there.

Half the battle is getting used to what a serving looks like. If you've allowed yourself three ounces of skinless chicken breast for lunch, make sure you know what a three-ounce portion looks like. Hint: It's not much bigger than a deck of playing cards or the palm of your hand.

You'll need a few tools of the trade: a kitchen scale (it's probably a better investment than a bathroom scale), measuring cups and spoons, and plenty of low-fat, low-calorie recipes that you should follow to the letter.

Don't turn your food diary into an obsession. Train your eye to remember what a reasonable portion looks like so you won't forever have to rely on scales or counters.

---

few days a week; and limit fats such as butter, margarine, and salad dressing. (See Fat in Part I for more tips on cutting back the fat in your diet.)

Anti-diet Backlash

There is a growing vocal minority of obese people who have decided to stay fat and be happy that way. They have decided that being fat is easier than enduring repeated attempts and failures at weight loss. Is that unhealthy? No one knows for sure, because it hasn't yet been proven whether the health risks associated with obesity are due to being fat or due to the repeated ups and downs in weight that obese people usually experience in a lifetime. In the absence of proof that dieting can provide permanent weight loss and long-lasting health benefits, even some health professionals say the medical community should reexamine the common practice of repeatedly subjecting people who are severely overweight to diets that simply don't work.

But it goes beyond that. Society puts demands on people to lose weight so they can be slim. And most overweight people try to comply. But, experts say, they wind up yo-yoing because biologically they're not meant to be thin. The result is tremendous physical and psychological stress. Moreover, some diet researchers say that the "dieter's mentality" of simply being on a diet is stressful and can cause you to overeat fattening "comfort" foods.

Should I Lose Weight?

That is definitely the "Double Jeopardy" question. But there is no right or wrong answer. If you're not overweight now, you should work at preventing weight gain by adopting healthy eating habits and a regular exercise program. If you have a high BMI, say 30 or above, experts say you should try to shed a few pounds. Even small losses of 10, 15, or 20 pounds can have tremendous health benefits, including lowering blood pressure and normalizing blood sugar levels in Type II diabetics.

However, keeping in mind that repeated ups and downs in your weight can carry their own health risks, avoid the "lose-ten-pounds-in-ten-days" type of dieting. Rapid weight loss is inevitably followed by a rapid weight gain, sometimes to an even higher weight than before you began dieting.

Unfortunately, no one seems to agree whether healthy, moderately overweight people need to lose weight for health reasons. If you fit this description, try to avoid any additional weight gain that could push you over the edge into a high-risk category. But if the body of your dreams seems elusive, the experts say you may just have to accept your less-than-slender shape. That may be the healthiest move for you.

If you are very overweight and you decide to give weight loss a go, bear in mind that you may have to treat your weight problem just as someone with diabetes or hypertension treats their disease—for life.

STROKE

Many of us worry about getting heart disease or cancer, but few of us lose sleep over whether we're going to suffer a stroke. Better wake up, because about 150,000 people die each year from strokes. And stroke is the leading cause of serious disability in the United States. Though it's seldom talked about, stroke is the third most frequent cause of death among adults after heart disease and cancer. Your risk rises steeply with age, and in the United States, more blacks die from stroke than do whites.

A stroke can be devastating. But do the right thing and you just may be able to prevent becoming the next statistic. A stroke occurs when a blood vessel carrying oxygen and nutrients to the brain bursts or is clogged by a blood clot. Because of the rupture or blockage, the brain isn't able to receive the oxygen-rich blood it needs. Deprived of oxygen, nerve cells in the brain die within minutes.

About 80 percent of strokes are due to clots. The rest are the result of hemorrhages; these "bleeding strokes" occur when vessels rupture, spilling blood into the brain. Your risk of dying is much greater with a bleeding stroke than it is with one due to a clot. In either type, brain cells may die, leaving the victim faced with possible permanent paralysis and loss of speech or memory.

By far the most powerful of all the risk factors for stroke is high blood pressure, the silent killer discussed previously (see High Blood Pressure). The lower your blood pressure, the lower your risk. But high blood pressure isn't the only cause of stroke. And, although stroke is usually thought of as a disease of old age, it can strike young people as well. Overweight, high blood-cholesterol levels, and high blood-glucose levels also contribute to the most common types of stroke in the United States. A history of rheumatic heart disease, a weakened blood vessel known as an aneurysm, the heart condition endocarditis (inflammation of the lining of the heart), or abnormal heart rhythms increase your risk regardless of your age.

The Most Striking Risk Factors for Stroke

The typical stroke is the result of the same process that causes most heart attacks—a blood clot that cuts off blood flow. So it's no surprise to find that the things that increase your risk of a heart attack are remarkably similar to those that put you at risk for stroke. Just as with heart attacks, risk factors can be divided into those you have some control over and those you don't.

Risk factors you can prevent or treat:

High blood pressure. It affects almost one out of every three American adults. According to researchers, high blood pressure is clearly the number one risk factor—even more important than age, which comes in second. One study found that the risk for stroke was progressively greater as systolic blood pressure (the top number in a blood-pressure reading) increased from below 140 to 160, regardless of the diastolic pressure (the bottom number in a blood-pressure reading). So, an elevated systolic blood pressure, even if your diastolic blood pressure is normal, increases your risk for stroke. You should have your blood pressure checked regularly. Get your blood pressure under control and you can significantly reduce your risk of having a stroke.

High blood cholesterol. High blood cholesterol often causes atherosclerosis, clogging of the arteries, which can raise blood pressure and trigger a stroke. It has also been shown that people with low HDL (high-density lipoprotein) levels are at greater risk for having stroke. Losing weight and eating less saturated fat and more soluble fiber can lower your cholesterol.

Overweight. Though being overweight increases your risk of stroke, in several studies the distribution of body fat was more strongly related to stroke than was total body fat. Risk of stroke doubles in people with apple-shaped bodies—those with a high ratio of abdominal fat to hip fat. (See Overweight for how to calculate your fat ratio.)

Heart disease. A diseased heart increases the risk of having a stroke. Regardless of their blood pressure, people with heart problems have more than twice the risk of stroke than people whose hearts function normally. The four major risk factors for heart attacks that you can control are cigarette smoking, high blood cholesterol, high blood pressure, and physical inactivity. Controlling these risk factors reduces your risk of heart disease and thus your risk of stroke.

Smoking. Inhaling cigarette smoke damages the cardiovascular system. Nicotine in tobacco smoke increases blood pressure. Carbon monoxide from smoke also gets in the blood, reducing the amount of oxygen supplied to the body. Cigarette smoke also causes platelets (blood cells that help blood to clot) to become sticky and clump together, making blood clot quicker and increasing blood thickness.

Heavy alcohol consumption. Drinking an average of two or more drinks per day increases the risk of high blood pressure, which by itself is a risk factor for stroke.

High red-blood-cell count. An increase in your red-blood-cell count is a risk factor for stroke. That's because an increased number of red blood cells thickens blood, allowing it to clot easily. The problem can be treated with blood thinners.

Risk factors you can't change:

Diabetes. People with diabetes are two to six times more likely to have a stroke than people who do not have diabetes. Even if your blood sugar is under control, if you are diabetic, you are still much more likely to suffer a stroke. This is even more true for women with diabetes than it is for men with diabetes. Diabetics who also have high blood pressure have an even greater risk.

Gender. The incidence of stroke is about 30 percent higher for men than for women.

Race. Blacks have about a 60 percent greater risk of death and disability from stroke than whites. This probably is because blacks have a much greater incidence of high blood pressure.

Previous stroke. The risk of stroke for someone who's already had one is several times that of someone who has not.

Age. Strokes are relatively uncommon before the age of 45. After age 55, the incidence of stroke more than doubles with each decade. Still, 28 percent of stroke victims are under the age of 65.

Heredity. Stroke risk is greater for people who have a family history of stroke.

An abnormality of the heart. Specifically, overdevelopment of the left side of the heart, what doctors call left ventricular hypertrophy, is a risk factor for stroke.

Geographic location. Strokes are most common in the southeastern United States. It's even sometimes referred to as the "Stroke Belt." The stroke-belt states are Alabama, Arkansas, Georgia, Indiana, Kentucky, Louisiana, Mississippi, North Carolina, South Carolina, Tennessee, and Virginia.

Season and climate. Stroke deaths occur more often in extreme temperatures, perhaps because this puts more strain on the heart and blood vessels.

Socioeconomic status. There's some evidence that strokes are more likely to occur among poor people.

Of all these risk factors, five stand out. Thirty percent of people who suffer strokes have all five:
- High blood pressure
- High blood cholesterol
- Abnormal glucose tolerance (See Diabetes.)
- Cigarette smoking
- Heart abnormality (Left ventricular hypertrophy)

Recognizing Stroke Signals

Signs that you've had a stroke are clear but are sometimes wrongly attributed to other things or are ignored. A stroke can come on suddenly; quick medical attention is essential. So learn to recognize the symptoms. They include:
- Sudden weakness or numbness of the face, arm, or leg on one side of the body

• Headache or stiff neck
• Dizziness, seizures, or convulsions
• Nausea and vomiting
• Sudden dimness or loss of vision, particularly in only one of the eyes
• Loss of speech, or trouble understanding speech

Treating a stroke may involve surgery, drugs, and/or physical therapy. Most recovery takes place within the first 30 days following a stroke. After that, about one-third of stroke victims will still need help caring for themselves.

Nutrition Prevention of Stroke

Some stroke victims recover completely, others are permanently disabled, and some do not survive. It's the risk of long-term disability or death that makes prevention crucial. The nutritional key to preventing strokes is as simple as eating lots of fruits and vegetables. Look at the list of stroke preventors below, and you'll see why.

Potassium. A high intake of potassium may prevent you from dying from a stroke. Research shows that an intake of 3,500 milligrams a day is beneficial. Some of the richest sources of potassium include dried fruit, lima beans, spinach, dried beans, potatoes, tomato juice, cantaloupe, orange juice, squash, and bananas.

Beta-carotene. Eating lots of carrots and spinach can dramatically lower the risk of having a stroke, at least for women. Researchers found that women who ate five or more servings of carrots a week were 68 percent less likely to suffer a stroke than those who ate no more than one serving a month. Eating spinach also appeared to protect against stroke, though not as much as carrots. The key here appears to be beta-carotene, a form of vitamin A that acts as an antioxidant in the body. Researchers believe that antioxidants may fight stroke by setting off a series of biochemical changes that prevent cholesterol from sticking to artery walls. Other rich sources of beta-carotene include cantaloupe, pumpkin, apricots, nectarines, mangoes, broccoli, and cooking greens.

Fruit fiber. Researchers have found that men who eat less than 12 grams of fiber a day are almost 60 percent more likely to develop high blood pressure—the chief risk factor for stroke—than those who eat more than 24 grams of fiber a day. Increased intake of fruit fiber was found to be most closely associated with a decrease in high blood pressure.

Omega-3 fatty acids. Research suggests that regular fish-eaters—at least one serving a week—have about a 50 percent lower risk of having a stroke compared to people who eat no fish. Fish is rich in omega-3 fatty acids, which act as natural blood thinners. Rich sources of omega 3s include salmon, herring, sardines, anchovies, tuna, and bluefish.

ULCERS

"Calm down, you're going to give yourself an ulcer," is something friends might say to you if you were getting angry and agitated. Though your friends might mean well, they would be perpetuating the myth that anger and anxiety lead to an ulcer. Experts no longer agree with this notion. Neither do they believe that there is such a thing as an ulcer-prone personality. And—hold on to your hat—it's now been discovered that while spicy foods such as chili, lasagna, or pepperoni pizza may aggravate ulcer symptoms in some people, they cannot cause you to develop an ulcer. Milk, that old-time ulcer remedy, may even make your ulcer worse! To put this changing view of ulcers into perspective, it's probably best just to begin at the beginning.

The Ulcer Profile

Ulcers, which affect about one of every ten people, can strike at any time, from infancy to old age. There are two kinds of ulcers: duodenal and gastric. Duodenal ulcers are the garden variety ulcer you hear about most often. Though you usually think of ulcers as being in the stomach, this most-common type actually forms in the duodenum, the part of the small intestine next to the stomach. Gastric ulcers, on the other hand, are true stomach ulcers that occur when stomach acid eats away at the stomach's lining.

The unpleasant symptoms of either type of ulcer can include a loss of appetite, pain, nausea, or vomiting. The pain is usually just below the breastbone, and the area can be sensitive to the touch. You will probably experience temporary relief each time you eat. But later you can almost feel the digestive juices churning away.

In the past, many theories have been suggested as to what makes the lining of the intestine or the stomach vulnerable to ulcer formation in some people, but not in others. Now, researchers think they know the secret.

Recent research seems to confirm that a high percentage of all ulcers are caused not by diet, stress, or a "Type A" personality, but by bacteria called *Helicobacter pylori*. Though almost everyone carries the bacteria in their digestive tracts, only ten percent of people actually develop ulcers.

It's believed that *H. pylori* bacteria somehow alter the tissue lining of the digestive tract, making it more likely, in some people, that an ulcer will develop. Genetics may play a role in determining who is most sensitive to the bacteria. People who have family members with ulcers are more likely to develop one themselves.

Certain drugs can also promote ulcers. Aspirin and ibuprofen, both commonly taken for arthritis, can irritate the stomach or intestinal lining enough to trigger an ulcer.

Undoing an Ulcer

An effective ulcer treatment remained elusive for years. Despite the fact that most ulcers heal within two to six weeks, regardless of the type of treatment given, there was no permanent cure. About one-half of ulcer sufferers had a recurrence, usually within two years.

Then the bacterial connection was uncovered in the early 1980s. It was contrary to everything that was known about ulcers before. In essence, it revolutionized the treatment of ulcer disease.

Currently, ulcer drugs such as Tagamet, which suppresses acid secretion in the stomach, are still used. In fact, Tagamet is one of the most widely prescribed drugs in the United States. It is often prescribed as the first line of defense against ulcers.

In addition, you may be tested for *H. pylori*. If you test positive, the regimen typically prescribed to eliminate the bacteria includes a combination of antibiotics such as tetracycline or amoxicillin, plus metronidazole (Flagyl) and bismuth subsalicylate (Pepto-Bismol) four times a day for two weeks. Once the *H. pylori* bacteria are eliminated, the recurrence rate is very low.

Banish Bland Diets

Now that we know that it's nasty bacteria, and not the food you eat, that sets an ulcer in motion, there's no longer much reason to eat a bland diet. No one has uncovered evidence that the long-recommended bland ulcer diet helps at all. If, however, you find that certain foods seem to aggravate your ulcer symptoms, you might want to limit them.

BAN YOUR ULCER BURN

• If ulcer symptoms persist, despite the antibiotics, try eliminating extra-spicy foods or foods high in fat from your diet. Everyone has individual tolerance levels to spicy foods. You'll have to find out which foods, if any, are troublesome for you.

• Spices in moderation are OK, with the exception of black pepper and chili powder, which do irritate the gastrointestinal tract.

• Though it was once common advice to eat small, frequent meals instead of three meals a day, now experts say different. Food stimulates acid production, so regular, well-spaced, moderate-sized meals are the order of the day.

• Stop smoking. Experts agree that smoking not only irritates stomach ulcers but may delay healing.

• Stop taking "nonsteroidal anti-inflammatory" medications such as aspirin, ibuprofen, and other drugs used to treat arthritis. Check with your physician for alternatives.

• Don't eat close to bedtime. Late-night eating stimulates the secretion of stomach acid during the night.

• If you're a coffee drinker, limit your consumption (including decaf) to one cup after meals.

• Cut out alcohol. It irritates the lining of the digestive tract. If you must drink alcohol, dilute it with water, soda, or juice and eat food along with it to decrease the acid-stimulating properties of alcohol.

• Forget about milk as an ulcer reliever. While it may feel soothing at first, it stimulates increased acid secretion.

• Experiment with different over-the-counter antacids to find the one that works best for you.

HEALTH-WISE EATING

Good health comes from good habits. And good nutrition is just one of them. There are lots of other influences on your health, including heredity, level of physical activity, and personality, as well as the medical care you receive and the environment in which you live. But what you eat is a powerful determinant of what you are—especially of what your health will be as you age. So what's the best approach?

You've probably heard it a million times: Eat a variety of foods. You may think that's boring advice. But even with all the scientific discoveries of late, we have yet to improve on that advice. In fact, it may be proving more true than we ever imagined. And when you think about it, what could be less boring than being told you can eat some of everything? The key is moderation.

Also, remember, it's the little things that are important. It's making small changes in everyday habits. It's relying on whole foods instead of processed frozen dinners. It's taking the time to choose, store, and prepare food in ways that maximize nutrition and minimize the hazards of food poisoning. It's knowing what new developments are worth listening to and which are just hype. It's being confident, above all, that if you eat lots of different foods in moderation, you will be eating more healthfully.

Keep in mind that any food can fit into a healthy diet; none is taboo. But some foods are clearly healthier than others. Eating well means balancing these foods so that the healthiest ones take center stage, while the less-than-admirable ones play a minor role. It also means being physically active enough to allow you to eat enough food—and garner the benefits of their nutrients—without gaining excess weight.

You may be surprised to learn there really is a consensus on what basic nutrition guidelines we should be following. We'd like to show you how to embrace them while ensuring variety, balance, and moderation in your choices.

Once you've got the basics down pat, we'll tackle the harder issues: how to store and prepare your food for best nutrition and prevention of food poisoning; what hidden dangers are lurking in your food; and the burgeoning "natural" movement and what it means in the real world.

The most important take-home message from this section is that it's up to you how you combine the foods in your diet and whether you take care to keep them safe from contamination and from spoilage. We'll give you guidance from the experts on how to strike the right balance amongst the foods in your diet. The first step toward this goal is to ensure that you're eating a safe and healthy diet. Read on to find out how you can do that.

GUIDELINES FOR HEALTHY EATING

Medical science—nutrition in particular—has a bad reputation for flip-flopping on advice, with one arm of government contradicting the views of another arm of government. That's what many people think of nutrition advice—that no one agrees on anything. But is that the reality? Nothing could be further from the truth.

In reality, the major health organizations—government and private—offer amazingly similar advice on what we should eat to be healthy and to decrease our risk of chronic diseases, including such killers as coronary heart disease, cancer, diabetes, and high blood pressure.

Sure, some groups offer specific numbers to aim for, while others prefer to word their advice in more general terms. But there are no major differences of opinion amongst the organizations. All of them urge Americans to eat a variety of foods; maintain a healthy weight; limit fat and salt; emphasize fruits, vegetables, complex carbohydrates, and fiber; and not worry too much about protein and sugar. Alcohol and dietary cholesterol are minor worries for most people. Calories are a concern if you're overweight.

The reason people may have an impression of conflicting nutrition advice is because that advice has changed over the years as our knowledge has grown—and for good reason. Not so long ago, just getting enough calories and protein to survive was a major concern. Before antibiotics were discovered, bacterial infection was a major killer. And the more calories people ate, the more nutrients they ingested to fight infection. People didn't live long enough to develop the chronic conditions we acquire as we age today—cancer, heart disease, diabetes, cataracts. Now we have a different nutrition agenda, which requires different priorities. Here's the lowdown on what's important and what's not.

The Dietary Guidelines Shine the Way

Almost all of the recommendations from the various health organizations are summarized neatly in the Dietary Guidelines for Americans, issued jointly by the Department of Agriculture (USDA) and the Department of Health and Human Services (HHS).

Eat a variety of foods. Although most foods provide many different nutrients, no single food supplies them all in the amounts needed. Because you require more than 40 nutrients for good health, you need to eat a variety of foods, even if you take a multivitamin/mineral supplement. Any food can be part of a nutritious diet. Your total day's diet, not a particular food, is what's important. (See Variety, Balance, and Moderation.)

It's also important to note that you need to consume enough food to meet your nutrient requirements. That's where physical activity can play a vital role in a healthy lifestyle. Physical activity allows you to take in more calories—increasing your likelihood of meeting your nutrient needs—without gaining weight than you can if you are sedentary.

Maintain a healthy weight. Your chances of health problems increase if you weigh too much or too little. How healthy your weight is depends, in part, on how much of your weight is fat and where it's located. (See Eating Disorders and Overweight in Part II.)

Choose a diet low in fat, saturated fat, and cholesterol. If your diet is high in total fat, you increase your risk of heart disease, stroke, diabetes, obesity, gallbladder disease, and, possibly, certain cancers. If your diet contains a lot of saturated fat and cholesterol, you increase your risk of heart disease and stroke.

Average Americans get more than 35 percent of their calories from fat. Most experts advise lowering that to 30 percent or less. And some think it should be much lower—less than 25 or 20 percent. Saturated fat should account for no more than ten percent of calories—better yet, keep it to seven percent. Dietary cholesterol is less important; if you cut down on fat and saturated fat, your dietary cholesterol will drop also. (See Fat in Part I and the individual diseases in Part II.)

Choose a diet with plenty of vegetables, fruits, and grain products. If you follow this guideline, you will succeed in upping your intake of complex carbohydrates and fiber. Both are important for reducing risk of a variety of diseases and conditions, including cancer, heart disease, and diabetes, as well as gastrointestinal complaints such as constipation, diverticular disease, and hemorrhoids. Sources of both soluble and insoluble fiber should be included in the diet. (See Carbohydrate and Fiber in Part I and the chapters on the individual diseases listed above in Part II.)

Fruits and vegetables, by themselves, have been singled out as protective factors against several cancers, high blood pressure, cataracts, and heart disease. The National Cancer Institute recommends we eat five to nine servings a day of a wide variety of fruits and vegetables. Ideally, this would include selections rich in vitamin C, beta-carotene, and fiber, as well as a cruciferous vegetable twice a week.

Use sugars only in moderation.

The only disease sugar is guilty of causing is dental caries—what kids call cavities. But sugar can instigate trouble when it's combined with fat in sweets. Consume too many of these and you're likely to gain weight. And although diabetics can eat some sugar if it is eaten with other foods, too much sugar can wreak havoc with their blood-sugar levels.

Another good reason for not eating too much sugar is that it provides "empty calories," taking the place of other more nutritious foods. So a diet with too much sugar is rarely a healthy one. (See Carbohydrates in Part I and the chapters Dental Disease, Diabetes, and Overweight in Part II.)

Use salt and sodium only in moderation.

Because we can't predict who will develop high blood pressure, and who among those folks is sensitive to sodium, it's wise for everyone to moderate their salt and sodium intake. This is especially true when you consider that high blood pressure often has no symptoms and is a direct contributor to heart disease and stroke. (See High Blood Pressure in Part II.)

If you drink alcoholic beverages, do so in moderation.
Although one or even two drinks of alcohol a day may not be harmful—indeed some research suggests it

may even be beneficial to your heart—more than this is not a good idea. Gram for gram, alcohol supplies your body with even more calories than sugar. Besides providing no nutrients to go with those calories, alcohol increases urinary excretion of some minerals and decreases the absorption of some vitamins. Chronic, heavy use of alcohol can cause liver disease and cancer and may contribute to high blood pressure and stroke.

Alcohol is not recommended in any amount for: women who are pregnant or are trying to conceive; anyone who plans to drive or operate machinery within five hours; anyone taking medicine, whether prescription or over-the-counter; alcoholics or recovering alcoholics; children and adolescents.

DIETARY GUIDELINES FOR AMERICANS

- Eat a variety of foods.
- Maintain a healthy weight.
- Choose a diet low in fat, saturated fat, and cholesterol.
- Choose a diet with plenty of vegetables, fruits, and grain products.
- Use sugars, salt, and sodium only in moderation.
- If you drink alcoholic beverages, do so in moderation.

FOODS *VS.* INDIVIDUAL NUTRIENTS

So far, the spotlight has been on nutrients. We've spent a lot of pages telling you why you need to slash the fat and add more fiber to your diet; how vitamin C may protect you from infection, while beta-carotene bolsters your anticancer defenses. We've told you who needs more calcium and iron, and who doesn't. We've told you when you might need more folic acid. We've even told you what foods are rich in beta-carotene and vitamin C, and where to find folic acid and zinc.

Now we'd like to switch the focus to foods. There's a popular nutrition maxim that you eat foods, not nutrients. After all, that's where nutrients are found. And if you eat a balanced variety of foods, you'll get them all.

Wouldn't it just be easier to get all this in a pill? Easier—yes. Possible—no. Here's why.

THE SULFORAPHANE SAGA

For a number of years, researchers urged us to eat more cruciferous—or cabbage family—vegetables to fight cancer. Only recently have we found a clue as to why these foods appear to be beneficial. A researcher at the Johns Hopkins University School of Medicine in Baltimore isolated a chemical—called sulforaphane—from broccoli. This chemical jump-starts the activity of protective enzymes—called phase II enzymes—in cells. These enzymes disarm dangerous substances in the body, including carcinogens.

It's thought that sulforaphane is particularly helpful in preventing cancer because it stimulates phase II enzymes without triggering their counterculture cousins, phase I enzymes. Phase I enzymes do just the opposite of phase II enzymes by provoking carcinogens into action. In many foods, the actions of these two competing enzyme systems simply cancel each other out. But by stimulating the virtuous enzymes without sparking the sinister ones, we may give ourselves an extra clip of ammunition in the dogfight against cancer.

The Johns Hopkins researchers found that quinone reductase, just one of the beneficial phase II enzymes, was coaxed into action most easily by broccoli and brussels sprouts.

Identifying the Unknown

First of all, there are a lot of substances in foods we don't know much about, and probably many more we haven't even identified yet. Scientists used to think we might find more vitamins. That's unlikely. It is plausible we may discover that certain minerals are more essential to life than we thought.

The big discoveries in the future, however, are likely to concern chemicals that are not essential to life, as vitamins and minerals are, but that enhance certain body processes and defenses, making them critical for optimal health. These substances have been dubbed "phytochemicals," a word coined to describe any chemical produced by plants. Researchers have identified 14 classes of phytochemicals.

Active phytochemicals are found in fruits, vegetables, and grains. There are literally hundreds or thousands of individual, interacting chemicals in each bite of apple or swallow of orange juice you take. And each individual phytochemical is unique and plays a different role in the body.

A few years ago, the National Cancer Institute (NCI) instituted a project dubbed the "Experimental Foods Program." Its original mission was to study and isolate disease-fighting phytochemicals that could eventually be concentrated and added to foods—so-called "designer foods."

The program has since been scaled back, but its lofty goals remain. At its heart is the concept that plants produce chemicals to help them survive. It's not too far-fetched to assume that one of the survival values of these phytochemicals might be that they stop cell division. If phytochemicals have this same effect in humans, they may be able to arrest the proliferation of cancer cells. Hence, the excitement.

So far, the government has only studied six specific types of foods to find the way the combination of phytochemicals in them fights disease. These six promising food groups include citrus fruits, flax, garlic, licorice, soybeans, and umbelliferous vegetables (carrots, celery, parsley, and parsnips).

The common thread among all the phytochemicals is that we still know very little about them and how they interact. What appears to be effective in the test tube or even in animals may not always prove to be of importance in humans.

Some of the chemicals scientists have been able to isolate from foods show remarkable properties, and, indeed, have been used for years in folk medicine. Many are substances that stimulate or block the body's production of protective enzymes. The allylic sulfides in garlic, for example, can stimulate an enzyme that fights cancer.

Genistein, a chemical found in soy products—tofu, miso, and tempeh—and cabbage, was recently shown to block the proliferation of new blood vessels that are needed to feed the growth of solid tumors such as those in the brain, breast, and prostate. Genistein has estrogenlike properties and serves to inhibit the cell cycle in tissues that have a high turnover rate. People who eat a traditional Japanese diet of soy products have 30 times as much genistein in their urine as those who eat a traditional Western diet. Whether this translates into a lower incidence of tumors isn't yet known, but it's been suggested that it might.

Other phytochemicals, such as the tannins in tea and some berries, may act directly as antioxidants. This may help prevent the formation of carcinogens as well as prevent other chronic conditions, such as heart disease and cataracts. Resveratrol is a chemical isolated from red grapes, red wine, and grape juice. It's believed to be the compound responsible for wine's apparent ability to lower blood cholesterol.

And some phytochemicals deactivate prostaglandins and estrogens that can cause cells to multiply in an uncontrolled way—the characteristic prelude to cancer. Cabbage, brussels sprouts, and broccoli contain a chemical known as indole-3-carbinol. This chemical shunts estradiol, a precursor to estrogen, to a biochemical pathway that produces a harmless form of estrogen, instead of a form that's associated with breast cancer.

We could go on and on. But even if the specifics are still sketchy and their significance arguable, few experts now doubt that one day we will have a greater appreciation of the wide array of these disease-fighting chemicals found naturally in foods. It's an exciting glimpse into what the future may hold as the science of nutrition makes the transition from a study of how to prevent nutrient deficiencies to a search for how to optimize our health.

The Mysterious Mix of Nature

Besides all the as yet unidentified chemicals in foods we'd be missing if we were to rely on supplements, there's the additional problem of achieving the right balance. You may remember in the chapter on Minerals, we talked about how important it is to get minerals in the right proportion to each other. One classic example is calcium and phosphorus—too much of one, and the other's absorption suffers. Likewise, take too much zinc, and copper absorption suffers. How about those B vitamins? They must all be present in the body in correct proportion or they can't do their job processing proteins, carbohydrates, and fats. The list of interrelationships of nutrients goes on.

For all we know, it may be just as important for all the unknown phytochemicals in foods to be present in certain combinations, too. That's why researchers are studying foods, not individual phytochemicals. And it's a good reason why you, too, should concentrate on eating foods rather than taking supplements.

Since we don't know yet what the proper phytochemical combinations are, or even what chemicals are present, we certainly can't duplicate it in a pill. So be sure to include these foods in your diet regularly. Mother Nature will do the rest.

How can you be sure you're getting all the good stuff? Easy. Eat a variety of foods.

VARIETY, BALANCE, AND MODERATION

No one food is blessed with all the nutrients needed for life. Even "nature's perfect food"—breast milk—is only perfect for the first six months. Even before that, however, an infant may need vitamin C, vitamin K, iron, and fluoride. And after the first six months, an infant needs a source of iron. So how do you get all the nutrients you need? Eat a lot of different foods—and eat all of them in moderation.

By different, we mean even subtle differences. So you think an apple is an apple is an apple? Until recently, so did nutritionists, because the nutrient breakdown is the same no matter the color. But in terms of phytochemicals, they're quite different. Red apples contain cancer-fighters that yellow apples don't. And green and yellow apples contain beneficial substances that red apples don't.

The same goes for sweet peppers and grapefruit. With these two, even the nutrient contents are not the same. Red sweet peppers contain nine times more beta-carotene than green sweet peppers. And did you know that pink or red grapefruit provides almost 100 times the beta-carotene you'll get from a white grapefruit?

But it goes beyond that. Even plants that look alike can be very different underneath. National Cancer Institute (NCI) researchers have found that different varieties of Chinese licorice root have extremely dissimilar phytochemical profiles. More baffling—the same variety grown in another region differs substantially. Why? Researchers point out that these wide variances in the amount of phytochemicals from one specimen to the next arise from diverse growing conditions: soil composition, weather patterns, water availability, and even the plant's position relative to the sun.

Perhaps someday we'll know the phytochemical "finger-print" of every food, and therefore be able to eat more of exactly those that benefit us the most. Or, researchers will be able to concentrate these protective substances and add them to foods. But until then, the only way to get it all is to eat it all.

You'll notice we feature more than 80 healthy foods in this book. We don't just give you six categories of foods or limit it to 20 or even 50 foods. You may be surprised to know there are that many top-notch foods that are wise additions to your diet. But there are, and we urge you to take advantage of them all. Only by eating moderate amounts of a variety of foods—including those cataloged here—will you be able to get all the substances you need in the correct proportions to live healthfully. What's more, with such a wide variety to choose from, you can select foods to suit your individual tastes, needs, and lifestyle.

There are other advantages to eating a variety of foods. It's also a defensive tactic. In the upcoming chapter Hidden Dangers, you'll find out about natural toxins and synthetic pesticides in foods. The best defense against these rather minor risks is to eat a variety of foods. That way, you don't get too much of any one harmful substance.

Nutrition: The Great Balancing Act

OK, so now you are eating lots of different foods. But how much of each should you eat? Aren't some better than others? Well, yes. We've tried to highlight the healthiest foods. Of course, there are other foods out there, and you may wonder how they fit into the big picture. Even the foods in this book need to be chosen with the right balance for a healthy diet.

Enter the Food Guide Pyramid—one of your greatest tools for improving your diet. The U.S. Department of Agriculture (USDA) adopted this graphic shape to represent the relative amounts of each type of food you should be eating. They scrapped the old Basic Four Food Groups you may have grown up with, because the concept didn't address the fact that some groups were more equal than others. The Food Guide Pyramid gives you useful guidelines for getting the foods and nutrients you need while allowing room for individual choices, preferences, and lifestyles.

Check out the Pyramid on the opposite page. You'll see that more space is devoted to those foods that are most important. Grains—the bread, cereal, rice, and pasta grouping—should form the basis upon which the rest of your diet is built. Fruits and vegetables are next and are equally important, so they take up equal space on the same level of the Pyramid.

Protein sources are not so important—at least for adult Americans, because most adults get so much protein already—so they are not as prominent on the Pyramid. They should not be the focus of your meals; rather, they should serve only to complement the bulk of your diet—grains. What is not clear on the Pyramid is that dry beans are a preferred source of protein over meats, because they are low in fat and high in fiber. And low-fat dairy products are preferred over their full-fat cousins.

Fats and sweets are at the top, not because they are the pinnacle of your diet, but because they should only contribute a tiny portion of your calories.

How Many Servings for You?

You'll notice the Pyramid gives a range of servings for each group. This is because some of us need more calories than others. Most women and older adults will do best with the lowest number of servings from each group. If you choose low-fat and lean foods from these groups and use fats and sweets sparingly, this will provide about 1,600 calories.

Active women, most men, children, and teenage girls should aim for a number in between the lowest and highest number of servings listed. With low-fat choices, this will approximate 2,200 calories. Most active men and teenage boys can eat the maximum servings listed to provide about 2,800 calories, assuming low-fat choices.

FOOD GUIDE PYRAMID

A Guide to Daily Food Choices

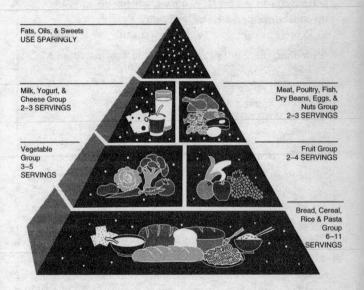

Fats, Oils, & Sweets
USE SPARINGLY

Milk, Yogurt, &
Cheese Group
2–3 SERVINGS

Meat, Poultry, Fish,
Dry Beans, Eggs, &
Nuts Group
2–3 SERVINGS

Vegetable
Group
3–5
SERVINGS

Fruit Group
2–4 SERVINGS

Bread, Cereal,
Rice & Pasta
Group
6–11
SERVINGS

KEY

● Fat (naturally occurring and added)
▼ Sugars (added)

These symbols show fats, oils, and
added sugars in foods.

241

WHAT IS A SERVING?

The Food Guide Pyramid indicates how many servings of each food group we should aim for, but what kind of serving are they talking about? Here's what they mean:

Bread, Cereal, Rice, and Pasta (Grains)
1 slice bread
1 oz. ready-to-eat cereal (see package for cup equivalent)
½ cup cooked cereal, rice, or pasta

Fruit
1 medium piece of raw fruit (an apple, banana, orange, peach, or plum, for example)
½ cup of cut-up raw fruit
½ cup of canned fruit
¾ cup of fruit juice

Vegetable
1 cup raw, leafy vegetables
½ cup cut-up raw vegetables
½ cup cooked vegetables
¾ cup vegetable juice

Meat, Poultry, Fish, Dry Beans, Eggs, Nuts
2-3 oz. cooked, lean meat, poultry, or fish
May substitute for 1 oz. meat:
    ½ cup cooked dry beans
    1 egg
    2 tbsp. peanut butter

Milk, Yogurt, Cheese
1 cup milk or yogurt
1½ oz. natural cheese
2 oz. processed cheese

Fats/Sweets
Use sparingly

GOOD FOOD GONE BAD

Which of these food problems do you think poses the greatest risk to your health—pesticide residues or bacterial contamination? If you guessed pesticide residues, you're wrong. Surprised? Don't feel bad. Though pesticide residues found in food pose potential problems, bacteria that find their way into your food pose the most immediate threat to your health. What too many of us fail to realize is that food poisoning can be downright deadly.

Older people, infants and young children, and people with faltering immune systems—those receiving cancer treatment and people with AIDS—are most at risk of becoming seriously ill or dying as a result of food poisoning. Aging and many of the diseases common to older people weaken the immune system. In addition, as the body ages, the stomach produces less acid, limiting the body's ability to kill bacteria in food.

But it's not all doom and gloom. The good news is that most food poisoning can be avoided if you simply take the proper food-safety precautions. That's what this chapter is all about: letting you in on a lot of simple steps that will dramatically cut your risk of suffering food poisoning.

But first, you should know your enemies. The following are some of the most common bugs.

Salmonella: It is the most common cause of food-borne illness, causing an estimated four million illnesses a year—most of which go unreported. Foods most likely to be contaminated with salmonella are poultry, eggs and egg products, meat, and sausage. Rat, mouse, and human feces are all likely to contain salmonella. That's why washing your hands in hot, soapy water is so important before handling foods and between handling raw meat or poultry and handling other foods. Food left on a counter to thaw is a common cause of salmonellosis (salmonella infection) because warm temperatures allow salmonella to multiply rapidly. Thawing foods in the refrigerator and promptly refrigerating leftovers can slow the growth of bacteria. Thorough cooking at normal cooking temperatures will kill the bacteria.

Nearly half of the reported salmonella infections require hospitalization. One to two percent of the 40,000 cases that are reported each year result in death. The symptoms of salmonella poisoning range from none to serious illness. But the most common are flulike symptoms that include fever, headache, abdominal pain, diarrhea, and vomiting that last from one to eight days. Symptoms may show up as quickly as six hours after eating the contaminated food or may be delayed for up to 36 hours. Even low levels of salmonella, even a single organism, can trigger symptoms.

Campylobacter: It is the leading cause of acute gastroenteritis (inflammation of the stomach and intestines). Raw milk and poultry are the most common causes. No wonder the Food and Drug Administration (FDA) has banned the interstate sale of raw milk. But campylobacter bacteria has also been found in cake icing, eggs, beef, and even municipal drinking water, usually as a result of fecal contamination. Within two to five days of consuming a contaminated food or drink, you can develop severe, even bloody, diarrhea, cramping, nausea, vomiting, fever, and headache that last from two to seven days.

Campylobacter is destroyed at normal cooking temperatures and with freezing. Salt doesn't destroy the bacteria, but it does prevent it from multiplying. The usual causes of illness are undercooked or raw animal-based foods. Prevention is just a matter of avoiding raw milk and raw-milk cheeses, and cooking meat, poultry, and fish thoroughly.

Escherichia coli (E. Coli): This bacteria, which exists naturally in the human intestinal tract, is the most common cause of diarrhea in infants and travelers. One uncommon strain of *E. coli,* called 0157:H7, sets the stage for two life-threatening conditions: hemorrhagic colitis (marked by severe abdominal cramps followed by bloody diarrhea) and hemolytic uremic syndrome (the leading cause of acute kidney failure in children). These illnesses have been linked with raw and undercooked ground beef, raw milk, and unchlorinated water.

Ingestion of the bacteria can cause bloody diarrhea, abdominal cramping, and vomiting that can last a week. In about ten percent of cases, it progresses to anemia and kidney failure. Children under five years of age are especially vulnerable. Antibiotics are not effective. The bacteria can be controlled by cooking meat thoroughly and avoiding cross-contamination of raw food. Be sure to cook meat and meat patties until the center is gray or brown and until the juices run clear, with no trace of pink. Ground beef is most susceptible because any bacteria present is mixed throughout the meat when it is ground. A steak has bacteria only on the outer surfaces. As long as the exterior reaches a temperature high enough to kill bacteria, the interior should be safe. A medium-rare steak offers minimal risk, but stay away from steak tartar.

Staphylococcus: Staphylococcus is found in the nose and throat and on the skin of healthy people, as well as on infected cuts, boils, burns, scratches, and pimples. Staphylococcus is also found in raw milk from both cows and goats and in cream and cheese made from raw milk.

The bacteria multiply rapidly at warm temperatures. They produce a toxin that can make you violently ill but is not seri-

TELLTALE TOXINS

You may kill bacteria in fish by cooking it thoroughly, but that doesn't touch toxins that sometimes lurk in fish. These toxins can cause diarrhea, vomiting, tingling, numbness, rashes, and even respiratory paralysis and death. Here are the top three culprits:

Ciguatera: It occurs mainly in Hawaii, Puerto Rico, the Virgin Islands, Guam, and Florida. You're most likely to get it from amberjack, grouper, goatfish, barracuda, and snapper. Don't eat these fish in these locals.

Scromboid poisoning: It's caused mainly by improperly handled mahimahi, tuna, and bluefish.

Paralytic shellfish poisoning: It is primarily a problem in the New England coastal states and in Alaska, California, and Washington state. Most poisonings have involved mussels, clams, and scallops that have been illegally harvested in waters that are off-limits.

ous enough to require hospitalization. Thorough cooking can kill "staph," but the toxin is resistant to mild heat, refrigeration, and freezing.

Once enough toxin is produced and the bacteria is consumed, symptoms begin two to six hours later. They include violent vomiting, abdominal pain, diarrhea, and, occasionally, collapse. The horrible episode is usually over within 24 hours. A distinguishing feature is that food poisoning from staph does not produce a fever.

Controlling staph is largely a matter of not touching cooked food with your bare hands and washing your hands frequently while preparing food and after wiping your nose or going to the bathroom. Wash your hands and utensils before preparing or serving food, and promptly refrigerate leftovers in shallow, covered containers that will cool to a safe temperature quickly.

Listeria: These bacteria are common characters in your everyday environment. Most people exposed to listeria experience only mild, flu-like symptoms. But listeria can be deadly to fetuses and newborns and to people with weakened immune systems. Pregnant women who become infected are likely to develop chills, fever, back pain, headache, and diarrhea. Usually, the infection will become life-threatening to the fetus. Listeria is estimated to cause at least 1,700 serious infections and contribute to about 450 deaths and 100 stillbirths each year.

Contaminated milk products, including soft cheeses, have been the most commonly traced cause of listeria outbreaks. Outbreaks are most likely to occur in the summer months. The bacteria can grow at refrigeration temperatures and can survive mild heat. Most people who are exposed to listeria develop no infection and have no symptoms.

There's not much you can do at home to prevent listeriosis (listeria infection) except to stay away from raw milk. Preventing listeria in the food supply is the job of commercial dairies.

Yersinia: One type of yersinia is deadly—it is the cause of "the Plague." Another type has been linked to food-borne illness. The symptoms are often mistaken for appendicitis. Yersinia can grow at refrigeration temperatures, but it is usually destroyed by mild heat. Pasteurization destroys any yersinia found in milk. The yersinia strains that cause illness in people are most frequently found in pork but are easily killed by cooking.

Clostridium botulinum (C. botulinum): This is a tough and dangerous bug. Its spores survive cooking and can grow without oxygen, allowing them to survive in cans and other airless environments. *C. botulinum* is naturally found in meat, soil, vegetables, and fruits.

Botulism has typically been linked to canned sources—sometimes identifiable by bulging lids. However, outbreaks have also been linked more recently to potato salad, sauteed onions, chopped garlic, raw cabbage, and hazelnut yogurt. Infant botulism, a very serious disease, can be caused by honey, which often contains botulinum bacteria. *Never give honey to an infant under one year old.* Infants are more susceptible to botulism than others because they haven't yet developed mechanisms to inhibit the growth of botulinum bacteria in the intestinal tract.

Botulism is very rare, but the overall fatality rate is high—about eight percent—so it demands our attention. Unlike the usual gastrointestinal symptoms of food poisoning, botulism causes atypical fatigue, muscle weakness, headache, and dizziness that begin twelve hours to four days after eating contaminated food. There usually is no fever. Initially, diarrhea may be a symptom, but constipation is more common. After that, the nervous system is affected, appearing as a loss of vision and slurred speech. If untreated, death often occurs within eight days due to paralysis of the muscles that control breathing. Fortunately, there is an antidote, called antitoxin. To be most effective, however, it must be given soon after initial symptoms begin. The survivor of severe botulism may need several months to recover.

Food-poisoning Preventors

Keeping food poisoning at bay is actually easy. But you have to know what to do and then do it! Here are some guidelines that can help you keep these unwelcome guests away:

• Don't buy bulging canned foods—this could be an indication of *C. botulinum* contamination. Do not taste food from such cans; even a small amount can be deadly. Do not buy

WHAT IF FOOD IS MOLDY?

If a food is moldy, don't even smell it. You may inhale some of the toxins that molds produce. But you don't have to throw away everything that has a moldy spot. Here are some guidelines:

• Cut away small moldy spots from hard cheese, salami, and firm fruits and vegetables like cabbage, bell peppers, and carrots. Keep your knife out of the mold and cut out at least one inch around and below the spot. Store the food in a clean container, and use it as soon as possible.

• Invisible mold spores can easily penetrate soft foods, no matter how small the moldy spot. That's why you should toss certain foods whenever you spot mold, such as individual slices of cheese, any soft cheese, cottage cheese, cream, sour cream, yogurt, bread, cake, rolls, pastry, corn on the cob, nuts, flour, whole grains, rice, dried peas and beans, and peanut butter.

dented or leaky cans, either, as these can increase the risk of contamination of the food.

• Make sure refrigerated foods are cold to the touch. If they feel warmer than usual, it could mean there's a risk of bacterial growth.

• Don't buy foods past the freshness date that is stamped on the package or container. Keep in mind that you generally cannot see, taste, or smell the bacteria that cause food-borne illnesses.

• Shop for cold foods last, just before going to the checkout lane. Then refrigerate the foods as soon as you get home.

• Throw out or return to the store any food that, upon opening, has an "off" odor or looks unusual to you. Do not taste even a tiny bit. Most hazardous bacteria will not make the food taste different.

• Wash your hands thoroughly before, during, and after handling of raw and cooked foods and after pet cleanups, diaper changes, nose wipes, and trips to the bathroom.

• Wash vegetables thoroughly before cooking or serving.

• Be sure your refrigerator and freezer are set to proper temperatures—40 degrees Fahrenheit or below for the refrigerator and 0 degrees Fahrenheit or below for the freezer.

• Keep hot food hot (internal temperature of above 140 degrees Fahrenheit) and cold foods cold (below 40 degrees Fahrenheit). Bacteria multiply rapidly in food that is at or near room temperature. After only two hours, there may be enough bacteria to make you sick.

The following food-specific tips were developed with freshness and safety in mind:

Dairy Products

• Powdered milk should be used within three months for maximum freshness, but it is safe to use, if stored dry, for months.

• Use milk before the freshness date on the carton.

• Hard cheese, if properly wrapped, will keep for six months.

• Soft cheese should be used within a week or two.

• Avoid raw milk and products made from raw milk.

Meat, Poultry, and Fish

• Never leave meat at room temperature for longer than two hours, even if still partially frozen.

• Most meats keep well in the refrigerator for three to five days—but no more.

• Hamburger and ground chicken and turkey present a greater risk of spoilage. They should be used within one to two days after purchase or should be frozen.

• Thoroughly clean all surfaces and equipment, including your hands, before and after contact with raw meat.

• Reserve a separate cutting board for preparing meat, fish, and poultry.

• Cook meat until the juices run clear. Say no to rare burgers.

• Avoid recipes that call for slow cooking after the heat is off, such as preheating the oven to 500, inserting a dish, and then turning off the heat.

• Use a meat thermometer for meat and poultry more than two inches thick. For ground meat and for meat and poultry less than two inches thick, look for clear juices and lack of pink in the center as signs of doneness.

• Don't put cooked meat or poultry back on a plate containing raw juices.

• Don't thaw or marinate poultry on the kitchen counter. Instead, to minimize the risk of bacterial growth, thaw or marinate in the refrigerator. You can also thaw poultry under cold

WOOD OR PLASTIC?

For years, the U.S. Department of Agriculture (USDA) has preached the gospel of plastic cutting boards. Wooden boards were off limits, we were told, because bacteria from contaminated meat and poultry could hide in wood's porous surface, making them hard to shake—even with soap and water.

But new research has turned that conventional wisdom on its ear. It seems that it's actually the plastic boards that are hard to get clean. Wooden boards seem to have uncanny powers to kill bacteria on contact.

What to do? Toss any cutting board, plastic or wood, if it's splintered or scarred with knife marks. If your plastic board is still in pretty good shape, clean it in the dishwasher after every use. If that's not practical, toss it and buy a wooden board. But, whichever type you use, there's no substitute for cleaning it well with soap and hot water after each use.

water. It's OK to thaw meat and poultry in the microwave, but it must be cooked promptly.

• Don't baste with uncooked marinade when the food is close to being done. Boil the marinade first.

• Stuff raw poultry just before cooking, never the night before. Remove stuffing from poultry as soon as it comes out of the oven. Better yet, cook poultry and stuffing separately. Refrigerate leftover stuffing as soon as dinner is done; it should not sit out more than two hours.

• Wash your cutting board well with hot, soapy water after each use. (See "Wood or Plastic?")

• Buy fish with clear, bulging eyes; clean, not slimy, scales; and bright red gills. Fresh fish does not smell "fishy."

• Clams, oysters, and mussels should have tightly closed shells, or the shells should close when you touch them. When steamed, they should open. If they do not, don't eat them.

• Refrigerate fish immediately, and use it within one to two days.

• Avoid raw shellfish. It is sometimes harvested from waters contaminated with human sewage.

• Cook fish thoroughly, until it flakes easily with a fork. That means eight to ten minutes per inch of thickness at 400 degrees Fahrenheit or higher.

Eggs

• Don't buy eggs that aren't refrigerated.

• Open the carton in the store and inspect each egg. If any of the eggs is cracked, pick another carton.

• Don't wash eggs in the shell, and avoid using the shells to separate the whites from the yolks.

• Cook eggs thoroughly to kill salmonella bacteria. You can trust the egg is safe when it is cooked until the white is completely firm and the yolk begins to thicken.

• Use raw eggs in the shell within five weeks of purchase— one week for peak freshness.

• Don't eat raw eggs or foods containing raw eggs, such as Caesar salad, hollandaise sauce, or homemade eggnog, ice cream, or mayonnaise. Commercial versions of these products are probably OK, because they usually contain pasteurized eggs.

• Never leave hard-cooked eggs out of the refrigerator for more than two hours. Despite popular belief, they are even more likely than raw eggs to be contaminated because they've lost all of their protective coatings.

• Store eggs in the original carton, not in the egg rack in the refrigerator door.

Breads, Crackers, Rice, and Cereals

• Store preservative-free breads and those made with whole grains in the refrigerator to prevent mold growth and rancidity.

• Store brown rice in the refrigerator. It is likely to become rancid if stored at room temperature.

• Check flour regularly for bugs. If you store it at room temperature, tiny insect eggs, found in all flour, are quicker to hatch.

WHEN GOOD OILS GO BAD

That obnoxious odor you detect in oils, butter, or margarine that you kept too long is due to rancidity. All fats and oils become rancid given enough exposure to air, sunlight, and heat. But unsaturated fats like vegetable oils are most prone to it. Still, any food that contains fat, including crackers, popcorn packaged with oil, nuts, and peanut butter, can go bad if kept too long or stored improperly. The best advice? If in doubt, throw it out. Though eating rancid foods won't make you sick like eating food contaminated with bacteria will, rancid fats contain chemicals that can damage cells, maybe even cause cancer, and may even be partly responsible for clogging arteries. So why chance it?

Be sure to store whole-grain flours in the refrigerator to prevent rancidity.

• Cold cereals can be stored in a cool, dry place. However, if you have a cereal with a high-fat content, such as high-fat granola, store it in the refrigerator.

• Be sure to use crackers by the "use by" date given on the package. High-fat crackers can become rancid if stored for a long period at room temperature, but they may become soft if you store them in the refrigerator—so only buy what you can use quickly.

Butter, Margarine, Mayonnaise, and Salad Dressings

• Once opened, keep mayonnaise and salad dressings refrigerated and tightly sealed. If an "off" odor develops, throw it out. It could be rancid. (See "When Good Oils Go Bad.")

• Put butter, margarine, and spreads in the refrigerator immediately. Follow the "use by" dates. Freeze them if you buy more than you can use in a few months.

• Store all protein-rich salads or sandwich mixtures, including those made with mayonnaise, in the refrigerator or over ice at 40 degrees Fahrenheit or below. Despite what you may have heard, mayonnaise is not the villain in dishes like tuna salad, egg salad, chicken salad, or potato salad. It's the protein-rich meat, poultry, egg, or fish that's mixed with mayo that creates a risky situation if it's not refrigerated properly. The acidic mayo actually helps protect it, but it still needs to be kept cold.

HIDDEN DANGERS IN FOOD

As concerned as you are about eating the right foods, chances are you're just as concerned about avoiding the wrong ones. You've probably heard that even nutritious foods carry hidden dangers. Among them: food additives, pesticides, preservatives, and natural toxins. Should you be concerned?

What foods should you avoid? Is it even possible to avoid all these hidden dangers? Read on—we think you'll be surprised at some of the answers.

Ten or fifteen years ago, most consumers cited food additives and preservatives among their top nutritional concerns. Times have changed. Today, many people view pesticides as the most worrisome components of the food supply. Natural toxins are rarely, if ever, mentioned. Yet, it's wise to develop an awareness of what all of these are, what they do, and why they are in our foods. Let's start with food additives and preservatives, those alleged bad guys of a decade ago.

Food Additives and Preservatives

Would you buy a food labeled "additives and preservatives have been added to provide better flavor, brighter color, and longer shelf life?" Chances are, you'd pass this one by. Foods boasting "no additives, no preservatives" are generally thought of as being superior to those containing such inventions of food technology as guar gum and diglycerides. But eliminating additives or preservatives does not improve a food's nutritional value.

There are somewhere in the neighborhood of 3,000 different government-approved additives, ranging from sugar and salt to BHT and MSG. Even vitamins and minerals are considered additives if a food has been enriched or fortified. Excluding salt and sugar, Americans consume, on average, about five pounds of additives per year. Though concerns are constantly raised over strange chemicals added to food, surprisingly, it's the boringly familiar salt, sucrose, corn syrup, pepper, baking soda, mustard, and vegetable colors that account for 98 percent, by weight, of all food additives in this country.

Is That Additive Safe?

Since 1958, all new additives must be proved safe before they can be added to foods. Under current regulations, known as the Delaney clause, any additive that causes cancer in animals or humans must be banned from the food supply (saccharin, however, is an exception to this rule).

Despite Food and Drug Administration (FDA) assurances that food additives are safe, their presence in foods has long been a concern. Is it a justifiable concern? Most experts say no. Their contention is that the benefits of food additives far outweigh the small risks, especially when compared to other risks we deal with in our lives. And indeed, overall, the U.S. food supply is one of the safest in the world.

Without many of the food additives commonly used today, bread would mold before a loaf was finished, salt would become lumpy, ice cream would resemble ice more than cream, and soft candies such as marshmallows would quickly be transformed into rocks. Consider the shelf life of baked products such as cookies, muffins, or crackers: Without preservatives to retain their freshness, these foods would become stale or moldy within days.

That's not to say that all additives should be given a clean bill of health without question. Some long-used additives such as red dye #2 were banned because of newly discovered health risks. But before demanding a blanket ban of the more than 3,000 food additives used today, experts urge us to take a close look at the benefits they provide and weigh them against the small risks they carry. Still, many additives currently used have not been tested for safety because they were accepted as safe under a "grandfather clause" of the Food Additive Amendment. If they had caused no problems before the amendment was passed, they were deemed GRAS, or Generally Recognized As Safe.

Of all the food additives, food colors and dyes have caused the most concern. Most recently, red dye #3 was banned for use in cosmetics and topical drugs because it was found to cause cancer in rats, but no decision has been made whether to ban its use in foods. Tartrazine, also known as yellow dye #5, is known to cause allergic reactions in some people who are sensitive.

Here's a list of some of the most common additives and the concerns that have been voiced about them:

Aluminum compounds (aluminum sulfate, sodium aluminum phosphate, aluminum chloride): These are used most often as leavening agents in baking soda and breads. There has been some concern over aluminum contributing to the development of Alzheimer's disease, but experts say the amount of aluminum ingested from foods is minimal—about 15 milligrams per day. Some antacids and buffered aspirin supply a thousand times more aluminum than do foods. The FDA considers it a safe food additive.

BHA (butylated hydroxyanisole): This is a preservative used in dry cereals, shortenings, and dry yeasts and in beverages made from mixes. Without BHA, food quickly becomes rancid. Though there was once concern about a possible connection between BHA and cancer, there is no evidence that consumption of BHA increases the risk of developing cancer. In fact, some research suggests that, acting as an antioxidant, it may actually protect against cancer.

BHT (butylated hydroxytoluene): Like BHA, BHT is a preservative used to prevent rancidity in dry cereals and shortenings as well as instant potatoes. However, unlike BHA, BHT has been found both to cause and prevent cancer in animals depending upon whether it is consumed before or after other cancer-causing agents. Many consumer advocates recommend avoiding it, but the scientific consensus is that it does not cause cancer in people.

Caramel: Caramel adds color to foods such as soft drinks, beer, and baked goods. Caramel is a natural product that is made when sugar or starch is heated, and it is generally considered to be a safe additive.

Carrageenan: Carrageenan is extracted from seaweed and is used to stabilize foods such as ice cream, hot cocoa, and infant formulas to prevent fats and proteins from separating. It is also the ingredient being used in McDonald's McLean Deluxe Burger to lower the fat content. Research with animals has proved it to be safe.

Guar gum: Guar gum is a thickening agent taken from the guar plant, which is similar to the soybean plant. It is used in ice cream, salad dressings, and puddings. Guar gum is considered a safe food additive.

Lecithin: Lecithin is naturally found in soybeans and eggs. It's also synthesized in the body and is naturally present in human cells. As a food additive, it is used in mayonnaise, margarine, chocolate, and vegetable-oil sprays to prevent blended ingredients from separating and fats from becoming rancid. The FDA says lecithin is a safe additive.

Modified food starch: This additive is exactly what it says—food starch from potatoes or tapioca that has been chemically modified. While regular starch may separate or clump when heated, modified starch is more stable, producing a creamy product. It is sometimes used in confectioner's sugar or baking powder to absorb moisture and prevent caking and in puddings and spaghetti sauces as a thickener. Its presence in baby foods caused the most controversy a while back. However, most baby-food manufacturers have stopped using modified food starch, though some toddler foods still contain it. It is not digested by the body, and therefore doesn't provide calories. Some consumer groups say its safety is questionable, but the FDA considers it to be safe.

Mono- & *Diglycerides:* These are types of fats used to provide a smooth texture in baked goods. They can be found in a wide variety of products from frozen entrees to low-fat muffins. Though they provide the same nine calories per gram as triglycerides, they contribute few calories because they are used in such small amounts—usually about one percent of the fat in a food product. They are considered safe.

Red dye #3: This is an artificial color that currently carries a question mark about its safety because it is under suspicion as a possible carcinogen. It was banned from use in cosmetics and topical drugs in 1989 and may eventually be banned from use in foods. It is currently used to color maraschino cherries, gelatin desserts, red-shelled pistachio nuts, and powdered beverage mixes.

WHEN SULFITES MAKE YOU SICK

Sulfites—including sodium sulfite, bisulfite, metabisulfite, and sulfur dioxide—have long been used to prevent fruits and vegetables from turning brown when exposed to air. They also help preserve dried fruit, shrimp, and wine. But after the deaths of several people found to be sulfite-sensitive, the FDA banned its use on fresh fruits and vegetables in 1986. However, sulfites may still be found on fresh-cut potatoes. People with severe asthma are most at risk for having life-threatening reactions to sulfites.

All wines contain some sulfites. They are a natural byproduct of processing. But those that have sulfites added and that were bottled after 1988 in the United States must be labeled.

Other foods that sometimes contain sulfites include olives, relishes, vinegar, crabs, lobsters, avocado mixes, dried vegetables, dry soup mixes, dried fruit, trail mixes, and beer.

Sodium nitrite: Sodium nitrite is used in cured and processed meats such as bacon, bologna, ham, hot dogs, and salami to impart their characteristic pinkish color and to prevent spoilage from the deadly botulinum bacteria. Sodium nitrite has generated much controversy because of its ability to be converted to carcinogenic compounds called nitrosamines. Much higher levels of sodium nitrite were used in the past, but bowing to consumer demands and updated U.S. Department of Agriculture (USDA) regulations, manufacturers have in the last few years reduced the levels of sodium nitrite in their products, specifically bacon, by as much as 50 percent. It's best to keep your consumption of foods containing sodium nitrite to a minimum.

Yellow dye #5: This dye adds color to foods such as cake, powdered beverage mixes, candies, and pudding mixes. Though it is safe for most, yellow dye #5 can cause severe allergic reactions in some people—particularly those allergic to a related compound, aspirin. Because of potential sensitivity, manufacturers are required by law to clearly state if yellow #5, also known as tartrazine, is present.

Pesticides on Parade

Concern over the dangers of pesticides in the food we eat has reached a fevered pitch. From Alar in apples to DDT in celery, each new headline fuels our growing paranoia. Pesticides are synonymous with poison. Consumer advocates admonish us to "go organic" or suffer the health consequences. So, what's the deal? Is the food supply truly riddled with poisonous pesticides, or have things just gotten out of hand?

We'll cut to the chase on this one. The bottom line is that the risk from not eating fruits and vegetables is greater than the risk from pesticides applied to them. That's not to say that there is no cause for concern. To the contrary, several organizations, including the National Academy of Sciences and the

Environmental Working Group, a nonprofit consumer group based in Washington, D.C., have attacked current government pesticide regulations as being inadequate and have called for reform.

Several of the 200-plus pesticides currently available for use on crops have been linked with cancer, and they are frequently found in the fruits and vegetables you buy at the supermarket. But many experts believe that pesticides rank low on the list of health risks that face the average person. Other risks such as smoking, drinking, and eating a fatty diet are more hazardous to your health. Still, you should be concerned about regulating your intake of pesticides, especially if you have children.

One of the biggest concerns health experts have voiced is that of children's exposure to pesticides. Because children generally consume more produce, relative to their size, than adults do, they're at greater risk of overexposure to pesticides that have been identified as causing cancer. In fact, it's been estimated that one-third of a child's lifetime exposure to some pesticides will occur by age five.

Here's how the pesticide-in-produce picture looks now, according to a recent random sampling by the USDA:

Apples: 77.3% tested positive for at least one pesticide residue
Bananas: 22.2% tested positive for pesticide residues
Celery: 79.2% had detectable pesticide residues
Green beans: 66% contained pesticide residues
Grapes: 79.1% contained pesticide residues
Peaches: 82.4% tested positive for pesticide residues
Potatoes: 74.8% tested positive for pesticide residues

But experts insist the situation is not as scary as it sounds. Almost all pesticides were found in amounts well below currently set tolerance levels. Some groups, however, argue that the tolerance levels are set too high. Don't despair: Pesticide reform is sure to come soon. The Environmental Protection Agency, the USDA, and the FDA are working together to come up with new, more stringent regulations concerning the use and misuse of pesticides in the United States. You can look for new, improved pesticide regulations in the not-too-distant future.

Protecting Yourself Against Pesticides

While we're waiting for stricter pesticide regulations to take effect, here are a few things you can do to reduce your exposure now:

• Wash all your produce well. For best results, dilute a drop of mild dish detergent in water and wash the produce in it. Be sure to rinse the produce thoroughly.

• Scrub vegetables such as potatoes and carrots with a vegetable brush, especially if you plan to eat the skin.

• Shop at farmers' markets. The produce is often treated with fewer pesticides since they aren't needed to help crops survive travel over long distances.

• Avoid imported produce. They may contain pesticides that have been banned in this country.

• Buy produce that's in season. It is less likely than out-of-season produce to have been heavily doused with pesticides to retain its appearance and freshness.

• Peel fruits and vegetables such as cucumbers and apples that have a waxy look to them. Peeling removes some pesticides that are sealed in with a coating of wax used to keep these foods fresh.

• Eat a variety of foods. Because pesticide use varies from crop to crop, variety helps minimize exposure to any one pesticide.

No Way to Say No to Natural Toxins

It's been estimated that the risk associated with eating the natural toxins contained in a peanut-butter sandwich is 1,000

ARE YOU PART OF THE PESTICIDE PROBLEM?

If you demand the best—ruby red tomatoes, blemish-free apples, perfectly hued oranges, and lettuce free of any marks—then you're also demanding overuse of pesticides. It's a contradiction to call for fewer pesticides on the one hand while demanding picture-perfect produce on the other. If and when pesticide use is cut, both farmers and especially consumers will have to lower their high aesthetic standards.

---

times greater than the risk from an average exposure to ethylene dibromide (EDB), a pesticide used on grains. Sound bizarre? It's not really as far out as it sounds. Almost all plant foods contain "natural" pesticides, or toxins, that ward off pests and therefore help plants protect themselves. A few have been shown to cause cancer in animals.

Here are a few common natural toxins found in foods:

Aflatoxin: This is a mold-produced toxin found most often in peanuts, peanut butter, and corn. It can cause cancer and cirrhosis of the liver and impair immune function. Monitoring by state agencies helps keep aflatoxin levels in storage grains and legumes below the toxic range.

Canavanine: Canavanine is found naturally in alfalfa sprouts. It is toxic to monkeys. It's not known if it causes harm to humans.

Glucosinolates (goitrogens): These can interfere with normal thyroid function if they make up a major part of the calories in the diet. They are found in cabbage, broccoli, brussels sprouts, cauliflower, turnips, kale, mustard greens, kohlrabi, and rutabaga.

Alkyl benzene compounds: These compounds cause cancer in rats. They are found in herbs and spices such as sweet basil, tarragon, black pepper, and cloves.

Glycoalkaloids: These chemicals are produced by potatoes as a defense against insect invaders. When exposed to light, one type of glycoalkaloid, solanine, leaves a green hue on the surface of the potato skin. Cut off small green areas; if green areas are extensive, toss the potato.

Hydrazines: Hydrazines are natural toxins found in white mushrooms. They can cause cancer in animals.

Nitrites and Nitrates: These are found in nature as well as being added to some foods. They are found naturally in beets, celery, lettuce, spinach, radishes, and rhubarb and are known to be cancer triggers.

Don't Panic

Should you avoid all the foods that contain these natural toxins? Definitely not. You would be eliminating some of the best natural cancer preventors in your diet—fruits and vegetables. That lends a certain logic, once again, to the admonition to practice "variety and moderation." Eat a variety of foods without overdosing on any one, and you eliminate the risk of overdosing on any natural toxin or man-made pesticides.

"NATURAL" FOODS

Natural. The word is inherently appealing. Who wouldn't want to eat natural foods? If something is "natural," the implication is that it's nutritious. This is not always true. Nor is it always true that something not labeled as natural is less nutritious than a product that is. As you can see, you have to be careful.

Fortunately, the word "natural" on food labels had its heyday in the 1970s, and has since been largely replaced by more specific claims, such as "low-fat" or "low-sodium," or even by the bold claim "healthy," most of which now have government controls over their use.

Don't get us wrong. We believe that it's best to center your diet around what we call "whole" foods—unprocessed foods such as fresh fruits and vegetables and whole grains. What we would like to caution you about in this chapter is all the meaningless hype and needless expense associated with some other so-called "natural" foods that are usually found in health food stores.

How Healthy Is "Natural"?

Health food stores boast they offer only "natural" foods. But like the "natural" label, that doesn't always mean much. Often, health food stores are schizophrenic places to browse. On the one hand, they offer some hard-to-find whole foods that are indeed healthy additions to your diet (see "What Is Worth Buying at the Health Food Store"). But all too often they overhype and overprice what they sell, some of which is no healthier than the fare in your local supermarket.

Take raw milk, for instance. Nothing could be more natural, right? Maybe so, but it's also full of natural bacteria, which can make you very sick. In fact, there are lots of "natural" foods that contain natural toxins, which may or may not pose a hazard (see "Hidden Dangers in Food").

Butter is natural, right? But does that make it healthy? Of course not. It's full of the saturated fats we all know we should limit. Yet you can find "homemade" butter in nearly all health food stores, dispelling any notion that you only find healthy foods there.

Another case of natural not always being better is natural peanut butter. A recent survey of peanut butters revealed that the highest levels of aflatoxin—a natural cancer-causing substance produced by mold that grows on peanuts—were found in natural, fresh-ground peanut butters. On average, they contained more than ten times the aflatoxin found in national brands.

How about sea salt? Isn't salt that's naturally from the sea better than the salt in grocery stores? After all, it costs two to four times more. But, surprise, there's no advantage; the two are virtually the same in taste and nutrition. Most of the minerals in sea salt are lost during the processing that concentrates the salt. And who decided salt from the sea is more natural than salt from the earth anyway?

Maybe you think brown eggs are a healthier choice? Nope. Brown isn't always better. White and brown eggs are exactly the same nutritionally. The color of the egg depends on the breed of the chicken.

Surely honey and "raw" sugar (turbinado sugar) are better for you than refined white sugar? Sorry. The minuscule amounts of minerals in raw sugar offer no benefit. And you're more likely to be getting contaminants and insect fragments in turbinado sugar, even though it has been washed and partially refined (true raw sugar is not sold for human consumption). Brown sugar is no health bargain either; it's simply refined sugar sprayed with insignificant amounts of molasses for color and taste. And your body? It treats all sugars the same.

Likewise, health-food versions of cookies and cakes may seem more nutritious, but it's just wishful thinking. Many "natural" sweets brag they contain "no sugar." Instead, they're sweetened with concentrated fruit juices, like white grape juice or honey. But there's little nutritional difference between the sugar in concentrated juices or honey, and the cane sugar or corn syrup in traditional sweets. The natural sweets may even be higher in calories, or may contain more fat.

The fat in packaged foods is one area where health food store products may be a legitimate step ahead. Many of the foods on their shelves contain no hydrogenated or partially hydrogenated oils. So although the total fat content of the products may not be any lower, they often contain less saturated fat.

All this comes at a price, however. Surveys of health food stores reveal they may charge up to five times as much for similar products found in a supermarket. Sometimes even the same brand name product costs more at the health food store. Foods found exclusively at the health food store—except the items sold in bulk—typically cost more. Why? Part of the reason is that many of the products are made by small companies that must charge more; the stores can't buy the large quantities supermarket chains can because they stock less; and because many items are free of preservatives, they have a shorter shelf life.

What "Organic" Means

The word "organic" on a label can mean many things. It's most meaningful if the product is labeled as "certified organic." This means any one of several organic foods associations have certified the product as having been grown on land that has been free of chemicals for at least one year, and has been processed without the use of artificial colors or preservatives. But certification only assures that an organic method has been used; it doesn't guarantee that the product being sold is free from pesticides.

It's possible even for "organic" produce to contain "stubborn" chemicals. For example, long-banned DDT still shows up in soil samples today. And sometimes pesticides sprayed on one plot of land can drift onto an organic farm, or contaminated water can run off where it wasn't intended. Conversely, up to half of conventionally grown crops show no trace of pesticides. For both these reasons, studies in the past have revealed that organically grown and conventionally grown crops often contain remarkably similar amounts of pesticide residues.

For extra peace of mind, you may want to choose products that are certified as three-year organic instead of just one year; some are labeled this way. You may also want to consider IPM-grown crops, which may or may not be advertised. Integrated Pest Management—or IPM—is a program that relies heavily on natural predators of pests, crop rotation, and various other "low-

WHAT IS WORTH BUYING AT THE HEALTH FOOD STORE

A few of the foods we feature in Part IV may be hard to find at your local supermarket. You may have more luck at a health food store if you're looking for unusual grains like millet. And because health food stores often sell grains and dry beans in bulk, they may be cheaper than at the supermarket, which may only offer small, expensively packaged versions. You'll probably also find a better selection of whole grain breads and ready-to-eat cereals.

Less common produce—arugula, dandelion greens, guava, kohlrabi—may be more plentiful and fresher at the natural food store or at a farmer's market.

As for packaged products, you may find it easier to avoid those made with hydrogenated oils or additives by shopping in health food stores. But read labels carefully to avoid surprises.

If you've decided to buy only organic foods, you will most certainly end up shopping at a natural food store.

Anyone who is truly allergic to wheat or other common ingredients may need to turn to a health food store.

If you like to be on the cutting edge, health food stores often offer unusual foods before they hit mainstream markets. They certainly were ahead of the game when they sold yogurt, acidophilus milk, wheat bran, oat bran, rice cakes, soy burgers, and granola. You can find all these now in almost every supermarket.

tech" methods to fight off pests. Pesticides are not taboo but are only used as a last resort, and sparingly.

The result is produce with much lower levels of pesticides, if any at all. You need to realize, though, that IPM-grown produce may be less attractive. There's nothing wrong with it, and it's just as nutritious.

Then there are products certified as containing "no detectable residues." This means the product's ingredients were not necessarily grown on organic fields, but the final product has been tested for certain pesticides, and none were found. Be aware also that some products may contain one or two ingredients that are "certified organic," but that doesn't mean the product itself is organic, since other ingredients in the product may not be.

The bottom line? You will certainly be eating fewer pesticides if you buy organic, but there's no guarantee your food will be free of all pesticides, or that you've gained any measurable health benefit. You will, however, be spending more money.

What to Do

We aren't trying to discourage you from visiting health food stores. They often offer items you can't find elsewhere and usually have a superior selection of organic produce, if that's your choice (see "What 'Organic' Means"). But we do think you're wasting money if you shop there exclusively. Don't assume you can't find certain products in the grocery store; it might just take a little searching or a special request to the store manager.

Try doing your own price and label comparison between the packaged foods in your area supermarkets and those in the health food store. Don't overlook upscale markets; many offer a wonderful selection of produce—even organic produce—at lower prices than a health food store. Above all, check out whether there's a farmer's market near you. If so, drive on down without delay; it probably offers the freshest value for your money.

WHAT GOOD NUTRITION CAN AND CAN'T DO

At this point, you may be looking for a guarantee of good health, but we can't give you one. We can't even promise you'll live an extra day if you do all we've suggested. That's because there are lots of other factors besides nutrition that affect your health. In a book on foods and nutrition, it's easy to lose sight of the fact that nutrition isn't everything. But improving your eating habits can certainly push the odds in your favor. And we can be fairly certain that you will have a better quality of life, however long it may be.

Understanding Your Genetic Connections

Almost every chronic disease that has a nutrition component also has a genetic component. Cancer, diabetes, heart disease, high blood pressure, obesity, osteoporosis—the odds of developing any of them are strongly influenced by your family history as well as your eating habits. While you can improve your diet, you have no control over your family tree. And there's no way to know how much of your health is influenced by what you eat versus who you are—genetically speaking.

Everyone is genetically unique, down to their taste buds. It's true. Your food likes and dislikes are partly predetermined. It's thought, for example, that the preference for strongly flavored vegetables like broccoli, cabbage, cauliflower, and spinach may be inherited. How? The ability to detect phenylthiocarbamide, a chemical found in these vegetables, is inherited. To most people, it tastes bitter, but some people can't tell it from water.

Faulty genes are to blame for some nutrition-related diseases called inborn errors of metabolism. They occur when critical enzymes, such as those needed to digest specific proteins or carbohydrates, are missing. A special diet is often required so an excess of the offending substance doesn't build up in the bloodstream. Examples include PKU, or phenylketonuria, in which the body can't handle the amino acid phenylalanine; the inherited forms of hypercholesterolemia,

ARE YOU FATED TO BE FAT?

The blame for being overweight has shifted away from our eating habits and toward our genes. But it's really somewhere in between—probably about half and half. It's been estimated that as many as 80 percent of children with two obese parents will become obese; only 14 percent of those with two parents of desirable weight will. Of course, some of that can be attributed to the eating habits of parents rubbing off on their children. But not all. A watershed study in Denmark looked at adults who had been adopted as children. The study showed that their weights resembled their biological parents' weights more closely than their adoptive parents' weights.

A perfect example of the influence of genes versus environment was demonstrated in research at Laval University in Canada with 12 pairs of identical twins who were deliberately overfed. There was remarkable individual variation in how much weight was gained and whether the excess calories were stored as fat. Most important, there was a significant similarity in weight gain between twins, but a great difference in weight gain between them and other twins.

So if your parents are overweight, are you tied to the same fate? Definitely not. You inherit only a vulnerability to gain weight. Whether you actually become overweight depends on your eating and exercise habits.

in which blood cholesterol soars sky high; and even the less serious condition lactose intolerance, in which the body can't adequately digest the sugar in milk products.

But unlike these inborn errors of metabolism, most of the major chronic diseases are not etched in stone in your genes. You give yourself a fighting chance to fend off these killers when you live the healthiest life you possibly can.

Let's look at a few examples of diet-related diseases that may be lurking in your gene pool. By checking your medical family tree, you'll have a better idea if you're vulnerable. This may give you incentive to make lifestyle changes. Because, remember, your diet may play the most significant role in determining whether these disease-carrying genes end up calling the shots.

Cancer: A few cancers are totally the result of heredity. And a few result mostly from exposure to environmental carcinogens. But, more commonly, cancers result from the interplay of your genes with your environment, including diet. There's little doubt this is true for cancers of the breast, colon, lung, prostate, and stomach. Scientists think you can inherit the gene for a certain type of cancer, but it may take an environmental "insult"—diet, chemical carcinogen, smoking—for that gene to be turned "on," causing cancer cells to grow. So simply inheriting the gene does not seal your fate. (See Cancer in Part II.)

Diabetes: Most people know that if diabetes runs in your family, you are much more likely to develop it yourself, especially the non-insulin-dependent type II that you develop later in life. But you can lower your risk if you can keep your weight under control. (See Diabetes in Part II.)

Heart disease: The inherited component of heart disease is undeniable but not well understood because it is complex and intertwined with environmental influences. Even identical twins who inherit the same tendency do not necessarily both develop heart disease to the same degree. It's estimated that a major reason why blood-cholesterol levels vary from person to person is due to who our parents are. It's even thought that how well we respond to a cholesterol-lowering diet may also be partly genetically determined. And all the other diseases that affect our susceptibility to heart disease— diabetes, high blood pressure, obesity—are also determined, to some extent, by family history. (See the Heart Disease profile in Part II.)

High blood pressure: Almost half the people with high blood pressure have a parent with the disease. Your susceptibility to the disease may depend partly on whether you have inherited salt-sensitivity. But environment—mostly smoking and diet—is thought to influence half your risk for high blood pressure. (See High Blood Pressure in Part II.)

Obesity: No single genetic defect is thought to explain why some people gain weight more easily than others, and why, for some, it becomes a health problem. Clearly, we are not all born with an equal response to the food we eat. Experts think some people are genetically predisposed to store more body fat than others. This may be a holdover from our origins, when this trait was a survival tactic for food shortages. That may explain why being overweight is so common a problem today in times of plenty. A slow metabolism may also be an inherited tendency, as may be the way your fat is distributed—upper body versus lower body. (See Overweight in Part II.)

Osteoporosis: Your bone-mineral content and bone density are likely to be similar to those of your parents. And if you are a woman, you are at considerably more risk for developing osteoporosis if your mother also suffered from the disease. But many experts think you can improve your chances of delaying or preventing osteoporosis through diet and exercise when young and even, to some extent, after menopause. (See Osteoporosis in Part II.)

Altering Your Habits

Your habits are the things you can change that affect your susceptibility to disease. Your eating habits are one of them—but only one. Other habits can enhance or detract from your nutritional efforts. To give yourself the best chance to fight chronic diseases, you should try to modify all your bad habits. Let's focus on the two most important ones.

Smoking: This is number one on the hit list. By now, everyone surely knows what a health hazard smoking is. Quitting is, by far, the best thing you can do to improve your chances of not developing high blood pressure, heart disease, stroke, and lung cancer. Smoking is also a major factor in oral cancers. Smoking combined with alcohol is particularly hazardous to your health.

Inactivity: Good nutrition should go hand in hand with regular exercise. Doing both together beats either one alone in keeping you at a healthy weight, which is important for avoiding so many chronic conditions, including heart disease, high blood pressure, and infections. But almost 60 percent of Americans qualify as "couch potatoes" because of their physical inactivity. And only 22 percent get enough exercise to gain a health advantage.

Fortunately, keeping fit doesn't have to mean "no pain, no gain." A new standard of how much physical activity is needed to improve health was agreed upon in mid-1993 by the Centers for Disease Control and Prevention (CDC) and by sports groups, including the American College of Sports Medicine.

The groups recommend 30 minutes or more of moderate activity at least five days a week.

The key word in that advice is moderate. That's good news for sedentary Americans who have no desire to run a marathon or sweat it out at the gym. The CDC defines "moderate" as the equivalent of brisk walking at three to four miles an hour. That's something that most people should be able to do. What's especially gratifying is the new thinking that accumulated activity is comparable to one sustained workout. So doing simple things like taking the stairs instead of the elevator and parking far from the mall entrance can indeed add up to a more fit you.

Tipping the Scales

What all this means is that you may inherit a tendency to develop certain diseases, but whether you actually develop them may depend on how you live your life. Certain factors, like smoking, a high-fat diet, exposure to carcinogens, a stress-filled lifestyle, and being overweight, may act as triggers that set into motion your inherited tendency. So you see, not everything is inevitable. You do have some control—maybe enough to tip the scales in your favor. The odds are good enough to give it a try.

FOODS FOR HEALTHIER LIVING

It's time to present our top food choices for healthier living. You may be surprised there are so many. To be honest, there are more, but we had to stop somewhere. So if your favorite food isn't here, that doesn't necessarily mean it's not good for you or you shouldn't eat it. It just didn't make our list.

Could you exist on these foods alone? Yes, quite nicely, thank you. But that's not the point. There are other foods you'll want to eat, as well. And that's fine. We just urge you to take advantage of as many of these whole foods as you can. By including many of them in moderation in your menus, you'll assure yourself a healthy, varied diet—one that offers an arsenal of nutrients and phytochemicals that can help to decrease your risk of disease and keep you in tip-top nutrition shape.

How should you approach this section? It's easy to flip to your favorite foods, because we've presented them alphabetically, but we think you'll be better off reading this section as a whole, from apples to yogurt. That way, you'll get a sense of all the foods outside your usual circle of selections. You'll see what health benefits they offer, how to select and store them, and how to prepare and serve them. Best of all, you'll discover new, taste-tempting recipes that you'll want to try out in your kitchen.

Some foods—such as dry peas and beans, salad greens, lemons and limes, and oranges and tangerines—are grouped together. That's because they share similar characteristics.

In nearly all of the profiles, we've listed the nutrients in a typical serving of the feature food (or a representative food). The first nutrient grouping—the major nutrients—is standard for every food. The second grouping lists only those vitamins that the food is particularly high in, while the third grouping does the same for minerals. We've also included nutritional information for the recipes; these nutritionals refer to one serving of the recipe.

You'll notice that some foods have a long list of key nutrients, while others have only one or two. Don't assume a food with fewer listed nutrients is not worth eating. It may be a critical source for the one or two nutrients it is rich in. Likewise, for many of these foods, we've listed only the nutrients that the food is particularly rich in; it may provide smaller amounts of various other nutrients, as well. Remember, each food included here has qualities that make it a valuable addition to your diet. And no one food has it all. That's why we've embraced so many—to emphasize variety and moderation. Include as many different types of food as you can so that you get a wide range of nutrients.

APPLES

Chances are, you've only tasted three or four of the thousands of varieties of apples that exist. Red Delicious is the most popular variety in the United States—probably more for its waxed look than its taste. Also widely available are Golden Delicious, McIntosh, Cortland, and Granny Smith.

Health Benefits

Apples are not bursting with nutrients like some fruits, but they do provide some vitamin C and lots of fiber. The pectin in apples contributes much of the fruit's soluble fiber, which helps keep blood-sugar and blood-cholesterol levels down. It also counteracts diarrhea (apple juice has the opposite effect). Apples also stimulate your gums and promote saliva producttion, making them nature's toothbrush.

NUTRIENT INFORMATION			
Apple, fresh		Fat	0.5 g
Serving Size: 1 small		Saturated	0.1 g
		Cholesterol	0
Calories	81	Dietary Fiber	2.8 g
Protein	0.3 g	Sodium	1 mg
Carbohydrate	21.1 g		
		Vitamin C	7.8 mg

Selection and Storage

A few varieties—like Cortland, Jonathan, and Winesap—are all-purpose apples, but, in general, you're better off choosing apples for their intended purpose. Golden Delicious and Cortland work well in salads such as Waldorf, because they don't turn brown when cut. For baking, try Golden Delicious, Rome Beauty, York Imperial, Cortland, Northern Spy, or Rhode Island Greening. They'll offer the best flavor and keep their shape when cooked. You can't beat tart Macouns or the award-winning Empire for munching.

Although available year-round, apples are best in autumn, right from the orchard if possible. The pesticide Alar is no longer used by apple growers. Apples in stores often have a waxy coating that may include a fungicide. To avoid the wax, you have to peel the apple, losing some fiber in the process.

To keep their crunch as long as possible, apples should be refrigerated. They're already ripe when picked, so at room temperature they only go bad. Apples like a very cold, humid spot, like the crisper drawer of the refrigerator. Keep them in a plastic bag with holes punched in the bag for ventilation. Well-refrigerated, some varieties will keep until spring, though most will get mealy in a month or two. Enjoy Golden Delicious right away; their skins shrivel after a few weeks.

Here's an old trick: Place an apple in a paper bag along with unripe fruit. The apple produces a gas that speeds ripening of other fruit.

Preparation and Serving Tips

Wash and scrub apples well before eating or cooking. Cut out any bruised spots. To prevent browning, sprinkle a little lemon or pineapple juice on cut surfaces.

Homemade applesauce is a cinch to make. Just core and quarter the apples, then cook until mushy over low heat in just enough water to prevent burning. Process in a food mill, to separate out the skin. Stir in sugar to taste. Serve warm or cold.

LEMON-GINGER APPLE CRISP

6   cups peeled apple slices
¼   cup plus 2 tablespoons packed brown sugar, divided

3 **tablespoons all-purpose flour, divided**
2 **tablespoons lemon juice**
1 **teaspoon grated lemon peel**
½ **teaspoon ground ginger**
¼ **cup quick-cooking rolled oats**
1 **tablespoon margarine, melted**

Preheat oven to 350°F. Toss apples with ¼ cup brown sugar, 1 tablespoon flour, lemon juice, lemon peel and ginger in 2-quart ovenproof, microwave-safe baking dish; set aside.

For topping, combine remaining 2 tablespoons brown sugar, 2 tablespoons flour, oats and margarine in small bowl; mix well. Sprinkle evenly over apple mixture.

Microwave at HIGH (100% power) 12 to 15 minutes or until mixture begins to bubble. Bake 15 to 20 minutes or until apples are tender and topping is golden brown.

Makes 6 servings

NUTRIENTS PER SERVING:

Calories	179.2	Sodium	26.41 mg
Protein	1.19 g	Vitamin C	7.89 mg
Carbohydrate	38.11 g		
Dietary Fiber	2.71 g	DIETARY EXCHANGES:	
Fat	2.54 g	Fruit: 1.5	Bread: 1
Saturated Fat	0.48 g	Fat: 0.5	
Poly Fat	0.81 g		
Mono Fat	0.92 g	% OF CALORIES FROM:	
Cholesterol	0 mg	PRO: 3%	CARB: 85%
Sugar	28.65 g	FAT: 13%	
Calcium	20.67 mg		
Potassium	217.2 mg		

APRICOTS

If you think apricots only come in cans, think again. A fresh apricot is a treat for its aroma alone. Native to China, and a relative of the peach, the apricot is smaller, more yellow, and more delicate. Its season is short and sweet.

Health Benefits

Apricots are brimming with beta-carotene. That's the prominent antioxidant member of the vitamin A family. Researchers have linked foods rich in beta-carotene to a reduced risk of certain cancers (especially lung cancer), cataracts, and heart disease. Like many fruits, apricots contribute some vitamin C, another antioxidant. They're particularly rich in fiber for their size.

Canned apricots are not the nutritional equivalent of fresh. Not only does the added sugar double the calories, but canned apricots contain only half the beta-carotene and vitamin C of the fresh fruit. When fresh apricots aren't available, choose water-packed or juice-packed varieties.

Dried apricots, like all dried fruit, are a concentrated source of nutrients and calories, because you tend to eat more of them than you would the fresh fruit. One-half cup of dried apricots packs in triple the fiber of three fresh apricots, but also triple the calories and less vitamin C; there's little difference in the beta-carotene contents. Dried apricots are also a good source of iron.

NUTRIENT INFORMATION		Cholesterol	0
Apricots, fresh		Dietary fiber	2.6 g
Serving Size: 3 medium		Sodium	1 mg
Calories	51		
Protein	1.5 g	Vitamin A	2,769 IU
Carbohydrate	11.8 g	Vitamin C	10.6 mg
Fat	0.5 g		
Saturated	0	Potassium	313 mg

Selection and Storage

Most apricots consumed in the United States are grown in California and are available fresh only from late May to early August. You may be able to find imported apricots in winter.

The apricot is a delicate fruit and must be handled carefully or it will bruise. To avoid damage when shipped, growers pick apricots before they are ripe. But don't choose any tinged with green; they were picked too soon. Avoid pale yellow fruit also. For best flavor, look for plump, golden-orange apricots. Surface blemishes are harmless, but avoid those with soft spots or broken skin. Apricots should be fairly firm or yield just slightly to thumb pressure.

You'll need to ripen apricots for a day or two at room temperature before eating. Try ripening them in a paper bag, but don't pile them up or they'll bruise. Once ripe, they should be refrigerated.

Preparation and Serving Tips

When washing apricots, be gentle; they bruise easily. They are difficult to peel, but it can be done if you dip them in boiling water for 30 seconds, then peel right away under running cold water with a sharp knife. To prevent browning, sprinkle slices with lemon juice. Apricots are great in desserts and also make pleasing appetizers.

GOLDEN APRICOT MUFFINS

    1 cup all-purpose flour, divided
    1 cup whole wheat flour
   ¼ cup sugar
   ¼ teaspoon salt
    1 teaspoon baking powder
    1 teaspoon baking soda
    1 cup plain low fat yogurt
   ½ cup puréed apricots
    2 tablespoons vegetable oil
    1 cup diced apricots

Preheat oven to 400°F. Paper-line 12-cup muffin pan or coat with nonstick cooking spray; set aside.

Reserve 1 tablespoon all-purpose flour. Combine remaining all-purpose flour, whole wheat flour, sugar, salt, baking powder and baking soda in medium bowl; mix well. Combine yogurt, puréed apricots and oil in small bowl; mix well. Add yogurt mixture to dry ingredients; stir just until moistened.

Toss diced apricots with reserved flour. Gently stir diced apricot mixture gently into batter. Spoon batter into muffin cups, filling ¾ full.

Bake 20 to 25 minutes or until wooden toothpick inserted in center of muffin comes out clean. Immediately remove from pan; cool on wire rack.　　　***Makes 12 muffins***

NUTRIENTS PER SERVING:			
Calories	124.9	Potassium	131 mg
Protein	3.6 g	Sodium	154.3 mg
Carbohydrate	21.93 g	Vitamin C	1.33 mg
Dietary Fiber	1.76 g		
Fat	2.9 g	DIETARY EXCHANGES:	
Saturated Fat	0.4 g	Fruit: 0.5	Bread: 1
Poly Fat	0.81 g	Fat: 0.5	
Mono Fat	1.47 g		
Cholesterol	1.17 mg	% OF CALORIES FROM	
Sugar	6.30 g	PRO: 11%	CARB: 68%
Beta-Carotene	184.3 RE	FAT: 20%	
Calcium	46.19 mg		

ARTICHOKES

You have to really like artichokes to go through the trouble of eating one. And in Monterey County, California, they do. The artichoke is now the county's official vegetable.

Artichokes have been cultivated for thousands of years. And for good reason. They're very nutritious, if you can resist dipping the leaves into butter.

Health Benefits

Artichokes are so fibrous, it's probably no surprise to learn they are indeed full of fiber. That's a bonus for your digestive tract, as well as your heart, blood pressure, and blood-sugar level. They're also a super source of folic acid, which is especially important for women of childbearing age, as researchers are now convinced this vitamin helps prevent neural-tube birth defects.

NUTRIENT INFORMATION			
Artichoke, fresh, cooked			
Serving Size: 1 medium			
Calories	53	Vitamin C	8.9 mg
Protein	2.8 g	Folic Acid	53.4 µg
Carbohydrate	12.4 g		
Fat	0.2 g	Iron	1.6 mg
Saturated	0	Magnesium	47 mg
Cholesterol	0	Manganese	0.3 mg
Dietary Fiber	6.2 g	Potassium	316 mg
Sodium	79 mg		

Selection and Storage

Although there are many varieties of artichokes, only one—globe—is grown in the United States. It differs from European varieties in that it is entirely green, while its European cousins often have purplish-red leaves. Baby artichokes are artichokes from a side thistle of the plant. Artichoke hearts are the meaty base of an artichoke. A Jerusalem artichoke is not an artichoke at all (nor does it come from Jerusalem); it's an unrelated root vegetable.

You can find this delicacy year-round in the supermarket, though there are two peak seasons—spring and fall. Look for heavy artichokes with a soft green color and tightly packed, closed leaves. Watch out for moldy or wilted leaves. Bronzed or frosted leaf tips are a sign of a particularly tender, flavorful artichoke.

Store artichokes in a plastic bag in the refrigerator; add a few drops of water to prevent them from drying out. (Do not wash before storing.) Although best if used within a few days, they'll keep for a week or two if stored this way and handled gently.

Preparation and Serving Tips

Before cooking, wash artichokes under running water. Pull off the outer, lower petals and cut the stems. To cook, stand them in a pan and boil for 20 to 40 minutes or steam them for 25 to 40 minutes. They're done when a center petal pulls out easily.

How to eat an artichoke? Pull off a leaf and dip in low-fat yogurt sauce (see below). Then, holding on, put the leaf in your mouth, curved side down. As you pull it out, use your bottom teeth to scrape the flesh off.

Artichokes can be served hot, at room temperature, or cold. They're best served as appetizers so they can be enjoyed alone. That's important, because they command all your attention, and because they contain a chemical that makes other foods taste sweeter. For a healthy dip, use low-fat yogurt with garlic or stick to plain lemon juice.

ARTICHOKE-VEGETABLE STIR-FRY

- 10 whole baby artichokes∗
- ¼ cup lemon juice
- 1 teaspoon olive oil
- 2 cups oyster mushrooms *or* shiitake mushrooms, sliced
- 1 cup diagonally sliced celery
- 1 cup diagonally sliced green onions
- ¼ cup defatted low sodium chicken broth∗∗
- 2 teaspoons dried thyme leaves, crushed
- 1 teaspoon garlic salt
- ¼ teaspoon pepper
- 2 cups packed torn stemmed washed spinach
- 8 ounces vermicelli or thin spaghetti, cooked according to package directions and drained
- 1 teaspoon minced parsley

To prepare artichokes, cut off stems and tough outer leaves. Cut off top third of artichokes. Cut artichokes lengthwise into halves. Place 4 cups water, artichokes and lemon juice in large saucepan; bring to a boil over high heat. Reduce heat to low. Simmer, uncovered, about 10 minutes or until artichokes are tender; drain.

Heat oil in large nonstick skillet or wok over medium-high heat. Add artichokes, mushrooms, celery, green onions, broth, thyme, garlic salt and pepper; cook 3 minutes or until heated through. Add spinach; stir-fry just until spinach is wilted.

Toss vegetables with hot cooked pasta; garnish with parsley.

Makes 4 servings

* Substitute 1 package (9 ounces) frozen baby artichokes for fresh. Thaw artichokes before using; omit preparation and simmering of artichokes.

** To defat chicken broth, skim fat from surface of broth with spoon. Or, place can of broth in refrigerator at least 2 hours ahead of time. Before using, remove fat that has hardened on surface of broth.

NUTRIENTS PER SERVING:

Calories	263.2	Magnesium	94.83 mg
Protein	12.32 g	Manganese	0.83 mg
Carbohydrate	48.34 g	Potassium	588.2 mg
Dietary Fiber	7.38 g	Sodium	645.1 mg
Fat	2.83 g	Vitamin C	23.57 mg
Saturated Fat	0.47 g	Vitamin K	74.55 µg
Poly Fat	0.9 g		
Mono Fat	1.04 g	DIETARY EXCHANGES:	
Cholesterol	0 mg	Veg: 1	Bread: 3
Sugar	0.67 g	Fat: 0.5	
Beta-Carotene	1,491 RE		
Calcium	96.15 mg	% OF CALORIES FROM:	
Folate	111.3 µg	PRO: 18%	CARB: 72%
Iron	4.77 mg	FAT: 9%	

ASPARAGUS

This vegetable has a reputation for being elitist, probably because it's rather expensive. But, like many people, you may swear it's worth it.

Asparagus, along with onions and garlic, is a member of the lily family. While it may spare your breath the odor of those vegetables, 40 percent of the population notices a distinct aroma to their urine after eating it.

Gourmet or not, you can't beat the nutrition you get for what asparagus "costs" calorie-wise. At less than four calories a spear, you can't go wrong. Just don't top it with a hollandaise sauce.

Health Benefits

Asparagus provides substantial amounts of two major antioxidants—vitamins A and C. But it truly shines as a source of folic acid, the nutrient newly discovered to help prevent neural-tube defects, a type of disabling birth defect.

NUTRIENT INFORMATION
Asparagus, fresh, cooked
Serving Size: 4 spears

Calories	15	Vitamin A	498 IU
Protein	1.6 g	Vitamin C	15.7 mg
Carbohydrate	2.6 g	Folic Acid	58.8 µg
Fat	0.2 g		
Saturated	0	Potassium	186 mg
Cholesterol	0		
Dietary Fiber	1.2 g		
Sodium	3 mg		

Selection and Storage

Spotting the first asparagus in stores is a sign of early spring. You may see it as early as February and can enjoy it all the way through July.

Look for fresh asparagus with a bright green color; stalks that are smooth, firm, straight, and round, not flat; and tips that are compact, closed, pointed, and purplish in color. Avoid sandy stalks, as the sand is very difficult to wash out. Thick stalks are fine; they don't indicate toughness. But do choose stalks of similar size, so they will cook at the same rate.

Keep fresh asparagus cold, or it will lose flavor and vitamin C. Wrap it loosely in a plastic bag. It will keep for almost a week, but it won't taste as good after a day or two. If you want to enjoy asparagus year-round, blanch it the day you buy it. Then wrap it tightly in foil and freeze for up to 12 months.

Preparation and Serving Tips

Snap off the whitish stem end, where it breaks easily. Try adding these to your soup stock instead of just tossing them. Whether you boil, steam, or microwave your asparagus, avoid overcooking it. When cooked to crisp-tender, it will still be bright green. When overcooked, it turns a dark, unappealing green and becomes floppy. To boil, simmer for three to five minutes only. For more even cooking, stand the stalks upright in boiling water, with the tips sticking out of the water, for five to ten minutes. This way, the tips will be steamed as the stalks cook. Microwaving will take two to three minutes in a dish with a quarter cup water.

You can serve cooked asparagus hot, warm, or cold. Try adding cut-up asparagus to your next stir-fry or pasta dish. Or, for a real change, buy imported white asparagus. It's grown underground to keep the sun from turning it green and has a slightly bitter taste.

ASPARAGUS SPEARS WITH SUN-DRIED TOMATOES

- ½ cup sun-dried tomatoes (not packed in oil)
- 1 clove garlic, minced
- 2 tablespoons balsamic vinegar
- 1 teaspoon sugar
- ¼ teaspoon dried oregano leaves, crushed
- ¼ teaspoon dried basil leaves, crushed
- ⅛ teaspoon pepper
- 1 pound asparagus, trimmed

Soak dried tomatoes in 1 cup boiling water 30 minutes; drain and coarsely chop. Process tomatoes and garlic in food processor or blender until smooth. Add vinegar, sugar, oregano, basil and pepper. Blend well; set aside.

Bring ½ cup water to a boil in large skillet over high heat. Add asparagus; return to a boil. Reduce heat to medium-low. Simmer, covered, about 5 minutes or until asparagus is crisp-tender. Drain. Serve hot or cold with tomato mixture.

Makes 4 servings

NUTRIENTS PER SERVING:			
Calories	48.82	Folate	135.5 µg
Protein	3.44 g	Magnesium	23.17 mg
Carbohydrate	7.57 g	Potassium	267.4 mg
Dietary Fiber	1.49 g	Sodium	20.49 mg
Fat	0.71 g	Vitamin C	33.85 mg
Saturated Fat	0.06 g		
Poly Fat	0.12 g	DIETARY EXCHANGES:	
Mono Fat	0.01 g	Veg: 2	
Cholesterol	0 mg		
Sugar	0.97 g	% OF CALORIES FROM:	
Beta-Carotene	1,196 RE	PRO: 27%	CARB: 60%
Calcium	23.88 mg	FAT: 13%	

BANANAS

Bananas come in their own perfect package. No mess, no fuss. No wonder they're so popular. They are, in fact, the most popular fruit in the United States. Actually, they're not a true fruit, but a berry. And the banana "tree" is really an herb.

Health Benefits

Bananas are so easily digested, they're often the first fruit given to infants. They're the perfect take-along snack, and many athletes treasure them as a concentrated energy source.

If you have been prescribed a potassium-losing diuretic, you may have been told to eat a banana every day, for its rich potassium lode. That serves a double purpose, since potassium is also thought to help prevent high blood pressure (diuretics are often prescribed as part of the treatment for high blood pressure). The magnesium in bananas may serve the same purpose.

The potassium story may be old hat to you, but you may not know that bananas are one of the best sources of vitamin B_6, a nutrient that many people don't get enough of. Vitamin B_6 is especially important for keeping your immune system performing at its peak.

NUTRIENT INFORMATION
Banana, yellow
Serving Size: an 8½-inch banana

Calories	105	Vitamin C	10.3 mg
Protein	1.2 g	Vitamin B_6	0.7 mg
Carbohydrate	26.7 g		
Fat	0.6 g	Magnesium	33 mg
Saturated	0.2 g	Manganese	0.2 mg
Cholesterol	0	Potassium	451 mg
Dietary Fiber	2.2 g		
Sodium	1 mg		

Selection and Storage

The familiar yellow banana in the supermarket is a Cavendish. There are also red bananas. Plantains are a different variety of banana that remain green and stay starchy.

Selecting the right banana depends a lot on whether you prefer it ripe or still green. Bananas ripen after being picked, and as they do, the starch in them turns to sugar. So the riper, the sweeter and easier to digest. But avoid choosing very ripe bananas; they tend to get mushy and may start to ferment. Look for plump, firm bananas with no bruises or split skins. Brown spots are just a sign of ripening.

To ripen, let sit at room temperature. Better yet, hang them to avoid bruising. Once ripe, you can refrigerate them for a few days; it will stop the ripening process, but it will also turn the bananas black. While this is unsightly, it's not harmful. Don't refrigerate unripe bananas, or they'll never ripen.

Preparation and Serving Tips

Yellow bananas are great plain or cut up into fruit salad or on cereal. Sprinkle lemon juice on banana slices to prevent darkening.

To salvage bananas that are too ripe, blend them with some orange juice and low-fat milk for a healthy treat.

For the kids, try frozen banana treats: Peel a banana, stick a wooden stick in it, dip the banana in orange juice, roll it in wheat germ to coat, then freeze.

Plantains must be cooked to be digestible. Try fried plantain chips.

BANANA COFFEE CAKE

½ cup 100% bran cereal
½ cup strong coffee
1 cup mashed ripe bananas
½ cup sugar
1 egg, slightly beaten
2 tablespoons canola *or* vegetable oil
½ cup all-purpose flour
½ cup whole wheat flour
2 teaspoons baking powder
1 teaspoon ground cinnamon
¼ teaspoon salt

Preheat oven to 350°F. Coat 8-inch square baking pan with nonstick cooking spray; set aside. Combine bran cereal and coffee in large bowl; let stand 3 minutes or until cereal softens. Stir in bananas, sugar, egg and oil.

Combine all-purpose flour, whole wheat flour, baking powder, cinnamon and salt in small bowl; stir into banana mixture just until moistened. Pour into prepared pan.

Bake 25 to 35 minutes or until wooden toothpick inserted in center of cake comes out clean. Cool in pan on wire rack.

Makes 9 servings

NUTRIENTS PER SERVING:			
Calories	168.7	Magnesium	36.96 mg
Protein	3.08 g	Potassium	199.7 mg
Carbohydrate	30.13 g	Pyridoxine (B₆)	0.3 mg
Dietary Fiber	2.55 g	Sodium	165.9 mg
Fat	4.09 g	Vitamin A	12.73 RE
Saturated Fat	0.5 g	Vitamin K	38.01 µg
Poly Fat	1.18 g		
Mono Fat	2.06 g	DIETARY EXCHANGES:	
Cholesterol	23.67 mg	Fruit: 1	Bread: 1
Sugar	11.38 g	Fat: 1	
Beta-Carotene	12.96 RE	% OF CALORIES FROM:	
Calcium	26.77 mg	PRO: 7%	CARB: 71%
Folate	14.89 µg	FAT: 22%	

BARLEY

This ancient Middle Eastern grain is chock-full of fiber and shouldn't be relegated simply to soups. But there's no rejoicing for beer drinkers—the fiber in hops is not brewed into the beer.

Health Benefits

You may be familiar with oat bran and its ability to lower blood-cholesterol levels, but barley also contains the soluble fiber beta-glucan, the same constituent that's in oat bran and dry beans. Barley, therefore, may have a similar action. Farmers are now growing varieties—such as hull-less, waxy barley—that are high in beta-glucan.

Barley is more than rich in soluble fiber; the whole, hulled form also contains more insoluble fiber than wheat. And that's of benefit to your digestive tract, because it may help ward off constipation, diverticular disease, hemorrhoids, even rectal and colon cancers.

NUTRIENT INFORMATION			
Barley, pearled, cooked		Niacin	1.6 mg
Serving Size: ½ cup			
Calories	97	Iron	1.1 mg
Protein	1.8 g	Manganese	0.2 mg
Carbohydrate	22.3 g		
Fat	0.4 g		
Saturated	0.1 g		
Cholesterol	0		
Dietary Fiber	3.9 g		
Sodium	2 mg		

Selection and Storage

Whole, hulled barley, the brown, unpearled form, is the most nutritious—with twice the fiber and more than twice the vitamins and minerals of pearled—but it may be difficult to locate. You may need to check a health food store if your regular grocery store does not stock it.

Scotch barley, or pot barley, is refined (pearled) three times. That's not as much as the pearled type, so part of the bran's goodness remains.

Pearled barley is the easiest to find. While it is nutritionally inferior to the other two types, it is certainly not nutritionally devoid. It still can boast of fiber and iron, despite missing the nutritious outer husk and bran layers that come off after five or six "pearlings."

Store barley in an airtight container in a cool, dark location. It will keep for several months this way.

Preparation and Serving Tips

Whole, hulled barley and Scotch (pot) barley require overnight soaking and longer cooking times than pearled barley. In general, whole barley more than doubles when cooked. Pearled barley quadruples when cooked.

To cook: Add one cup of pearled barley to three cups of boiling water (or one cup of whole barley to four cups of boiling water), and simmer, covered, for 40 to 50 minutes (50 to 60 minutes for whole barley).

As barley cooks, the starch in it swells, releasing pectin that absorbs water, making it soft and bulky. This contributes to its cholesterol-lowering properties, but also makes it the perfect thickener for soups and stews. Barley is delicious in soups, such as Scotch broth, but don't stop there. Barley can be successfully substituted for rice in almost any recipe. It's more flavorful than white rice but isn't as strong-tasting as brown rice—it's a perfect compromise that gives you both flavor and valuable nutrients.

BEEF BARLEY SOUP

Nonstick cooking spray
¾ pound boneless beef top round, excess fat trimmed, cut into ½-inch pieces
3 cans (about 14 ounces each) defatted low sodium beef broth＊
1 can (14½ ounces) no-salt-added tomatoes
2 cups ½-inch unpeeled potato cubes
1½ cups ½-inch green bean slices
1 cup chopped onion
1 cup sliced carrots
½ cup pearl barley
1 tablespoon cider vinegar
2 teaspoons caraway seeds, lightly crushed
2 teaspoons dried marjoram leaves, crushed
2 teaspoons dried thyme leaves, crushed
½ teaspoon salt
½ teaspoon pepper

Coat large saucepan with cooking spray; heat over medium heat. Add beef; cook and stir until browned on all sides. Add beef broth, tomatoes, potatoes, green beans, onion, carrots, barley, vinegar, caraway seeds, marjoram, thyme, salt and pepper; bring to a boil over high heat. Reduce heat to low. Simmer, covered, about 2 hours or until beef is fork-tender, uncovering saucepan during last 30 minutes of cooking.

Makes 4 servings

❋ To defat beef broth, skim fat from surface of broth with spoon. Or, place can of broth in refrigerator at least 2 hours ahead of time. Before using, remove fat that has hardened on surface of broth.

NUTRIENTS PER SERVING:			
Calories	447.3	Niacin (B₃)	10.84 mg
Protein	41.75 g	Potassium	1,556 mg
Carbohydrate	58.93 g	Pyridoxine (B₆)	0.83 mg
Dietary Fiber	8.88 g	Riboflavin (B₂)	0.51 mg
Fat	5.54 g	Sodium	431.8 mg
Saturated Fat	1.37 g	Vitamin A	874.6 RE
Poly Fat	0.59 g	Vitamin C	48.86 mg
Mono Fat	1.46 g	Vitamin K	41.36 µg
Cholesterol	76.04 mg	Zinc	5.45 mg
Sugar	6.41 g		
Beta-Carotene	5,242 RE	DIETARY EXCHANGES:	
Calcium	130.1 mg	Veg: 2	Bread: 3
Cobalamin (B₁₂)	2.29 µg	Meat: 3.5	
Folate	64.48 µg		
Iron	7.91 mg	% OF CALORIES FROM:	
Magnesium	104.7 mg	PRO: 37%	CARB: 52%
		FAT: 11%	

BEANS AND PEAS, DRY

If you had to pick one food to be stuck on a desert island with, beans would be a good bet. They'd provide you with almost complete nutrition, and you wouldn't have to worry about offending anyone. Yes, beans can be gassy. But there are ways around that. Don't let their "explosive" nature scare you away from some of the best nutrition around.

Health Benefits

Beans are one of your best sources of soluble fiber, even though all the headlines have highlighted oat bran. So, not only are beans low in fat and high in good quality protein, but they have the added bonus of soluble fiber's disease-fighting qualities.

The soluble fiber in beans becomes gummy in your intestines, trapping bile acids. This, in turn, tends to lower your level of damaging LDL cholesterol, especially if it was high to begin with, without lowering your level of protective HDL cholesterol. And by slowing down carbohydrate absorption, soluble bean fiber fends off unwanted peaks and valleys in your blood-sugar levels.

Beans also provide substansial amounts of insoluble fiber. That's good for combatting constipation and colon cancer.

By centering your diet around beans and other complex carbohydrates, you will automatically be eating a low-fat, high-fiber diet. The chances are good that, if you're overweight, you'll lose weight on such a diet. It helps that beans are satisfying enough to stave off hunger. And check out the bonanza of folic acid, copper, iron, and magnesium. Indeed, dry beans and peas generally are rich sources of iron, and that's good news for people who don't eat meat, especially females.

NUTRIENT INFORMATION
Black Beans, cooked
Serving Size: ½ cup

Calories	113	Thiamin	0.2 mg
Protein	7.6 g	Folic Acid	127.9 µg
Carbohydrate	20.4 g	Copper	0.2 mg
Fat	0.5 g	Iron	1.8 mg
Saturated	0.1 g	Magnesium	60 mg
Cholesterol	0	Manganese	0.4 mg
Dietary Fiber	6.1 g	Phosphorus	120 mg
Sodium	1 mg	Potassium	306 mg

There are lots of different kinds of beans, but their nutritional content is very similar to the black beans we've highlighted here. (Soybeans are in a class by themselves, however; see Tofu for more on them.) Exceptions? White beans have almost twice the iron of black beans, while kidney beans are somewhere in between. And fiber does vary (see "Fiber Content of Selected Dry Beans and Peas"). But most differences are minor.

FIBER CONTENT OF SELECTED DRY BEANS AND PEAS	
(per ½ cup serving, cooked)	Grams
Kidney beans	6.9
Butter beans	6.9
Navy beans	6.5
Black beans	6.1
Pinto beans	5.9
Broad (fava) beans	5.1
Great Northern white beans	5.0
Black-eyed peas	4.7
Chickpeas (garbanzos)	4.3
Mung beans	3.3
Split peas	3.1

Selection and Storage

Dry beans are available year-round, are inexpensive, and can be found in any well-stocked supermarket. Check the ethnic section. You may need to visit a health food store for more exotic varieties.

If you buy your beans packaged, you'll want bags that are strong and well-sealed, with no punctures. See if the beans inside look clean, not shriveled, and are uniformly sized with an even color and uncracked hulls. If you buy beans loose, sift through them, looking for these same features. Discard beans with pinholes, a sign of insect infestation.

If stored properly, beans will last for a year or more. Keep them in their unopened bag. Once open, store them in a dry, tightly closed glass jar in a cool, dark spot.

Some varieties of beans are available canned. They offer convenience—they only need heating—but are rather mushy and very salty.

Preparation and Serving Tips

When cooking with beans, it's best to plan ahead. They do not qualify as fast food. Before soaking or cooking, sort through the beans, discarding bad beans, pebbles, and debris. Then rinse the beans in cold water. It's best to soak your beans overnight, for six to eight hours. They'll cook faster and you'll get rid of gas-producing carbohydrates. But if you haven't planned far enough ahead, you can quick-soak for one hour. Quick-soak by putting the beans in water and boiling for one minute; then turn off the heat and let the beans stand in the same water for one hour. You'll end up with a less-firm bean, however.

If flatulence is still a problem after using the above techniques, then try this method suggested by the U.S. Department of Agriculture: Pour boiling water over the beans and let them soak for four to eight hours before cooking. (If all else fails, you might try Beano, a product which purports to eliminate the gas problem; just add a few drops to your first bite of food.) In addition, to help combat the gas problem, be sure to let your body get used to eating beans. Start slowly, eating only small amounts at first. Also, eat beans when you know you'll be active; it helps break up the gas.

After soaking, discard any beans that float to the top, then throw out the soaking water and add fresh water to cook in. Add enough water to cover the beans plus two inches. Bring to a boil, then simmer, covered, until tender—about one to three hours, depending on the bean variety. The beans are done cooking when you can easily stick them with a fork. Remember, cooked beans double or triple in volume; keep that in mind when choosing and filling your cooking pot.

Beans are notoriously bland-tasting, but that's what makes them versatile. They can take on the spices of any ethnic cuisine. Many other cultures have perfected the art of combining beans with grains or seeds to provide a complete protein. For instance, try Mexican corn tortillas with beans and tomatoes, or classic Spanish rice and beans, or traditional Italian pasta e fagioli (a pasta and bean soup). As an occasional treat, there's hummus, a popular Middle Eastern dip made from chickpeas, olive oil, and tahini, which is a sesame-seed paste; it's high in fat, but tasty. Try black beans in soup.

MARINATED BEAN AND VEGETABLE SALAD

- ¼ **cup orange juice**
- 3 **tablespoons white wine vinegar**
- 1 **tablespoon canola *or* vegetable oil**
- 2 **cloves garlic, minced**
- 1 **can (15 ounces) Great Northern beans, rinsed, drained**
- 1 **can (15 ounces) kidney beans, rinsed, drained**
- ¼ **cup coarsely chopped red cabbage**
- ¼ **cup chopped red onion**
- ¼ **cup chopped green bell pepper**
- ¼ **cup chopped red bell pepper**
- ¼ **cup sliced celery**

For dressing, combine orange juice, vinegar, oil and garlic in small jar with tight-fitting lid; shake well.

Combine Great Northern beans, kidney beans, cabbage, onion, bell peppers and celery in large bowl. Pour dressing over bean mixture; toss to coat.

Refrigerate, covered, 1 to 2 hours to allow flavors to blend. Toss before serving.   *Makes 8 servings*

NUTRIENTS PER SERVING:			
Calories	136	Iron	1.96 mg
Protein	7.39 g	Magnesium	32.94 mg
Carbohydrate	22.88 g	Niacin (B_3)	0.69 mg
Dietary Fiber	3.13 g	Potassium	394.2 mg
Fat	2.18 g	Sodium	180 mg
Saturated Fat	0.45 g	Vitamin C	20.83 mg
Poly Fat	1.26 g		
Mono Fat	1.75 g	DIETARY EXCHANGES:	
Cholesterol	0 mg	Veg: 1.5	Bread: 1
Sugar	2.21 g	Fat: 0.5	
Beta-Carotene	20.26 RE		
Calcium	51.06 mg	% OF CALORIES FROM:	
Copper	0.23 mg	PRO: 21%	CARB: 65%
Folate	60.5 µg	FAT: 14%	

BEEF, LEAN

You may think including beef in a book on healthy foods is a mistake, but we assure you it's not. Yes, beef can be high in fat. But you'll notice we specify lean beef. So unless you're a vegetarian, read on.

The trick is in choosing the right cut and grade, trimming visible fat, preparing it without adding fat, and eating only small amounts. Forget the half-pound steaks; three ounces of beef is enough. For visual aid, that's about the size of your palm or a deck of playing cards. That won't seem so paltry if you think of your meat as a side dish to accompany your main dish of grains or beans. Make meat more of a condiment and less the whole show.

Health Benefits

Beef shouldn't be revered so much for its protein; you can get that elsewhere. But beef is the most nutrient-dense source of iron and zinc—problem minerals for many Americans. While it is possible to get enough iron or zinc without eating meat, it's not easy. Eating lean meat is also a dandy way to get vitamin B12, niacin, and riboflavin. So, small amounts of lean beef in your diet can be nutritionally uplifting.

The iron in beef carries a double bonus. About half the iron in beef is heme iron, a highly usable form found only in animal products. And the absorption of the nonheme iron in meat is enhanced by the fact that it's in meat. Eating meat also enhances the absorption of nonheme iron from plant foods. The zinc in meat is absorbed better than the zinc in grains and legumes, as well.

You need iron, of course, to make red blood cells. Without it, you'd become anemic and listless. Zinc is crucial for a smooth-running immune system that fights infection. And cutting-edge research is exploring how niacin may protect against the cellular damage that often precedes cancer.

NUTRIENT INFORMATION Eye of Round, roasted (Choice, trimmed)			
Serving Size: 3 oz (4 oz uncooked)		Sodium	53 mg
Calories	143	Niacin	3.2 mg
Protein	24.6 g	Vitamin B12	1.8 µg
Carbohydrate	0		
Fat	4.2 g	Iron	1.7 mg
Saturated	1.5 g	Phosphorus	192 mg
Cholesterol	59 mg	Potassium	336 mg
Dietary Fiber	0	Zinc	4 mg

Selection and Storage

Here's where we get down to business: selecting a cut and grade of beef. First, stick to U.S. Department of Agriculture (USDA) grade Choice or Select. They have the least marbling of fat throughout the meat. Prime grade does indeed melt in your mouth, but that's only because it is well-marbled with fat, which makes it so tender.

Next, choose from what's known as the "skinny six" cuts— eye of round, top round, sirloin, bottom round, top loin, and tenderloin—in order of fat content, from least to most. Even the tenderloin is surprisingly low in calories and fat. The fat and calories for the other four cuts are in between eye of round and tenderloin. Bottom line? If you choose from these cuts—or anything with round or loin in its name—you're off to a lean start.

If you visit your neighborhood butcher shop, they'll be glad to sell you ground round. It's the leanest ground beef you'll find; leaner than the "extra-lean" ground sirloin in supermarkets. Whatever you do, avoid regular ground chuck; it contains as much as 20 grams of fat in a three-ounce serving.

No matter what cut, choose meat that looks evenly red and not dried out. If it's turning brown, it's not fresh. Refrigerate all meat as soon as you get home. Place it on a plate so that the drippings won't contaminate other foods. If you don't plan to cook the meat within three to four days (one to two days for ground meat), freeze it.

It's best to freeze meat in heavy-duty freezer paper wrapped airtight to prevent freezer burn. But try not to handle meat much before freezing; this only adds to the bacteria population. Organisms don't grow in the freezer, but they don't die either; they hang around and start growing again once the meat is defrosted.

Preparation and Serving Tips

Defrost meat in the refrigerator, in the microwave, or sitting in cold water you change every hour. Never let it sit out at room temperature, which just invites bacteria to multiply.

Choose your cooking method to match your cut of beef. Lean cuts do better with a method that includes a liquid, such as braising or stewing. Grilling will work as long as you don't overcook the meat. But keep in mind the new cooking recommendation issued to help prevent food-borne illness from contaminated meat: Cook ground meat until the center is no longer pink and juices run clear.

Trim all visible fat from the meat before cooking. If you cannot buy ground meat as lean as you like, you can halve the fat by pouring boiling water over your cooked ground meat. Unfortunately, you do lose flavor in the process. But you can make up for that by using more seasonings.

To tenderize tough cuts, try marinating; it also adds zing to the flavor. Or do it the old-fashioned way and pound your meat with a mallet to break down the connective tissue.

To cut down on the amount of meat you eat at a meal, try dishes such as stir-fry that use lots of vegetables and just a little meat. Or use similar proportions of vegetables to meat in tortillas, taco shells, and pita bread. Experiment with salads that use beef almost as a garnish, or try kebabs loaded with veggies and just a chunk or two of beef.

STEAK FRITE

- 1 **pound boneless beef eye of round steak, trimmed**
- 2 **medium cloves garlic, minced**
- 1 **teaspoon salt, divided**
- ½ **teaspoon pepper, divided**
- 4 **medium Idaho potatoes**
  Nonstick cooking spray
- ½ **teaspoon paprika**
- ¼ **cup thinly sliced shallots or sweet onions**

Pound beef with meat mallet until ½ inch thick. Rub both sides with garlic, ½ teaspoon salt and ¼ teaspoon pepper. Place in glass baking dish; refrigerate, covered, 20 to 30 minutes.

Preheat oven to 400°F. Cut potatoes lengthwise into ¼-inch-thick slices; then cut slices lengthwise into ¼-inch-wide sticks. Arrange potatoes in a single layer in jelly-roll pan. Spray generously with cooking spray; sprinkle with paprika and toss to coat.

Bake about 25 minutes or until potatoes are lightly browned and crisp, turning 1 or 2 times during baking. Sprinkle with remaining ½ teaspoon salt and ¼ teaspoon pepper.

Coat medium skillet with cooking spray; heat over medium heat. Add shallots. Cook and stir shallots about 3 minutes or until tender. Remove shallots; set aside until ready to serve. Add beef to skillet; cook over medium to medium-high heat to desired degree of doneness, about 5 minutes on each side for medium. Serve with shallots and potatoes.

Makes 4 servings

NUTRIENTS PER SERVING:			
Calories	331.9	Iron	3.05 mg
Protein	36.29 g	Magnesium	73.16 mg
Carbohydrate	36.09 g	Niacin (B₃)	6.51 mg
Dietary Fiber	3.84 g	Potassium	1,107 mg
Fat	4.18 g	Pyridoxine (B₆)	0.95 mg
Saturated Fat	1.49 g	Sodium	613.4 mg
Poly Fat	0.23 g	Zinc	5.9 mg
Mono Fat	1.69 g		
Cholesterol	78.71 mg	DIETARY EXCHANGES:	
Sugar	2.99 g	Bread: 2	Meat: 3.5
Beta-Carotene	845.4 RE		
Calcium	24.88 mg	% OF CALORIES FROM:	
Cobalamin (B₁₂)	2.46 µg	PRO: 44%	CARB: 44%
Folate	25.72 µg	FAT: 12%	

BEET GREENS

Like most greens, beet greens are a powerhouse of nutrients. It's too bad, then, that more people don't partake of their pleasures. In Roman times, the greens were eaten and the beets themselves were tossed or used for medicinal purposes. Today, we often do the opposite. Nutritionally, that makes little sense, since beet greens offer, by far, more nutrients. So why not get in the habit of eating both? We'll start at the top and discuss beet greens here, then work our way down to the root of the beet in the next profile.

Health Benefits

The vitamin A in beet greens, as in other greens, is enough to knock your socks off. It comes mostly from beta-carotene and its carotene cousins, the anticancer antioxidants. Vitamin C, another antioxidant, is present in an admirable quantity as well. Together, these antioxidants do more than help to reduce the risk of cancer; they also help to combat cataracts and heart disease. Potassium is especially plentiful in this vegetable—good news for anyone trying to avoid high blood pressure. And this is one more respectable source of calcium, for anyone who does not, or cannot, eat dairy products.

NUTRIENT INFORMATION			
Beet greens, cooked			
Serving Size: ½ cup		Vitamin A	3,672 IU
		Vitamin C	17.9 mg
Calories	20	Riboflavin	0.2 mg
Protein	1.9 g		
Carbohydrate	3.9 g	Calcium	82 mg
Fat	0.1 g	Copper	0.2 mg
Saturated	0	Iron	1.4 mg
Cholesterol	0	Magnesium	49 mg
Dietary Fiber	0.7 g	Potassium	654 mg
Sodium	173 mg		

Selection and Storage

You're most likely to find beets with their greens attached in early summer—the beginning of beet season. The green tops should look fresh—crisp, not limp, and dark green, not yellow. Look for smallish leaves for the best flavor.

Snip off the greens from the beets once you get home, and refrigerate them in a plastic bag. They'll only keep for about a day or two before they're too wilted to use. You may be able to perk them up with a brief bath in ice-cold water.

Preparation and Serving Tips

Wash the greens to remove any sand. To cook, you can boil beet greens, but steaming will preserve more nutrients. Just don't overcook them. Add lemon juice and herbs.

Beet greens are also a popular addition to any soup. They add flavor while boosting the nutritional value. You can even make a soup with just beet greens as the main ingredient, as you would kale or broccoli. Don't add much extra salt, though. Beet greens are naturally high in sodium.

For a change, try eating fresh, raw beet greens. They can be combined with other greens for a tasty, nutritious salad. When used this way, stick to greens from young beets in the spring.

Lemon Garlic Greens

1½   **pounds beet greens**
  2   **teaspoons olive *or* canola oil**
  ¼   **cup finely chopped onion**
  3   **cloves garlic, minced**
  2   **tablespoons lemon juice**
  ¼   **teaspoon salt**
  ¼   **teaspoon pepper**

Wash beet greens. Drain but do not pat dry; leave some water clinging to leaves. Remove stems; coarsely chop.

Heat oil in large saucepan over medium heat. Add beet greens, onion and garlic; cook and stir 5 minutes. Stir in lemon juice, salt and pepper; continue cooking about 5 minutes or until greens are wilted and onion is tender. Serve warm.   *Makes 4 servings*

NUTRIENTS PER SERVING:			
Calories	75.2	Iron	3.35 mg
Protein	4.68 g	Magnesium	117.9 mg
Carbohydrate	11.64 g	Potassium	1,581 mg
Dietary Fiber	5.43 g	Sodium	543.5 mg
Fat	2.62 g	Vitamin C	47.36 mg
Saturated Fat	0.38 g	Vitamin E	3.40 mg
Poly Fat	0.32 g		
Mono Fat	1.72 g	DIETARY EXCHANGES:	
Cholesterol	0 mg	Veg: 2	Fat: 0.5
Sugar	0.47 g		
Beta-Carotene	863.2 RE	% OF CALORIES FROM:	
Calcium	201.6 mg	PRO: 21%	CARB: 52%
Folate	27.26 µg	FAT: 27%	

BEETS

Beets have only been appreciated as a root vegetable in modern times. In years past, they were valued more for supposed medicinal powers than for their sugary sweet taste. It was beet greens that were prized for eating. Maybe, back then, people were put off by the red urine and red stools that can appear for a few days after eating beets. Some of us inherit an inability to break down the red pigment in beets, and it passes right through the body. It's harmless enough, but you may want to lay off the beets a few days before your next doctor visit.

Health Benefits

Beets are particularly rich in folic acid, essential for preventing some anemias and neural-tube birth defects. Folic acid may even be of help in preventing cervical cancer. Beets also contain a wealth of fiber—about half soluble and half insoluble. That helps keep your intestinal tract running smoothly and your blood-sugar and blood-cholesterol levels on track, too.

```
NUTRIENT INFORMATION
Beets, fresh, cooked
Serving Size: 2 beets
```

Calories	31	Folic Acid	53.2 µg
Protein	1.1 g		
Carbohydrate	6.7 g	Magnesium	37 mg
Fat	0.1 g	Manganese	0.2 mg
Saturated	0	Potassium	312 mg
Cholesterol	0		
Dietary Fiber	2.6 g		
Sodium	49 mg		

Selection and Storage

Beets are in stores year-round, but their peak season is June through October. Your best bet is to choose small, firm beets that are well-rounded and uniformly sized for even cooking.

The skin should be deep red, smooth, and unblemished. A clue to tenderness is a thin taproot, the root that extends from the bulb of the beet. The freshest beets are those with bright, crisp greens.

Once home, immediately cut off the greens, because they suck moisture from the beet. Leave two inches of stem to prevent the beet from "bleeding" when it's cooked; don't trim the taproot. It's not essential to refrigerate beets, if they're kept in a cool spot. Refrigerated, they'll keep for a week or two.

Preparation and Serving Tips

Wash fresh beets gently, so you won't break the skin and allow color and nutrients to escape. Peel beets after they're cooked. Microwaving retains the most nutrients. Steaming is OK but takes 25 to 45 minutes. The beets are done when a fork easily pierces the skin. Beware beets' powerful pigment; it stains utensils and wooden cutting boards.

Beets have a succulent sweetness because, unlike most vegetables, they contain more sugar than starch. It makes them particularly well suited to being served cold, warm, or at room temperature. Cooked beets don't need fancy sauces to taste good; a little margarine, salt, and pepper is enough.

Canned beets will do in a pinch; they're more similar to fresh than most vegetables, because the sweetness hides the canned taste. Pickled beets can be homemade or bought ready-to-serve. Borscht, or beet soup, is an old-time favorite that's served cold.

SAVORY BAKED BEETS

- 1 **pound small beets, trimmed**
- 1 **large red onion, cut into 12 wedges**
- ¼ **cup balsamic vinegar**
- 2 **teaspoons olive** or **canola oil**
- 4 **cloves garlic, minced**
- 1 **tablespoon caraway seeds**

¼ **teaspoon salt**
¼ **teaspoon pepper**
1 **tablespoon minced parsley**

Preheat oven to 350°F. Bring 1½ quarts water and beets to a boil in large saucepan. Reduce heat to low. Simmer, covered, 15 minutes; drain. Peel beets; cut into halves.

Arrange beets and onion wedges on jelly-roll pan. Combine vinegar, oil, garlic, caraway seeds, salt and pepper in small bowl. Brush half of mixture on vegetables.

Bake 35 minutes or until vegetables are fork-tender, basting 2 times with remaining vinegar mixture during baking. Transfer to serving bowl; sprinkle with parsley. *Makes 6 servings*

NUTRIENTS PER SERVING:			
Calories	63.53	Magnesium	19.69 mg
Protein	1.46 g	Manganese	0.28 mg
Carbohydrate	11.21 g	Niacin (B₃)	0.31 mg
Dietary Fiber	2.16 g	Potassium	251 mg
Fat	1.79 g	Sodium	130.2 mg
Saturated Fat	0.24 g	Vitamin C	10.47 mg
Poly Fat	0.21 g		
Mono Fat	1.2 g	DIETARY EXCHANGES:	
Cholesterol	0 mg	Veg: 2	
Sugar	0.73 g		
Beta-Carotene	29.63 RE	% OF CALORIES FROM:	
Calcium	26.26 mg	PRO: 9%	CARB: 67%
Folate	55.41 µg	FAT: 24%	

BLACKBERRIES

Summertime in the country—anyone who's experienced it surely knows the joys of picking berries off brambles in the hot sun. And blackberries are as big as berries get.

Health Benefits

What a treasure trove of fiber you get from a bowl of blackberries. You can't get much better than this for a source of dietary fiber and also have it taste so good. Two-thirds of the fiber in blackberries is insoluble, the kind that keeps your digestive tract running smoothly. Much of the rest is pectin, a soluble fiber. The more tart the berry, the more pectin it contains. And that's good for keeping you full on just a few calories—in other words, blackberries are the perfect diet food. Pectin and other soluble fibers help keep blood-sugar levels on an even keel, too, which is especially helpful to diabetics.

NUTRIENT INFORMATION			
Blackberries, fresh			
Serving Size: ¾ cup			
Calories	56	Vitamin C	22.7 mg
Protein	0.8 g		
Carbohydrate	13.8 g	Manganese	1.4 mg
Fat	0.4 g	Potassium	211.5 mg
Saturated	0		
Cholesterol	0		
Dietary Fiber	3.7 g		
Sodium	0		

Selection and Storage

Blackberries are often confused with black raspberries or related berry hybrids. For example, the loganberry is a cross between a blackberry and a raspberry. The boysenberry is a cross between a blackberry, a raspberry, and a loganberry. Both are wine-colored and tart.

July and August are the best months for blackberries, although in some parts of the United States, you can find them in May and June. In the Northeast, where they flourish, they're still ripe for picking in September. Try to indulge when in season. Although never truly economical, they are less expensive in summertime.

Look for berries that are glossy, plump, deep-colored, firm, and well-rounded. The darker the berry, the riper and sweeter it is. As berries overripen and lose their moisture, they become dull and less plump. Avoid baskets of berries that have juice all over the bottom. It's a sure sign some of the berries have been crushed.

Refrigerate, but do not wash, blackberries until you're ready to eat them, or they'll get moldy. Use within a day; they do not store well. You can freeze them, however. Do it in single layers, then stack the berries, once frozen. If you like, layer sugar in between.

Preparation and Serving Tips

Do not overhandle blackberries; otherwise, their cells will break open, causing loss of juice and destruction of nutrients. Wash them under gently running water, then drain them well and pick through them to remove stems and too-soft berries.

Who can resist a simple bowlful of fresh berries, sprinkled with a little sugar if tart, and maybe splashed with milk?

Blackberries also make divine desserts, especially when paired with raspberries or apples. Or serve them over sorbet. And, of course, there's blackberry jam and pie. Both the loganberry and boysenberry hybrids make excellent pies, jams, and jellies.

BLACKBERRY STRUDEL CUPS

- 6 sheets frozen phyllo dough, thawed
  Nonstick cooking spray
- 1 pint blackberries
- 2 tablespoons sugar
- 1 cup thawed frozen reduced fat nondairy whipped topping
- 1 container (6 ounces) custard-style apricot *or* peach low fat yogurt
  Mint sprigs for garnish

Preheat oven to 400°F. Cut phyllo dough crosswise into 4 pieces. Coat 1 piece lightly with cooking spray; place in large custard cup. Coat remaining 3 pieces lightly with cooking spray; place over first piece, alternating corners. Repeat with remaining phyllo dough to form 6 strudel cups. Place custard cups on cookie sheet; bake about 15 minutes or until pastry is golden. Let cool to room temperature.

Meanwhile, combine blackberries and sugar in small bowl; let stand 15 minutes. Mix whipped topping and yogurt in medium bowl. Reserve ½ cup blackberries for garnish; gently stir remaining blackberries into whipped topping mixture. Spoon into cooled pastry cups. Garnish with reserved blackberries and mint sprigs.   ***Makes 6 servings***

NUTRIENTS PER SERVING:		Calcium	54.59 mg
Calories	125.3	Folate	19.57 µg
Protein	2.84 g	Manganese	0.62 mg
Carbohydrate	24.65 g	Sodium	21.78 mg
Dietary Fiber	2.98 g		
Fat	3.52 g	DIETARY EXCHANGES:	
Saturated Fat	0.25 g	Fruit: 1.5	Fat: 1
Poly Fat	0.11 g		
Mono Fat	0.15 g	% OF CALORIES FROM:	
Cholesterol	2.76 mg	PRO: 8%	CARB:
Sugar	8.73 g	70%	
Beta-Carotene	47.62 RE	Fat: 22%	

BLUEBERRIES

Blueberries are the king of fruits in Maine, where tiny, tart, wild blueberries are legend. The wild version looks more like the huckleberry than the cultivated blueberry most of us see in the stores (although the huckleberry has larger seeds and is even more tart). The one we're all familiar with is big, plump, firm, juicy, and sweet. Americans are loyal to their native son, the blueberry, especially for baking.

Health Benefits

Blueberries can't boast the nutrients other fruits can. But they provide more than their fair share of vitamin C, manganese, and fiber, most of which is insoluble, the intestinal-tract hero. So tossing some blueberries on your cereal every morning in the summer will boost the effectiveness of that bran. The manganese helps keep bones strong, while the vitamin C is a natural antioxidant and immune-system booster.

Selection and Storage

The good news is that blueberries have a longer season than other berries. You'll find them in stores from late May to October, with the best of the crop appearing in the middle of summer.

Look for plump, very firm, juicy-looking berries. The color should be dark purplish-blue underneath, covered with a whitish "bloom" that gives it a powdery appearance. This is a natural protective coating and should not be washed off until you're ready to eat them. Beware of packages that have a lot of moisture under the plastic wrap; the berries on the bottom may be moldy.

Pick through the berries when you get them home, discarding any that are moldy, crushed, shriveled, or soft, and pulling off stems. Refrigerate them right away, in a dry, covered, nonmetal container, without washing first. They'll keep at least a week—three to four times longer than other berries. You can freeze them in single layers on cookie sheets. Once frozen, transfer to a covered container or plastic bag. They'll keep for a few weeks, even months if your freezer is below zero degrees Fahrenheit. They won't be as firm after defrosting.

NUTRIENT INFORMATION Blueberries, fresh Serving Size: ¾ cup			
Calories	62	Dietary Fiber	1.4 g
Protein	0.7 g	Sodium	7 mg
Carbohydrate	15.4 g		
Fat	0.4 g	Vitamin C	14.2 mg
Saturated	0		
Cholesterol	0	Manganese	0.3 mg

Preparation and Serving Tips

Wash blueberries thoroughly just before using. Enjoy them by the bowlful, plain or in milk, for breakfast or dessert. If not sweet enough, add a sprinkle of sugar. Blueberries are ideal on cereal and in pancakes.

Blueberries are an American favorite in baking. Muffins, bread, coffee cakes, pies, cobbler—you name it, you can put blueberries in it. They're even good in jams—a flavor you won't find at your local supermarket. For jam, combine three parts berries to one part sugar, and cook gently for ten minutes.

BLUEBERRY PANCAKES WITH BLUEBERRY SPICE SYRUP

    1   cup all-purpose flour
    2   tablespoons sugar
    2   teaspoons baking powder
    ¼   teaspoon salt
    ¾   cup skim milk
    2   egg whites
    1   tablespoon margarine, melted
    ½   cup blueberries
        Blueberry-Spice Syrup (recipe follows)
        Nonstick cooking spray

Combine flour, sugar, baking powder and salt in medium bowl. Beat milk and egg whites in small bowl; stir in margarine. Add milk mixture to flour mixture, stirring until almost smooth. Gently fold in blueberries. Prepare Blueberry-Spice Syrup; set aside.

Coat large nonstick skillet with cooking spray. Heat over medium heat until water droplets sprinkled on skillet bounce off surface. Drop batter by ¼ cupfuls into skillet. Cook 2 to 3 minutes until bubbles appear at edges and bottoms of pancakes are lightly browned. Turn pancakes; cook until bottoms of pancakes are lightly browned. Serve with Blueberry-Spice Syrup.

Makes 4 servings

BLUEBERRY-SPICE SYRUP

- ½ **cup blueberries, divided**
- ½ **cup maple syrup, divided**
- ½ **teaspoon grated lemon peel**
- ½ **teaspoon ground cinnamon**
- ¼ **teaspoon ground nutmeg**

Bring ¼ cup blueberries and ¼ cup syrup to a boil in small saucepan over medium heat. Mash hot berries with fork. Add remaining ¼ cup blueberries and ¼ cup syrup, lemon peel, cinnamon and nutmeg. Cook and stir over medium heat about 2 minutes or until heated through. ***Makes 1 cup.***

NUTRIENTS PER SERVING:			
Calories	306.6	Potassium	239.4 mg
Protein	6.85 g	Riboflavin (B₂)	0.34 mg
Carbohydrate	63.09 g	Sodium	388.5 mg
Dietary Fiber	1.68 g	Vitamin A	66.6 RE
Fat	3.41 g	Vitamin C	5.58 mg
Saturated Fat	0.71 g		
Poly Fat	1.1 g	DIETARY EXCHANGES:	
Mono Fat	1.35 g	Fruit: 3.5	Bread: 1
Cholesterol	0.75 mg	Fat: 0.5	
Sugar	11.02 g		
Calcium	139.2 mg	% OF CALORIES FROM:	
Magnesium	19.77 mg	PRO: 9%	CARB: 81%
Manganese	0.37 mg	FAT: 10%	

BREAD, WHOLE-WHEAT

Just because your bread is brown doesn't mean it's whole wheat. And just because the label proudly boasts it is "wheat" bread and lists "wheat flour" as the first ingredient doesn't mean it's whole wheat, either.

"Wheat" refers to the grain the flour comes from. Anything made with the flour from wheat can be called "wheat" and can list "wheat flour" as an ingredient, even refined white flour. (The brown color often comes from caramel coloring.) Is this lying? No. Is it misleading? Yes, we think so. Now that you know the score, you won't be misled anymore.

Health Benefits

Whole-wheat bread is good for you for a number of reasons. It's high in complex carbohydrates, low in fat, adequate in protein, and a storehouse of nutrients and fiber—an exact microcosm of what your diet should be.

To understand what's so special about whole wheat, you need to understand the structure of wheat grain. There are three basic layers of the grain—the endosperm, the germ, and the bran. When whole-wheat flour is milled (refined) to make white bread, the germ and outer bran layer are removed, leaving only the inner endosperm.

Unfortunately, more than half the fiber is in the bran and germ, along with almost three-quarters of the vitamins and minerals. Besides nutrients, the milling process also removes nonnutrient components, such as phytoestrogens, phenolic acids, oryzanol, and tannins, that may have health benefits, including reducing the risk of cancer.

Enriched bread products add back some B vitamins—thiamin, riboflavin, and niacin—and iron. But lots of other nutrients, especially minerals, don't get added back. And that includes fiber. So if you eat white bread, you're definitely missing a fiber opportunity. (See Fiber in Part I for more on its benefits.) One of fiber's benefits is its role in weight loss.

Sadly, a lot of people still think bread is fattening. Not so. In fact, studies have proven that people who eat 8 to 12 slices of bread a day still lose weight as long as their total diet is low in fat and calories. That's the trick—keeping yourself from slathering that hearty bread with butter or margarine.

Selection and Storage

The key to buying whole-wheat bread is to be sure it clearly says "100% whole wheat." Without the word "whole," you're not getting all the goodness of the bran and germ of the wheat berry.

What about whole-grain or multigrain breads? They sound and look healthy, but refined wheat (in other words, white) flour still may be the primary ingredient. Your only defense is to carefully read labels. If you want 100 percent whole wheat, then whole wheat should be the only grain listed.

If you like the taste of multigrain breads, pick one that lists whole wheat first in the list of ingredients. That way, you know it's the predominant grain. And check the fiber content.

Cracked-wheat breads are not always 100 percent whole cracked wheat. Again, check bread labels carefully.

NUTRIENT INFORMATION Whole-wheat bread Serving Size: 1 slice			
Calories	61	Thiamin	0.1 mg
Protein	2.4 g	Niacin	1 mg
Carbohydrate	11.4 g		
Fat	1.1 g	Chromium	14 µg
Saturated	na	Copper	0.1 mg
Cholesterol	0	Iron	0.9 mg
Dietary Fiber	1.6 g	Magnesium	23 mg
Sodium	159	Manganese	0.6 mg

Pumpernickel bread looks hearty but is really just a form of rye bread with caramel or molasses added. Both rye and pumpernickel breads are usually made from refined rye flour that has had the bran and germ removed, because 100 percent rye bread is very dense. If you can find it, look for rye bread made from "unbolted" rye and whole wheat.

After comparing ingredient labels, check the expiration date of the bread you buy. Whole-wheat breads may not have preservatives added. To prevent your bread from going stale, leave out at room temperature only as much as you'll eat in the next day or two; keep it tightly closed in a plastic bag. Freeze the rest. It defrosts quickly at room temperature if you take out one or two slices as you need them. Or you can put one slice in the microwave on the defrost cycle for about 30 seconds, two slices for 40 seconds, or four slices for a minute. But don't refrigerate your bread—it only goes stale faster.

Mold on bread usually starts as a whitish bloom. If you see it, throw the bread out. You can't salvage bread that is moldy, because mold spores spread quickly throughout soft foods. Do not even smell inside the bag, as you can inhale mold spores. In fact, you should throw away all the bread that's in the wrapper, as well as the bag itself.

Preparation and Serving Tips

Of course, you don't have to resort to stalking the aisles, investigating ingredient labels, for the perfect loaf of bread. You can make it yourself. Nothing could be fresher or taste better. Not knowing how to bake bread or not having the time are no longer excuses if you have one of the new bread-making machines. And you get to use just the ingredients you want. Look for whole-wheat bread flour, which contains more gluten, for perfect rising. Add nonfat dry milk powder for more protein and calcium. Add wheat germ for extra fiber plus a hefty dose of nutrients.

Try using a hearty whole-wheat bread next time you make French toast—a great way to get the goodness of eggs without overdoing it. If you cook on a nonstick skillet, you don't have to add any fat. Then top with reduced-sugar syrup or fresh fruit or jam.

If your bread is stale, use it for toast, crush it for bread crumbs on top of a casserole, or make your own croutons to enjoy on salads.

WHOLE WHEAT FOCACCIA

1   teaspoon olive oil
1   cup chopped onion
3   cloves garlic, chopped
¼   cup chopped red bell pepper
½   teaspoon paprika
2   teaspoons canola *or* vegetable oil
2   cups whole-wheat flour
½   cup all-purpose flour, divided
1   package (¼ ounce) quick-rising yeast
½   teaspoon sugar
¼   teaspoon salt
1   cup warm water (105° to 115°F)
2   teaspoons dried oregano leaves, crushed
¼   to ½ teaspoon coarsely ground black pepper

For topping, heat olive oil in large nonstick skillet over medium-low heat. Cook and stir onion, garlic, bell pepper and paprika 5 minutes or until tender. Set aside.

Brush 12-inch pizza pan with canola oil; set aside. Combine wheat flour, 2 tablespoons all-purpose flour, yeast, sugar and salt in large bowl. Stir in warm water until well mixed.

Sprinkle kneading surface with 1 tablespoon all-purpose flour. Turn out dough onto surface; knead 3 minutes or until smooth, adding up to 2 tablespoons all-purpose flour to prevent sticking if necessary. Cover with inverted bowl or clean towel; let stand 10 minutes. Place oven rack in lowest position; preheat oven to 425°F.

Knead dough on lightly floured surface about 3 minutes or until smooth and elastic, adding remaining 3 tablespoons all-purpose flour to prevent sticking if necessary. Roll out dough into 13-inch round; transfer to prepared pan. Crimp edge of dough to form rim.

Spread topping on dough; sprinkle with oregano and black pepper. Bake 15 to 20 minutes or until rim of crust is lightly

browned. Remove from pan; let cool on wire rack 5 minutes
before cutting into wedges.   *Makes 8 servings*

NUTRIENTS PER SERVING:			
Calories	161.6	Folate	56.21 µg
Protein	5.72 g	Magnesium	48.02 mg
Carbohydrate	31.27 g	Niacin (B₃)	2.81 mg
Dietary Fiber	4.75 g	Riboflavin (B₂)	0.16 mg
Fat	2.44 g	Sodium	69.44 mg
Saturated Fat	0.29 g	Vitamin K	18.56 µg
Poly Fat	0.7 g		
Mono Fat	1.17 g	DIETARY EXCHANGES:	
Cholesterol	0 mg	Veg: 0.5	Bread: 2
Sugar	1.51 g		
Beta-Carotene	67.01 RE	% OF CALORIES FROM:	
Calcium	25.14 mg	PRO: 13%	CARB: 74%
		FAT: 13%	

BROCCOLI

This vegetable wins hands down, nutritionally, for vegetable of the year and of the decade—maybe even of all time. Lucky for us so many of us like it. It's now the second most popular vegetable, after potatoes. What's not to like? You can eat it raw or cooked, dressed up or down. Even kids like it.

Health Benefits

You simply can't get a bigger dose of more nutrients eating any other vegetable, especially for so few calories. Particularly noteworthy are its contributions of vitamin C, vitamin A (mostly as beta-carotene), folic acid, calcium, and fiber.

While the calcium content doesn't equal that of milk, for people who don't consume dairy products, broccoli provides a large dose of the mineral that's hard to find elsewhere and is key to preventing osteoporosis.

Beta-carotene and vitamin C are important antioxidants that have been linked to a reduced risk for numerous conditions, including cataracts, heart disease, and several cancers.

Broccoli is a fiber find. Not only is it a rich source, but half of its fiber is insoluble and half is soluble, helping meet your needs for both types of fiber. So it may play a helpful role in preventing constipation, hemorrhoids, diverticular disease, and colon cancer, as well as diabetes, heart disease, and obesity.

Besides the exhaustive list of nutrients shown here, experts also cite broccoli as a good source of chromium, a little-appreciated mineral we may not get enough of. Reliable values, however, are not available to give you.

But the story doesn't end with the rich array of nutrients. Broccoli provides a health bonus in the form of protective substances that may shield you from disease. Botanically, broccoli belongs to the cabbage family, collectively known as cruciferous vegetables. Numerous organizations, including the National Cancer Institute and the American Cancer Society, have singled out cruciferous vegetables, recommending that we include them in our diet several times a week. Why? They seem to be associated with lower rates of cancer, leading researchers to conclude that these vegetables contain some compounds that may help protect against cancer. No one really knows the whole story yet.

NUTRIENT INFORMATION

Broccoli, fresh, cooked		Vitamin A	1,099 IU
Serving Size: ½ cup chopped		Vitamin C	49 mg
Calories	23	Riboflavin	0.2 mg
Protein	2.3 g	Vitamin B6	0.2 mg
Carbohydrate	4.3 g	Folic Acid	53.3 µg
Fat	0.2 g		
Saturated	0	Calcium	89 mg
Cholesterol	0	Iron	0.9 mg
Dietary Fiber	2.4 g	Magnesium	47 mg
Sodium	8 mg	Manganese	0.2 mg

Some light has been shed on broccoli, however. As a cruciferous vegetable, broccoli naturally contains indoles and isothiocyanates—thought to be cancer protectors. Just recently, researchers at the Johns Hopkins University School of Medicine in Baltimore isolated from broccoli an isothiocyanate called sulforaphane, which increases the activity of a group of enzymes that quash carcinogens.

Selection and Storage

Broccoli is available year-round, mostly from California. You'll notice a decline in quality and higher prices in summer, however. It's easy to tell a bunch of fresh broccoli from broccoli past its prime. Look for broccoli that's dark green or even purplish-green, but not yellow (yellowing means it's old). The florets should be compact and of even color. The leaves should not be wilted, and the stalks shouldn't be too fat and woody. The better it looks, the more nutritious it is. This is one vegetable where the greener it is, the more beta-carotene it has.

Be sure you buy broccoli that's kept cold. Some stores like to make a special display of their broccoli, on a stand that's not refrigerated. Steer clear of it, and search out the stash in the back, or ask the produce manager to get you some from cold storage. It'll taste better and contain more nutrients.

Keep broccoli cold at home, too. When not refrigerated, the sugar in broccoli is converted into a fiber called lignin, which is what makes old broccoli taste woody and fibrous. Store broccoli in the crisper drawer, in a plastic bag, but not sealed tight. Do not wash it before storing. Use it within a few days.

Preparation and Serving Tips

Wash broccoli carefully, just before eating or cooking. Cut off part of the stems, if you like; they contain fewer nutrients than the florets anyway. Steaming is the method of cooking that'll preserve the most nutrients.

Preventing broccoli's unpleasant sulfur odor is easy—just don't overcook it. And don't cook it in an aluminum pan. It also helps if you take the cover off the pot, briefly, near the beginning of cooking, to let the smell escape. Steam only until crisp-tender, while the stalks are still bright green. Five minutes is usually long enough. You'll save nutrients that way, too.

Try this trick to get the stems and florets done at the same time: make one or two long cuts up through the stem. This will help the stems cook as fast as the tops.

When serving broccoli, unless you want to undo its natural low-fat, low-calorie image, skip the cheese sauce. Keep it simple, with a squeeze of lemon and a dusting of cracked pepper. Children may find it more to their liking with a sprinkle of Parmesan cheese.

Broccoli florets are perfect for boosting the nutrition, flavor, and color of any stir-fry dish. Broccoli makes wonderful soup; try low-fat cream-of-broccoli. And raw broccoli tossed into salads makes a big nutritional difference.

Broccoli is a great finger food when served raw. Many children love it this way, perhaps because the flavor isn't as strong raw as it is when cooked; maybe just because it's fun. Double the fun by giving them a sauce to dip it in, such as a fat-free ranch dressing.

BROCCOLI ITALIAN STYLE

1¼ **pounds broccoli**
2   **tablespoons lemon juice**
1   **teaspoon olive oil**
1   **clove garlic, minced**
1   **teaspoon chopped parsley**
    Dash pepper

Trim broccoli, removing tough part of stems. Cut into florets with 2-inch stems. Peel remaining broccoli stems; cut into ½-inch-thick slices.

Bring 1 quart water to a boil in large saucepan over high heat. Add broccoli florets; return to a boil. Reduce heat to medium-high. Cook, uncovered, 3 to 5 minutes or until broccoli is fork-tender. Drain; arrange evenly in serving dish.

Combine lemon juice, oil, garlic, parsley and pepper in small bowl. Pour over broccoli, turning to coat. Let stand, covered, 1 to 2 hours before serving to allow flavors to blend.

Makes 4 servings

NUTRIENTS PER SERVING:			
Calories	44.01	Calcium	53.23 mg
Protein	3.37 g	Folate	56.9 µg
Carbohydrate	6.53 g	Sodium	29.07 mg
Dietary Fiber	3.15 g	Vitamin A	155.6 RE
Fat	1.52 g	Vitamin C	86.35 mg
Saturated Fat	0.22 g	Vitamin E	0.79 mg
Poly Fat	0.28 g		
Mono Fat	0.86 g	DIETARY EXCHANGES:	
Cholesterol	0 mg	Veg: 1.5	
Sugar	0.19 g	% OF CALORIES FROM:	
Beta-Carotene	181.6 RE	PRO: 25%	CARB: 49%
		FAT: 26%	

BRUSSELS SPROUTS

No one seems to really know the origin of brussels sprouts, although everyone assumes they originated in Belgium. Today, they are especially popular in England and France, where they are called brussels cabbage. That's a particularly appropriate name, since they look like miniature cabbages and, indeed, belong to the cabbage family.

Health Benefits

Like broccoli and cabbage—fellow cruciferous vegetables—brussels sprouts are thought to protect against cancer, through their indole content. They are particularly rich in the antioxidant vitamin C.

Unlike most vegetables, brussels sprouts are rather high in protein, accounting for more than a quarter of their calories. Although the protein is incomplete—meaning it doesn't provide the full spectrum of essential amino acids—it can easily be complemented with whole grains to make it complete.

NUTRIENT INFORMATION
Brussels sprouts, fresh, cooked
Serving Size: ½ cup

Calories	30	Vitamin A	561 IU
Protein	2 g	Vitamin C	48.4 mg
Carbohydrate	6.8 g	Folic Acid	46.8 µg
Fat	0.4 g		
Saturated	0	Iron	0.9 mg
Cholesterol	0	Manganese	0.2 mg
Dietary Fiber	3.8 g	Potassium	257 mg
Sodium	17 mg		

Selection and Storage

You can find fresh brussels sprouts in the fall and winter, when other produce is not so readily available. Most of it is grown in California and New York. Look for those with a pronounced green color and tight, compact, firm heads. The fewer yellowed, wilted, or loose leaves there are, the better.

As with many fruits and vegetables, you're better off choosing smaller heads; they'll be more tender and flavorful. Pick ones that are the same size for even cooking.

Store sprouts in the refrigerator in the cardboard container in which they're usually sold. Or keep them in a loosely closed plastic bag. They should last a week or two.

Preparation and Serving Tips

Dunk sprouts in ice water to debug them, then rinse under running water. Pull off any loose or wilted leaves; trim the stem end just a little. Cut an "X" in the bottom of the stem, so it will cook as fast as the leaves.

Steaming is your best cooking bet. The sprouts will stay intact, their odor will be minimized, and you'll preserve nutrients.

As with broccoli and cabbage, the odor of brussels sprouts is most pronounced when overcooked. Don't be afraid to leave your sprouts a bit on the crisp side. Too mushy means too strong a flavor. They'll also lose valued vitamin C when over-cooked. So as soon as you can barely prick them with a fork, they're done—anywhere from 7 to 14 minutes, depending on their size. Hint: Take the cover off for just a moment soon after cooking starts to help diminish the sulfur smell.

Brussels sprouts are delicious served plain, with just a squeeze of lemon. Or try a full-flavored mustard sauce. When planning meals, remember that sprouts go best with hearty foods like beef and potatoes.

BRUSSELS SPROUTS WITH LEMON-DILL GLAZE

- 1   pound Brussels sprouts
- 2   teaspoons cornstarch
- ½   teaspoon dried dill weed
- ½   cup defatted low sodium chicken broth∗
- 3   tablespoons lemon juice
- ½   teaspoon grated lemon peel

Trim Brussels sprouts. Cut an X in stem ends. Bring 1 cup water to a boil in large saucepan over high heat. Add Brussels sprouts; return to a boil. Reduce heat to medium-low. Simmer,

NUTRIENTS PER SERVING:			
Calories	58.12	Folate	75.66 µg
Protein	3.37 g	Iron	1.59 mg
Carbohydrate	13.13 g	Potassium	410.2 mg
Dietary Fiber	4.82 g	Selenium	10 mg
Fat	0.69 g	Sodium	30.51 mg
Saturated Fat	0.13 g	Vitamin C	82.25 mg
Poly Fat	0.32 g	Vitamin E	1.2 mg
Mono Fat	0.05 g		
Cholesterol	0 mg	DIETARY EXCHANGES:	
Sugar	0.29 g	Veg: 2	
Beta-Carotene	101.4 RE		
		% OF CALORIES FROM:	
		PRO: 19%	CARB: 73%
Calcium	48.81 mg	FAT: 9%	

covered, 10 minutes or until just tender. Drain well; return to pan. Set aside.

Meanwhile, combine cornstarch and dill weed in small saucepan. Blend in chicken broth and lemon juice until smooth. Stir in lemon peel. Cook and stir over medium heat 5 minutes or until mixture boils and thickens. Cook and stir 1 minute more.

Pour glaze over the Brussels sprouts; toss gently to coat. Serve hot. ***Makes 4 servings***

✱ To defat chicken broth, skim fat from surface of broth with spoon. Or, place can of broth in refrigerator at least 2 hours ahead of time. Before using, remove fat that has hardened on surface of broth.

BUCKWHEAT

There's more to buckwheat than flapjacks. Eastern Europeans know roasted buckwheat groats as kasha and eat it like porridge. Despite its name, buckwheat is not a type of wheat—nor is it related to wheat. Buckwheat isn't even a grain; it's the fruit of a plant that's related to rhubarb, and it enjoys some nutritional advantage because of this.

Health Benefits

Buckwheat contains more protein than true grains and is not deficient in the amino acid lysine as most grains are, so the protein in buckwheat is more nutritionally complete. That makes it a particularly good choice for vegetarians. It's an excellent source of magnesium, which can be a boon to your blood pressure. Presumably, it's relatively rich in fiber, but exact values aren't available.

Selection and Storage

Most of our buckwheat comes from New York and carries a premium price, because so few farmers grow it. Look for it in health food stores or mail-order catalogs. In larger cities, check stores in Russian or Slavic neighborhoods.

Buckwheat is sold as groats, grits, or flour. Groats are pale buckwheat kernels without the hard, inedible outer shell. They come whole or cracked into coarse, medium, or fine grinds. Roasted groats—kasha—are dark kernels. Very finely cracked unroasted groats are buckwheat grits. They can be found as a hot cereal, often labeled "cream of buckwheat."

Buckwheat flour is also available, in light and dark versions. The darker type contains more of the hull, therefore more fiber and nutrients and a stronger flavor.

Keep buckwheat in a well-sealed container in a cool, dark location. At room temperature, it is more susceptible to turning rancid than are true grains, especially in warm climates. To avoid this, do not buy it in large quantities. Better yet, keep it in the refrigerator or freezer.

NUTRIENT INFORMATION
Buckwheat groats, roasted,
   cooked (kasha)

Serving Size: ½ cup			
Calories	91	Cholesterol	0
Protein	3.4 g	Dietary Fiber	na
Carbohydrate	19.7 g	Sodium	4 mg
Fat	0.6 g	Iron	0.8 mg
Saturated	0	Magnesium	51 mg

Preparation and Serving Tips

You either like buckwheat or you don't. If you do, take advantage of its intense, nutty flavor. If you don't care for kasha plain, mix it in with pasta, grains, potatoes, or winter vegetables. It makes a hearty meal. For pilafs, stuffing, and soups, use whole kasha. Save the medium and fine grinds for cereals.

To cook: Combine ½ cup whole groats with a cup of water, and simmer for 15 minutes. It will triple in volume. Or combine ½ cup of cracked kasha with 2½ cups of liquid and cook for 12 minutes, to yield 2 cups.

Buckwheat flour is superb for pancakes, but you can't make bread with it because it contains no gluten. But you can add ¼ to ½ cup of buckwheat flour into a bread recipe, as long as the primary grain is wheat or another high-gluten grain.

KASHA AND BOW TIE NOODLES WITH MUSHROOMS AND BROCCOLI

2	cups broccoli florets
2½	cups small bow tie pasta
2	teaspoons olive oil
½	pound fresh mushrooms, sliced ¼ inch thick
½	cup chopped onion
3	cloves garlic, minced
¾	cup uncooked kasha
1	egg
1½	cups defatted low sodium chicken broth✳
1	teaspoon marjoram leaves, crushed
¼	teaspoon black pepper
	Chopped red bell pepper for garnish

Bring 3 quarts water to a boil in large saucepan over high heat. Add broccoli florets; return to a boil. Cook, uncovered, over medium-high heat 2 minutes or until crisp-tender. Remove broccoli to large bowl with slotted spoon, reserving water.

Return water to a boil. Add pasta; return to a boil. Cook, uncovered, over medium-high heat 5 minutes or until just tender. *Do not overcook.* Drain; add pasta to broccoli and mix gently. Set aside.

Wipe saucepan with paper towel. Add oil, mushrooms, onion and garlic to pan; cook and stir 5 minutes or until onion is soft. Stir into broccoli mixture.

Add kasha and egg to saucepan; stir until blended. Cook and stir over medium heat 3 minutes or until kasha is dry and grains separated. Stir in chicken broth, marjoram and black pepper. Bring to a boil over medium-high heat. Reduce heat to low. Cook, covered, 10 minutes, stirring occasionally. Remove from heat; let stand, covered, 10 minutes. Gently mix with bow tie mixture. Garnish each serving with bell pepper.

Makes 4 servings

✱ To defat chicken broth, skim fat from surface of broth with spoon. Or, place can of broth in refrigerator to chill at least 2 hours ahead of time. Before using, remove fat that has hardened on surface of broth.

NUTRIENTS PER SERVING:			
Calories	278.1	Folate	72.69 µg
Protein	11.82 g	Magnesium	103.5 mg
Carbohydrate	47.96 g	Potassium	566.1 mg
Dietary Fiber	4.67 g	Sodium	51.58 mg
Fat	5.93 g	Vitamin K	78.89 µg
Saturated Fat	1.16 g		
Poly Fat	1.08 g	DIETARY EXCHANGES:	
Mono Fat	2.7 g	Veg: 2	Bread: 2.5
Cholesterol	75.75 g	Fat: 1	
Sugar	2.1 g		
Beta-Carotene	415.3 g	% OF CALORIES FROM:	
Calcium	57.61 mg	PRO: 16%	CARB: 66%
		FAT: 18%	

BULGUR

This Middle Eastern staple sounds more exotic than it is. Bulgur is simply a minimally processed form of cracked wheat. The wheat berries are partially cooked before they are cracked. Bulgur resembles rice and is often used like rice.

Health Benefits

Bulgur doesn't lose much from its minimal processing; it's still high in protein and minerals. It's a standout in terms of fiber content, just like whole wheat, and can be a positive factor in keeping your digestive tract healthy as a result. And because it's high in complex carbohydrates, the body digests it slowly, helping to keep your blood-sugar level on an even keel.

```
NUTRIENT INFORMATION
Bulgur, cooked
Serving Size: ½ cup
Calories            76          Dietary Fiber      4.1 g
Protein             2.8 g       Sodium             5 mg
Carbohydrate        16.9 g
Fat                 0.2 g       Iron               0.9 mg
   Saturated        0           Magnesium          29 mg
Cholesterol         0           Manganese          0.6 mg
```

Selection and Storage

You can buy bulgur in three grinds—coarse, medium, and fine. You may need to visit a health food store to find it. If you store bulgur in a screw-top glass jar in the refrigerator, it will keep for months.

Preparation and Serving Tips

One thing that makes bulgur so appealing is that, because it's already been partially cooked, it cooks quickly. And many people find its fluffiness appealing. In fact, you can use bulgur in place of rice for most recipes. You'll get a nutrition bonus if you do.

To cook: Combine ½ cup bulgur with one cup liquid and simmer for 15 minutes. Then let stand for another ten minutes before fluffing with a fork. It will triple in volume.

Bulgur that you plan to use in cold salads must be soaked before using. To soak: Pour boiling water over the bulgur, in a three-to-one ratio. Thirty to forty minutes of soaking time is usually sufficient. Then drain away any excess water. If you like your bulgur chewier, let it sit longer and it will absorb more water.

Coarse bulgur is usually used to make pilaf or stuffing. Medium-grind bulgur is often used in cereals. The finest grind of bulgur is especially suited to the popular cold Middle Eastern salad called tabbouleh. It combines bulgur with parsley, mint, tomato, olive oil, and garlic or onion. It is exceptionally tasty and nutritious, owing to the parsley and bulgur. If you make it yourself, you can cut back on the oil most recipes call for, without making it too dry.

Bulgur lends its nutty flavor to whatever it is combined with. Add leftover vegetables from your refrigerator. Don't forget onions or scallions for a nice bite. Mushrooms work well, as do celery, carrots, zucchini, peas, almost anything. Perhaps one of bulgur's most useful roles is as a meat extender. Mix two cups of cooked bulgur into a pound of ground meat. It will blend in well, without being obvious and without disintegrating into mush. Add some extra liquid if you're using very lean meat.

TABBOULEH

½ cup uncooked bulgur
¾ cup boiling water
¼ teaspoon salt
5 teaspoons lemon juice
2 teaspoons olive oil
½ teaspoon dried basil leaves, crushed
¼ teaspoon black pepper
1 green onion, thinly sliced
½ cup chopped cucumber
½ cup chopped green bell pepper
½ cup chopped tomato
¼ cup chopped parsley
2 teaspoons chopped mint (optional)

Rinse bulgur thoroughly in colander under cold water, picking out any debris. Drain well; transfer to medium heatproof bowl. Stir in boiling water and salt. Cover; let stand 30 minutes. Drain well.

Combine lemon juice, oil, basil and black pepper in small bowl. Pour over bulgur; mix well.

Layer bulgur, onion, cucumber, bell pepper and tomato in clear glass bowl; sprinkle with parsley and mint.

Refrigerate, covered, at least 2 hours to allow flavors to blend. Serve layered or toss before serving.

Makes 8 servings

NUTRIENTS PER SERVING:

Calories	48.82	Calcium	12.67 mg
Protein	1.44 g	Iron	0.56 mg
Carbohydrate	8.73 g	Magnesium	20.29 mg
Dietary Fiber	2.59 g	Manganese	0.31 mg
Fat	1.35 g	Sodium	70.81 mg
Saturated Fat	0.2 g		
Poly Fat	0.18 g	DIETARY EXCHANGES:	
Mono Fat	0.86 g	Veg: 0.5	Bread: 0.5
Cholesterol	0 mg		
Sugar	0.86 g	% OF CALORIES FROM:	
Beta-Carotene	196.4 RE	PRO: 11%	CARB: 66%
		FAT: 23%	

CABBAGE

Cabbage is the head of the cruciferous vegetable family, but it's gotten a bad rap. It's a vegetable few people appreciate. Just identifying the different varieties of cabbage is a challenge. We'll mention the types sold most often in the United States, but there are literally hundreds more.

Health Benefits

If you've already read the broccoli profile, you know the health bonus cruciferous vegetables offer you. If you eat from this family a few times a week, odds are you'll reduce your risk of suffering certain cancers, including colorectal cancers. The phytochemical in cabbage called indole is also being studied for its ability to shunt estradiol (which may play a role in the development of breast cancer) into a safe form of estrogen. That's powerful incentive to add cabbage to your diet.

From cabbage, you'll also enjoy a fiber boost and a respectable amount of vitamin C—all for practically no calories. Two types of cabbage—Savoy and bok choy—provide beta-carotene—more anticancer help. And bok choy makes an important contribution of calcium to the diet, which can help prevent crippling osteoporosis and aid blood-pressure control.

NUTRIENT INFORMATION Green cabbage, fresh, cooked Serving Size: ½ cup chopped		Bok choy, fresh, cooked Serving Size: ½ cup	
		Calories	10
Calories	16	Protein	1.3 g
Protein	0.7 g	Carbohydrate	1.5 g
Carbohydrate	3.6 g	Fat	0.1 g
Fat	0.2 g	Saturated	0
Saturated	0	Cholesterol	0
Cholesterol	0	Dietary Fiber	1 g
Dietary Fiber	2.9 g	Sodium	29 mg
Sodium	5 mg		
		Vitamin A	2,183 IU
Vitamin C	18.2 mg	Vitamin C	22.1 mg
		Calcium	79 mg
		Iron	0.9 mg
		Potassium	315 mg

Selection and Storage

The most popular cabbage in the United States is green cabbage, which is really three varieties: Danish, domestic, and pointed. All three sport the familiar pale green, compact head and are similar nutritionally, shining in fiber. Their cousin is red cabbage, which is best described as purplish red in color. The red variety has a bit more vitamin C than the green types.

More nutritious is Savoy cabbage, a pretty, dark-green, round head that's loose, ruffly, and prominently "veined." As its dark color suggests, it is much higher in beta-carotene than green or red cabbage. Savoy cabbage contains about ten times the vitamin A activity of green cabbage—almost 15 percent of recommended levels.

Napa cabbage, also known as celery cabbage or pe-tsai, is often incorrectly referred to as Chinese cabbage. It is long and slender, like Romaine lettuce, but is very pale green, almost white, with a flavor that's much more delicate than other cabbages. Nutritionally, it's equivalent to green cabbage.

Bok choy, or pak-choi, is true Chinese cabbage and, as far as nutrition is concerned, is the king of cabbages. It has broad, dark-green leaves and a distinct taste. Nutritionally, it's more similar to its look-alike, Swiss chard, than to its true cabbage relatives. Again, color clues you in to the fact that it provides almost half of your vitamin A requirement. It's a good source of potassium and a particularly well-absorbed nondairy source of calcium, providing about ten percent of a day's requirement. It only falls short in the fiber category.

Most cabbage is available year-round, but it's truly a fall/winter vegetable. That's when it's at its best. (That may be the only time you see Savoy.)When choosing cabbage, pick a tight, compact head that feels heavy for its size. It should look crisp and fresh, with few loose leaves. The leafy varieties will not be as compact; look for green leaves and firm stems.

Store cabbage, whole, in the crisper drawer of your refrigerator. Compact heads keep for a couple of weeks, if uncut, but leafy varieties should be used within a few days.

Preparation and Serving Tips

To prepare: Discard outer leaves if loose or limp, then cut into quarters and wash. When cooking quarters, leave the core in, so the leaves will stay together. If shredding cabbage for cole slaw, core the cabbage first. But don't shred it ahead of time; once you cut cells open, enzymes are hard at work destroying vitamin C.

Old-fashioned recipes, especially for corned beef and cabbage, rely on cooking in lots of water for what seems like an eternity. But that's only necessary for the beef, not the cabbage. More nutrients will be preserved and the cabbage will taste best if cooked only until slightly tender but still crisp—about 10 to 12 minutes for wedges, 5 minutes if shredded. Red cabbage might take a few minutes more to cook, while leafy varieties will be done sooner.

To solve cabbage's notorious stink problem, use the same trick recommended for broccoli and brussels sprouts: Steam (or boil if you must) in a small amount of water for a short time. Leave the cover off briefly, shortly after cooking begins, to release some of the sulfur smell. Do not cook in an aluminum pan, or the odor will intensify.

Bok choy and napa cabbage work well in stir-fry dishes. Cut on the diagonal and cook briefly, so they remain crisp. They also work well raw in salads, as does Savoy. You can tear the leaves and slice up the crunchy stems.

Combine red and green cabbage for a more interesting cole slaw. To keep the fat down, try a dressing made with low-fat yogurt, laced with poppy seeds. Cooked red cabbage goes well with full-flavored meals; try it with venison.

Savoy is perfect for stuffed cabbage dishes. Blanche it first, then roll up and cook. Cut down on the amount of meat in traditional stuffed-cabbage recipes, then use a grain like quinoa or buckwheat, instead of rice.

Sauerkraut, that traditional German version of pickled cabbage, is exceedingly salty. To reduce the sodium content, rinse it in water and drain before heating.

SWEET-SOUR CABBAGE WITH APPLES AND CARAWAY SEEDS

4 cups shredded red cabbage
1 large tart apple, peeled, quartered, cut crosswise into 1/4-inch-thick slices
1/4 cup packed light brown sugar
1/4 cup cider vinegar
1/4 cup water
1/2 teaspoon salt
1/4 teaspoon caraway seeds
   Dash pepper

Combine cabbage, apple, sugar, vinegar, water, salt, caraway seeds and pepper in large saucepan. Cook, covered, over medium heat 10 minutes.

Stir mixture. Cook, covered, over medium-low heat 15 to 20 minutes or until cabbage is crisp-tender and apple is tender. Serve warm or chilled. *Makes 6 servings*

NUTRIENTS PER SERVING:			
Calories	62.43	Folate	34.08 µg
Protein	0.78 g	Sodium	191.3 mg
Carbohydrate	15.86 g	Vitamin C	29.25 mg
Dietary Fiber	1.61 g	Vitamin K	89.43 µg
Fat	0.19 g		
Saturated Fat	0.03 g	DIETARY EXCHANGES:	
Poly Fat	0.07 g	Veg: 1	Fruit: 0.5
Mono Fat	0.02 g		
Cholesterol	0 mg	% OF CALORIES FROM:	
Sugar	12.85 g	PRO: 5%	CARB: 93%
Calcium	39.18 mg	FAT: 2%	

CARROTS

You probably have a bag of carrots sitting in the crisper drawer of your refrigerator right now. If you don't, you should, because they're anything but ordinary when it comes to nutrition. Carrots contain an uncommon amount of beta-carotene and are worth eating for that reason alone. Their numerous health benefits make us think that perhaps that well-known ditty should be amended to: A *carrot* a day keeps the doctor away.

Health Benefits

Carrots have few rivals when it comes to beta-carotene; indeed, its name reflects the fact that beta-carotene is found in such great amounts in carrots. A mere ½ cup of cooked carrots, or one raw carrot, packs a walloping four times the recommended daily intake of vitamin A in the form of beta-carotene.

The strongest evidence for beta-carotene's protective antioxidant effect is against lung tumors (avoiding tobacco is still your best defense against lung tumors, however), but beta-carotene may also help ward off cancers of the stomach, cervix, uterus, and oral cavity.

The National Cancer Institute is studying the whole family of umbelliferous foods, of which carrots are a member, for protective effects. Recent study results from the Harvard School of Public Health suggest that people who eat more than five carrots a week are much less likely to suffer a stroke than those who eat only one carrot a month.

Carrots also are a respectable source of dietary fiber, half of which is soluble calcium pectate fiber. As with other foods that are rich in soluble fiber, such as oats, barley, and dry beans, research shows that carrots may help to lower blood-cholesterol levels.

Finally, carrots do help your eyes, in more ways than one. The retina of the eye needs vitamin A to function; a deficiency of vitamin A will cause night blindness. Although extra vitamin A won't help you see better, its antioxidant properties may help reduce your risk of cataracts.

Eat too many carrots, however, and you invite a trip to the doctor because you look jaundiced. Relax, it's only the orange carotene pigment showing up in your skin from eating so many carrots. It may be unsightly, but it's harmless.

NUTRIENT INFORMATION			
Carrots, fresh, cooked		Vitamin A	19,152 IU
Serving Size: ½ cup		Vitamin (B6)	0.2 mg
Calories	35		
Protein	0.9 g	Manganese	0.6 mg
Carbohydrate	8.2 g	Potassium	177 mg
Fat	0.1 g		
Saturated	0		
Cholesterol	0		
Dietary Fiber	2 g		
Sodium	52 mg		

Selection and Storage

Baby new carrots are young carrots sold in early summer. They're often sold with the greens attached. Mature carrots are usually sold already in bags, without the greens. They are available year-round; their true season is summer to fall.

Look for firm carrots, with a bright orange color and smooth skin free of roots. Avoid limp-looking carrots or those with black near the top; they're not fresh. Choose medium ones that taper at the ends. The thicker ones will taste tough. In general, early carrots are more tender, but less sweet, than larger, mature carrots.

Clip the greens so they won't suck out moisture from the carrots, and store both (if you plan to use the greens in soup stock) in perforated plastic bags in your refrigerator crisper drawer. Carrots will keep for a few weeks, if cold enough, but greens only last a few days. Don't store next to apples or pears, which produce ethylene gas that will rot the carrots.

Preparation and Serving Tips

Thoroughly wash and scrub carrots to remove any soil contaminants. Being a root vegetable, carrots tend to end up with more pesticide residues than some other vegetables. But you can get rid of a lot of it by peeling the carrots and by cutting off and discarding ¼ inch of the top (fat end) of the carrot.

Carrots are a great raw snack, of course. But their true sweet flavor shines through when cooked. And rest assured that very little of their nutritional value is lost in cooking, unless you overcook them until mushy. In fact, the nutrients in lightly cooked carrots are more usable by your body than those in the raw version, because cooking breaks down carrots' tough cell walls.

Take advantage of the fact that most children love carrots raw and cooked. But avoid serving coin-shaped slices to young children; they can choke on them. You can cut carrots into quarters or julienne strips. For adult variety, try cutting carrots on the diagonal, to expose more surface area and flavor.

Steaming is your best bet for cooking carrots. They are delicious served with a mustard sauce, a little grated orange rind, or a classic orange-juice-and-honey glaze. Try nutmeg or ginger for a spicy alternative.

Carrot soup is a delicious, nutritious first course or light lunch. And it doesn't need cream or any dairy ingredient. The carrots themselves provide the thickness, aided by leeks. Add onions, chicken stock, and white pepper, and you're in business.

In fact, the soluble fiber in carrots can add thickness to lots of foods, like soups and sauces, taking the place of fattening butter and cream. Just add puréed carrots. The stronger the flavor of the soup or sauce, the more it will hide the carrot flavor. Don't forget to add carrot greens to your soup stocks. They impart great flavor.

Shred carrots into salads for a beta-carotene bonus. They make a great addition to cole slaw and Waldorf salad.

Versatile carrots can even be used in baking. Carrot cake is a favorite, but watch out—it's usually loaded with calories. Try a low-fat version if you have a hankering for it.

POLYNESIAN GINGER CARROTS

- **1 pound carrots, cut diagonally into ⅛-inch-thick slices**
- **1 can (6 ounces) unsweetened pineapple juice**
- **½ cup finely chopped onion**
- **1½ teaspoons cornstarch**
- **1 tablespoon water**
- **1 teaspoon reduced sodium soy sauce**
- **½ teaspoon ground ginger**
- **2 teaspoons toasted sesame seeds✳**

Combine carrots, pineapple juice and onion in medium saucepan. Bring to a boil. Reduce heat to low. Simmer, covered, 10 minutes or until carrots are crisp-tender, stirring once.

Blend cornstarch with water in small cup until smooth. Stir cornstarch mixture, soy sauce and ginger into saucepan with carrots. Cook and stir over medium heat until sauce boils and thickens. Cook and stir 1 minute more. Just before serving, stir in sesame seeds.   ***Makes 4 servings***

* To toast sesame seeds, cook in small nonstick skillet over medium heat 3 minutes or until golden brown, stirring constantly. Remove from skillet; let cool.

NUTRIENTS PER SERVING:			
Calories	91.91	Calcium	41.1 mg
Protein	2.07 g	Folate	24.43 µg
Carbohydrate	19.93 g	Magnesium	28.52 mg
Dietary Fiber	4.14 g	Potassium	468 mg
Fat	1.02 g	Sodium	85.11 mg
Saturated Fat	0.14 g	Vitamin A	3,189 RE
Poly Fat	0.4 g	DIETARY EXCHANGES:	
Mono Fat	0.27 g	Veg: 2.5	Fruit: 0.5
Cholesterol	0 mg		
Sugar	13.36 g	% OF CALORIES FROM:	
Beta-Carotene	19,139 RE	PRO: 8%	CARB: 82%
		FAT: 9%	

CAULIFLOWER

Cauliflower has been referred to as upscale cabbage but could also be thought of as pricey broccoli. All three are cruciferous vegetables and share a similar pungent aroma and taste. They also share some healthy characteristics.

Health Benefits

As a cruciferous vegetable, cauliflower may be a natural cancer fighter. Phytochemicals may be the key.

Cauliflower is rich in vitamin C, an antioxidant that also appears to help reduce the risk of cancer. After citrus fruits, cruciferae are your next best natural source of vitamin C. Cauliflower is also notable for its fiber, folic acid, and potassium.

Selection and Storage

Though it is a fall and winter vegetable, supermarkets typically carry cauliflower year-round. But you'll notice a lower quality and higher price when it's out of season. Spend wisely by choosing carefully. Look for any size head that is creamy white, with compact florets. Brown patches and florets that have opened are signs of aging.

Broccoflower, a cross between cauliflower and broccoli, provides some beta-carotene that cauliflower does not and has a slightly milder flavor.

Store cauliflower—unwashed, uncut, and loosely wrapped in a plastic bag—in the refrigerator crisper. Keep upright to prevent moisture from collecting on the surface. It'll keep about two to five days.

NUTRIENT INFORMATION			
Cauliflower, fresh, cooked		Vitamin C	34.3 mg
Serving Size: ½ cup		Folic Acid	31.7 µg
Calories	15		
Protein	1.2 g	Potassium	200 mg
Carbohydrate	2.9 g		
Fat	0.1 g		
Saturated	0		
Cholesterol	0		
Dietary Fiber	1 g		
Sodium	4 mg		

Preparation and Serving Tips

To prepare cauliflower, remove the outer leaves, then break off the florets. Wash well under running water. Trim any brown spots.

Cauliflower serves up well both raw and cooked. Raw, its flavor is less intense and more likely to be acceptable to kids. Many kids love to dip it in dressing; try fat-free ranch. Many adults like the crunch raw cauliflower adds to salads.

To cook cauliflower, steam it, but don't overcook it. It tastes better when it still has a bit of crunch, and overcooking destroys much of its vitamin C and folic acid. Overcooking also stinks up your kitchen and gives the cauliflower a bitter, pungent flavor. To prevent this, steam it in a nonaluminum pan over a small amount of water, just until your fork can barely pierce a floret—about five minutes. Remove the cover momentarily, soon after cooking begins, to release the smelly sulfur compounds.

Although cheese sauces are popular over cauliflower, they add a hefty dose of fat and calories. Why ruin a good thing? Better to serve cauliflower plain, with some dill weed and maybe a little margarine. Or try baking it with bread crumbs and lemon. For a real switch, add raw cauliflower, broccoli, and carrots to homemade spaghetti sauce and simmer for 15 minutes. Serve over whole-wheat pasta for a hearty dose of taste and nutrients.

CURRIED CAULIFLOWER RICE & VERMICELLI

- 1 teaspoon canola *or* vegetable oil
- ½ cup finely chopped onion
- 1 large clove garlic, minced
- 1 teaspoon curry powder
- ½ teaspoon ground coriander
- ¼ teaspoon salt
- ⅓ cup uncooked long-grain rice
- ⅓ cup vermicelli broken into 1-inch pieces
- 1 cup apple juice
- ½ cup water
- 3 cups ½-inch cauliflowerets
- 3 tablespoons golden raisins

Heat oil in large nonstick skillet over medium heat until hot. Add onion and garlic; cook and stir 2 minutes. Add curry powder, coriander and salt; cook and stir 1 minute. Stir in rice and vermicelli until coated with spices. Remove pan from heat.

Bring apple juice and water to a boil in small saucepan; pour over rice and vermicelli mixture. Bring mixture to a boil over high heat. Reduce heat to low. Simmer, covered, 15 minutes.

Set cauliflower and raisins on top of rice mixture. Simmer, covered, about 7 minutes or until water is absorbed. Stir cauliflower and raisins into mixture. Remove from heat; let stand, covered, 5 minutes or until cauliflower is crisp-tender. Fluff with fork before serving. *Makes 4 servings*

NUTRIENTS PER SERVING:			
Calories	206.6	Iron	2.15 mg
Protein	5.45 g	Sodium	187 mg
Carbohydrate	39.29 g	Vitamin C	81.61 mg
Dietary Fiber	3.08 g	Vitamin K	152.8 µg
Fat	3.99 g		
Saturated Fat	0.47 g	DIETARY EXCHANGES:	
Poly Fat	1.18 g	Veg: 1	Fruit: 1
Mono Fat	1.85 g	Bread: 1.5	Fat: 0.5
Cholesterol	0 mg		
Sugar	2.03 g	% OF CALORIES FROM:	
Calcium	48.2 mg	PRO: 10%	CARB: 73%
Folate	63.26 µg	FAT: 17%	

CHEESE, LOW-FAT

"Low-fat cheese" used to be an oxymoron. No more. Today, there are dozens of reduced-fat and fat-free versions of American, Cheddar, mozzarella, Swiss, and other cheeses. Fat in this new generation of cheeses has been cut anywhere from 25 to 100 percent. The average fat reduction is about 30 percent. Most have added gums and stabilizers to help simulate the creamy texture and rich taste of full-fat cheeses.

The taste and texture of reduced-fat cheeses vary considerably. Some people find them fine substitutes for the full-fat varieties, while others find they would rather do without than settle for a low-fat substitute. Cheese connoisseurs will probably never be true fans of reduced-fat cheeses, but for the rest of us trying to cut back on saturated fat and cholesterol, they do offer alternatives.

The one nutrition drawback of reduced-fat cheeses is that they are usually considerably higher in sodium than full-fat natural cheeses. An ounce of regular Swiss cheese, for example, contains only about 74 milligrams of sodium. A reduced-fat Swiss may contain 300 to 400 milligrams or more per ounce.

Also, bear in mind that just because a cheese is low in fat doesn't mean it's significantly lower in cholesterol. Regular cheese contains about 25 to 35 milligrams of cholesterol per ounce. Several reduced-fat cheeses provide 20 milligrams.

Are reduced-fat cheeses the answer for a diet hopelessly high in fat? Hardly. Unless you're a big cheese eater, chances are other elements of your diet—such as fatty meats, whole milk, buttery muffins and croissants, chips, and ice cream—are more in need of a little fat-trimming. But reduced-fat cheese can't hurt. When it comes to the war on fat, every gram counts. Here's how much fat you might save by using a reduced-fat cheese: In a recipe that calls for four ounces of cheese and makes four servings, substituting a one-third reduced-fat cheese saves 12 grams of fat or 108 calories—about 3 grams of fat per serving.

Health Benefits

Like their full-fat counterparts, low-fat and fat-free cheeses are great sources of hard-to-get calcium, the bone-building mineral that helps prevent osteoporosis. Many cheeses provide 200 to 300 milligrams per ounce.

Selection and Storage

For lower-fat cheeses, opt for varieties that provide no more than five grams of fat per ounce. Regular cheeses provide eight to nine grams per ounce. Brands vary a lot in taste and texture. Shop around until you find one that you like. You're better off choosing a reduced-fat cheese based on taste and then trying it in recipes. Remember, the less fat a cheese contains, the harder it is to use in cooking.

Because of their high moisture contents, reduced-fat and fat-free cheeses turn moldy more quickly than their full-fat counterparts. Keep them well wrapped in the refrigerator and use as soon as possible.

NUTRIENT INFORMATION

Reduced-fat Cheddar Cheese Serving Size: 1 oz		Fat-free American Cheese Serving Size: 1 oz	
Calories	80	Calories	45
Protein	9 g	Protein	7 g
Carbohydrate	0	Carbohydrate	4 g
Fat	5 g	Fat	0 g
Saturated	3 g	Saturated	0
Cholesterol	20 mg	Cholesterol	5 mg
Dietary Fiber	0	Dietary Fiber	0
Sodium	220 mg	Sodium	420 mg
		Vitamin A	500 IU
Riboflavin	0.1 mg	Riboflavin	0.1 mg
Calcium	250 mg	Calcium	200 mg

Preparation and Serving Tips

In general, the farther you get from a traditional cheese, in terms of fat content, the more careful you have to be about applying heat. It's the high fat content of regular cheese, generally about 70 percent of calories, that gives it its smooth, creamy texture and allows it to melt easily. When fat is reduced, cheese becomes less pliable and more difficult to melt. The lower the fat, the tougher the problem. Trying to make a cheese sauce with a reduced-fat cheese can be an exercise in futility because the product is prone to break down into a clumpy, stringy mess.

Nonfat cheeses are best served "as is" in sandwiches or in salads. They generally have milder flavors than regular cheeses, and they sometimes have what cheese lovers might describe as "off" flavors.

To lighten the calories and fat of recipes without dramatically altering the flavor or texture, replace one-half to two-thirds of a full-fat cheese with a reduced-fat variety. Grated cheese blends best. Or combine a small amount of full-fat, full-bodied cheese like extra sharp cheddar or Parmesan with a reduced-fat cheese. A little can go a long way toward improving flavor. Most reduced-fat cheeses melt smoothly when layered in a casserole. The layers serve as insulation and help prevent the cheese from separating or becoming stringy.

The lower the amount of fat in a cheese, the longer it takes to melt and the more likely it is to produce a "skin" and scorch when baked. Top casseroles and baked pasta dishes with reduced-fat cheese only near the end of the baking time, and heat until just melted. Serve immediately.

Meltability on top of dishes like casseroles or pizzas varies among varieties of reduced-fat cheeses just as it does among traditional cheeses. You may, for example, find a fat-reduced mozzarella melts much more smoothly than does a fat-reduced cheddar.

THIN-CRUST WHOLE WHEAT VEGGIE PIZZA

- ¾ to 1 cup all-purpose flour, divided
- ½ cup whole wheat flour
- 1 teaspoon quick-rising dry yeast
- 1½ teaspoons dried basil leaves, crushed, divided
- ¼ teaspoon salt
- 1 tablespoon olive oil
- 1 large clove garlic, minced
- ½ cup very warm water (120° to 130°F)
- 1 teaspoon yellow cornmeal
- ½ cup no-salt-added tomato sauce

1 cup thinly sliced mushrooms
½ cup thinly sliced zucchini
⅓ cup chopped green onions
1 large roasted red bell pepper,✳ cut lengthwise into thin
   strips or ¾ cup sliced, drained, bottled roasted red
   peppers
1 cup (4 ounces) shredded part-skim mozzarella cheese
¼ teaspoon crushed red pepper

Combine ½ cup all-purpose flour, whole wheat flour, yeast, 1 teaspoon basil and salt. Blend oil with garlic in small cup; stir into flour mixture with water. Stir in ¼ cup all-purpose flour until soft, slightly sticky dough forms, adding remaining ¼ cup all-purpose flour to prevent sticking if necessary. Knead dough on lightly floured surface about 5 minutes or until smooth and elastic. Shape dough into a ball. Cover with inverted bowl or clean towel; let rest 10 minutes.

Place oven rack in lowest position; preheat oven to 400°F. Spray 12-inch pizza pan or baking sheet with nonstick cooking spray; sprinkle with cornmeal and set aside. Roll dough into large circle on lightly floured surface. Transfer to prepared pan, stretching dough out to edge of pan. (Too much rolling makes crust heavy and dense; stretching dough to fit pan is best.)

NUTRIENTS PER SERVING:			
Calories	270.5	Calcium	217.8 mg
Protein	13.20 g	Folate	58.73 µg
Carbohydrate	36.17 g	Sodium	276.9 mg
Dietary Fiber	4.12 g	Vitamin C	25.76 mg
Fat	8.6 g	Vitamin E	1.99 mg
Saturated Fat	3.46 g		
Poly Fat	0.7 g	DIETARY EXCHANGES:	
Mono Fat	3.85 g	Veg: 1	Bread: 2
Cholesterol	15.97 mg	Meat: 1	Fat: 1
Sugar	1.96 g		
Beta-Carotene	426.3 RE	% OF CALORIES FROM:	
		PRO: 19%	CARB: 53%
		FAT: 28%	

Blend tomato sauce and remaining ½ teaspoon basil in small bowl; spread evenly over crust. Top with mushrooms, zucchini, green onions, roasted bell pepper and mozzarella; sprinkle crushed red pepper on top. Bake 20 to 25 minutes or until crust is golden brown and cheese melts.

Makes 4 servings

✳ To roast pepper, cut pepper lengthwise into halves, remove stem, membrane and seeds. Broil 3 inches from heat, skin side up, until skin is blackened and blistered. Place halves in small resealable plastic food storage bag. Seal; set aside 15 minutes. Remove pepper from bag. Peel off skin; drain on paper towel.

CHERRIES

Plump, firm, juicy cherries are one of nature's most delectable treats. But these tasty bites are only available three months of the year. Be sure to take advantage of this short but abundant summer season. For just a few calories, you'll get cherries' sweet offering of vitamin C and a healthy dose of soluble fiber.

Health Benefits

The fiber found in cherries is water soluble, the kind thought to help lower blood cholesterol. Cherries are a good source of vitamin C, and sour cherries are a good source of vitamin A. Moreover, cherries are one of a handful of fruits that have been identified as containing ellagic acid, a natural compound that appears to have cancer-preventive properties.

Selection and Storage

Sweet cherries should be plump and firm with a bright color that may be red, yellow tinged with red, or reddish-brown to black, depending on the variety. Cherries are ready to wash and eat when you buy them. But make sure they have been kept cool and moist. As storage temperatures rise, their flavor and texture suffer. Keep them refrigerated, and use within a few days.

The cherry season is quite short. In fact, cherries are one of the few fruits that are still truly seasonal, available only from mid-June to mid-August. Bing is the most common variety. But you'll find other varieties, including Lamberts and Vans, that are hard to distinguish from the more familiar Bing.

NUTRIENT INFORMATION			
Cherries, sweet raw		Dietary Fiber	3 g
Serving Size: 1 cup or 21 cherries		Sodium	0
Calories	90	Potassium	270 mg
Protein	1 g		
Carbohydrate	19 g		
Fat	1 g		
Saturated	na		
Cholesterol	0		

Check cherries at the market for cuts or sticky leaks. It generally means there are others in the batch that are going bad. One bad cherry will eventually ruin the whole bunch. Choose cherries that still have the stem attached. A missing stem makes the fruit more vulnerable to spoilage, and besides, cherries are easier to eat with the stem attached. The stem should be green and pliable, not brown and brittle.

Cherries deteriorate rapidly, so use them right away. If you don't, store in the refrigerator in a covered container. Check for cherries that have gone bad and toss them out.

Preparation and Serving Tips

Sweet cherries are great by themselves. A bowl of washed cherries makes a low-fat, low-calorie snack that's hard to beat. But sweet cherries are also good mixed in a fruit salad, as a topping for frozen desserts, or as an ingredient in a frothy blended fruit drink. Sour cherries that are used for baking pies and making sauces are too tart to be eaten out of hand, and sugar is always added to recipes that include them.

CHERRY SALSA

¾ pound dark or light sweet cherries
¼ cup finely chopped red onion
1 tablespoon chopped cilantro
2 teaspoons lime juice
2 teaspoons minced jalapeño pepper*
1 teaspoon minced fresh gingerroot

Remove stems and pits from cherries; cut into halves (about 2¼ cups). Combine cherries, onion, cilantro, lime juice, jalapeño and gingerroot in medium bowl. Refrigerate, covered, at least 1 hour to allow flavors to blend. Toss before serving. ***Makes 4 servings***

* Chili peppers can sting and irritate the skin; wear rubber gloves when handling peppers and do not touch eyes. Wash hands after handling chili peppers.

Note: Serve salsa with baked or grilled chicken breasts, pork tenderloin or hearty fish, such as tuna, mackerel or catfish.

NUTRIENTS PER SERVING:			
Calories	66.7	Calcium	16.5 mg
Protein	1.2 g	Sodium	21.51 mg
Carbohydrate	15.38 g	Vitamin A	25.89 RE
Dietary Fiber	1.48 g	Vitamin C	8.5 mg
Fat	0.85 g		
Saturated Fat	0.19 g	DIETARY EXCHANGES:	
Poly Fat	0.26 g	Fruit: 1	
Mono Fat	0.23 g		
Cholesterol	0 mg	% OF CALORIES FROM:	
Sugar	12.7 g	PRO: 6%	CARB: 83%
Beta-Carotene	156.2 RE	FAT: 10%	

CHICKEN, SKINNED

Chicken is often considered a healthy low-fat alternative to beef. But that's not true across the board. A piece of dark meat, such as a chicken thigh, with the skin on can carry a fat load as heavy as any piece of beef. In fact, some cuts of beef, such as eye of round, are actually leaner. You have to make the right chicken choices to really save on fat. Best bet? Skinless chicken breast. It's lowest in fat and calories. Removing the skin before you eat any piece of chicken saves fat and calories. But you quickly lose your low-fat advantage if you turn around and smother it in fatty sauces or gravies or cover it with melted cheese. Use fresh herbs and spices instead.

Health Benefits

If you're trying to cut back on fat, skinless chicken breast offers a great low-fat alternative to fattier beef and pork. And the fat it does contain is higher in heart-healthy monounsaturates (the type of fat found in olive and canola oils) than beef or pork. You should be aware, however, that chicken contains about the same amount of cholesterol per serving as beef. Chicken is also a generous source of some B vitamins that aren't as plentiful in beef. Chicken is a fair source of iron.

NUTRIENT INFORMATION			
Chicken Breast, skinned		Niacin	11.8 mg
Serving Size: 3 oz		Pantothenic Acid	0.8 mg
Calories	142	Vitamin B6	0.5 mg
Protein	26.7 g	Vitamin B12	0.3 µg
Carbohydrate	0		
Fat	3.1 g	Iron	0.5 mg
Saturated	0.9 g	Phosphorus	196.0 mg
Cholesterol	73 mg		
Dietary Fiber	0		
Sodium	63 mg		

Selection and Storage

When choosing a whole chicken, look for one that is plump and firm with a skin that looks moist and supple, not dry and shriveled. The skin should have a creamy white or yellowish color (color varies depending on what the chicken was fed), and the chicken should have no odor.

Free-range chickens are becoming increasingly popular. These free-range chickens have been allowed free reign of a farmyard rather than being cooped up in a chicken house. The result is a little tougher meat, but some say it also results in a better flavor. Free-rangers are no more nutritious than the chicken-house variety but may not have been given antibiotics, as traditionally raised chickens often are. However, you'll pay a premium price for these hens. The decision is up to you.

Chicken is a highly perishable food, and it presents a standing invitation to bacteria if it's not stored properly. If you buy fresh whole chicken, be sure to store it right away in the coldest part of your refrigerator and use it within two to three days. If you don't have plans to use it before then, wash it, dry it, cut it into parts, wrap it, and freeze it. It will keep for up to nine months. If you freeze a chicken whole, it will keep for one year.

Never leave chicken out to thaw at room temperature. Let it thaw in the refrigerator. And leave it on a plate to catch the drippings. A three-pound chicken should take about nine to twelve hours to thaw completely. It's OK to thaw chicken in the microwave, if you cook it immediately after it has thawed.

Preparation and Serving Tips

When you handle raw chicken, be sure to wash your hands thoroughly afterwards with soap and warm water before you touch any other food or utensil. And be sure to wash well the cutting board and utensils used during preparation. Skip this important food-safety step and you're risking cross contamination—transferring bacteria like *salmonella* from raw chicken to other foods served at the meal. Cooking kills *salmonella* bacteria, but if the bug is transferred to a raw salad, for example, food poisoning can result.

If you marinate chicken, do it in the refrigerator, not on the kitchen counter at room temperature. And don't use the marinade as a sauce for the cooked bird, unless you boil the marinade before serving.

Chicken is versatile and, if seasoned properly, it's delicious. Though fried chicken is an American favorite, especially the fast-food variety, it's also loaded with fat. Opt for lower-fat methods of preparation. Roasting is a good fat-saving cooking technique for whole chickens. Skinless chicken breasts are perfect for marinating in low-fat sauces or, when cut up and mixed with vegetables, for stir frying. Chicken breasts also work well on the grill. If you add a sauce, wait until the chicken is almost done. Otherwise it could scorch and burn before the breast is cooked all the way through.

No matter how you prepare chicken, be sure that it's cooked thoroughly. Here's how to tell: The meat should be white, not pink, and the juices should run clear.

Standard advice has long been to remove the skin of chicken before you cook it, to save fat calories. But a few years ago it was discovered that fat calories in a piece of chicken were about the same whether the skin was removed before or after the chicken was cooked. Removing the skin after cooking keeps the chicken juicy and moist and keeps flavor locked in.

GRILLED RASPBERRY-THYME CHICKEN

  4 boneless skinless chicken breast halves (4 ounces each)
  3 tablespoons plus 1 teaspoon red raspberry preserves, divided
  1 tablespoon lemon juice
  2 teaspoons reduced sodium soy sauce, divided
 ¾ teaspoon grated lemon peel
 ¾ teaspoon dried thyme leaves, crushed
 ¾ pound fresh spinach, washed, stemmed, torn
  1 small cantaloupe, thinly sliced, peeled
  6 ounces fresh raspberries
  2 tablespoons rice wine vinegar
  2 teaspoons canola *or* vegetable oil

Place chicken in small resealable plastic food storage bag. Blend 2 tablespoons raspberry preserves, lemon juice, 1 teaspoon soy sauce, lemon peel and thyme in small cup; pour into bag over chicken. Seal bag securely; turn bag several times to coat chicken with marinade. Refrigerate 1 hour.

Arrange spinach, cantaloupe and raspberries on serving platter. Cover with plastic wrap; refrigerate until ready to use.

For dressing, combine vinegar, remaining 4 teaspoons raspberry preserves, oil and remaining 1 teaspoon soy sauce in small jar with tight-fitting lid. Shake well; set aside.

Remove chicken from marinade; reserve marinade. Place chicken on grill 4 inches from medium-hot coals.✱ Grill 5 minutes. Brush top of chicken with marinade; discard remaining marinade. Turn chicken over; grill 5 to 7 minutes or until juices run clear and center is no longer pink. Cut each breast diagonally into 4 slices. Drizzle dressing over spinach and fruit; arrange chicken on top. ***Makes 4 servings***

✱ Chicken may be broiled instead of grilled. To broil, place chicken on rack in broiler pan. Cook 4 to 5 inches from heat 6 minutes. Turn chicken over; brush with reserved marinade. Cook 6 to 8 minutes longer or until juices run clear and chicken is no longer pink in center.

NUTRIENTS PER SERVING:

Calories	319.9	Magnesium	135.5 mg
Protein	27.09 g	Niacin (B_3)	13 mg
Carbohydrate	45.13 g	Pyridoxine (B_6)	0.92 mg
Dietary Fiber	7.86 g	Sodium	269.6 mg
Fat	5.61 g	Thiamin (B_1)	0.21 mg
Saturated Fat	0.92 g	Vitamin C	152.3 mg
Poly Fat	1.46 g	Vitamin E	3.03 mg
Mono Fat	2.22 g	Vitamin K	245.1 µg
Cholesterol	57.86 mg		
Sugar	3.27 g	DIETARY EXCHANGES:	
Beta-Carotene	3,473 RE	Veg: 1	Fruit: 2
Calcium	153.7 mg	Meat: 3	
Folate	179.8 µg		
Iron	4.5 mg	% OF CALORIES FROM:	
		PRO: 32%	CARB: 53%
		FAT: 15%	

COLLARD GREENS

Most often thought of as a strictly budget-conscious Southern dish, collard and its green cousins are gaining new respect as nutrition powerhouses, loaded with disease-fighting beta-carotene and offering a respectable amount of vitamin C and calcium. All these attributes make collard greens a wise choice for your diet.

Health Benefits

Collards are a superb source of vitamin A, mostly in the form of beta-carotene, which is believed to help protect against cancer. The outer leaves usually contain more beta-carotene than do the inner leaves.

These greens belong to the cruciferous family, which also includes cabbage and cauliflower. Research has shown that people who eat a lot of cruciferous vegetables are less likely to suffer cancer than those whose diets contain few foods from the cruciferous family.

NUTRIENT INFORMATION
Collard Greens, cooked
Serving Size: ½ cup

		Sodium	18 mg
Calories	56	Vitamin A	2,109 IU
Protein	1 g	Vitamin C	9 mg
Carbohydrate	2.5 g		
Fat	0.14 g	Calcium	74 mg
Saturated	na		
Cholesterol	0		
Dietary Fiber	0.4 g		

Selection and Storage

Choose collard greens that have smooth, green, firm leaves. Small, young leaves are likely to be the least bitter and most tender. Collard greens don't grow from a head; rather, they grow outward from individual inedible stems. The flavor of the leaves is relatively mild compared to most other greens.

Though collards are available year-round, the quality is usually best during the first five months of the year.

Collards store well for three to five days if you wrap them unwashed in a damp paper towel and put them in a sealed plastic bag. When you're ready to cook them, be sure to wash them well since most greens have sand and dirt still clinging to the leaves. Be sure to remove the tough stems; cook only the leaves. One pound of raw leaves will yield about ½ cup cooked collards.

Preparation and Serving Tips

Cook collards in a small amount of water to preserve the vitamin C content, and cook with the lid off to prevent the greens from turning a drab olive color. When you can, keep the cooking liquid for use in soups or stews since a lot of nutrients leach out into the cooking water.

If you want to eat them plain as a vegetable side dish, try simmering collards in seasoned water or broth for up to 30 minutes. For a little Southern flair, add a bit of bacon or a ham hock to the cooking water for flavoring.

ITALIAN-STYLE COLLARD GREENS

- ½ pound collard greens
- 1 teaspoon olive oil
- 1 cup coarsely chopped celery
- ¾ cup coarsely chopped onion
- 2 large cloves garlic, minced
- 1 can (14½ ounces) no-salt-added stewed tomatoes, undrained
- 2 teaspoons Italian seasoning
- 1 can (15 ounces) white beans (such as cannellini, Great Northern or navy), rinsed, drained

Remove discolored leaves and tough stems from greens. Wash greens thoroughly in sink of cold water to remove any sand; drain, pat dry and coarsely chop.

Heat oil in large saucepan over medium heat. Add celery, onion and garlic; cook and stir 5 minutes. Add chopped greens, stewed tomatoes and juice and seasoning, breaking up tomatoes and stirring until greens wilt. Bring to a boil over high heat. Reduce heat to low. Simmer, covered, 15 minutes. Add beans; simmer, covered, 5 minutes more.

Makes 4 servings

NUTRIENTS PER SERVING:			
Calories	147.5	Potassium	657.9 mg
Protein	10.13 g	Sodium	233.4 mg
Carbohydrate	31.66 g	Vitamin A	261.7 RE
Dietary Fiber	10.35 g	Vitamin C	34.09 mg
Fat	2.49 g		
Saturated Fat	0.26 g	DIETARY EXCHANGES:	
Poly Fat	0.37 g	Veg: 2.5	Bread: 1
Mono Fat	0.91 g	Fat: 0.5	
Cholesterol	0 mg		
Sugar	0.82 g	% OF CALORIES FROM:	
Beta-Carotene	682.7 RE	PRO: 21%	CARB: 67%
Calcium	44.16 mg	FAT: 12%	
Folate	23.52 µg		

CORN

Corn is a low-fat complex carbohydrate that deserves a regular place on any healthy table. Unfortunately, as with many other naturally low-fat foods, the American tendency is to smother it in oil and butter. But these high-fiber kernels of goodness are better left alone.

Health Benefits

This popular grain is high in fiber and a surprising source of several vitamins, including folic acid, niacin, and vitamin C. Except for the loss of some vitamin C, canned and frozen corn are just as nutritious as fresh.

NUTRIENT INFORMATION			
Corn, yellow or white		Sodium	13 mg
Serving Size: 1 ear			
Calories	83	Vitamin C	4.8 mg
Protein	2.6 g	Folic Acid	35.7 µg
Carbohydrate	19.3 g	Niacin	1.2 mg
Fat	1 g		
Saturated	0.2 g	Potassium	192 mg
Cholesterol	0		
Dietary Fiber	3 g		

Selection and Storage

Though it's most abundant during the summer months, corn is usually available year-round. When you shop for fresh corn, be sure it's being kept in a cool place. As the temperature rises, the natural sugar in corn turns to starch, and the corn loses some of its distinctive sweetness.

The husks should be green and the visible kernels should be plump and tightly packed on the cob. The corn silk should be soft to the touch and a golden color. To test for freshness, pop a single kernel with your fingernail. The liquid that spurts out should be milky colored. If it's not, the corn could be either immature or overripe.

When you get the corn home, put it in the refrigerator. Warmer temperatures cause corn to lose sweetness quickly.

Frozen corn is a fine substitute for fresh, unless it's been frozen with a butter sauce. The hefty dose of fat that usually comes with it defeats the purpose of eating this healthy food.

So-called "creamed" corn is not really creamed at all. In fact, it has no added fat—just sugar and cornstarch. The calorie count is higher than for plain fresh, frozen, or canned corn, but creamed corn contains no more fat.

Preparation and Serving Tips

Boiling is the traditional method for preparing fresh corn on the cob, though grilling or roasting, steaming, and even microwaving will get the job done. A couple of notes about boiling corn: Adding salt to the water toughens the corn; over-cooking also toughens the kernels. Cook the corn for the shortest amount of time possible—that usually means about five to ten minutes.

Though the typical way to serve corn is smothered in butter or margarine (often with a hefty dose of salt, as well), keep in mind that each pat you add carries with it four unnecessary grams of fat. Instead, try sprinkling on a favorite herb; fresh-squeezed lime juice; a ready-made, shake-on herb mixture; or a touch of oil and vinegar.

MUSHROOM CORN CHOWDER

- 2 medium ears fresh corn or 1 package (10 ounces) frozen corn
- 1 cup unsweetened apple juice
- 1 cup defatted low sodium chicken broth✻
- 1 cup sliced mushrooms
- ½ cup chopped onion
- ½ cup water
- 1 tablespoon chopped fresh basil or 1 teaspoon dried basil leaves, crushed
- 2 teaspoons chopped fresh thyme or ½ teaspoon dried thyme leaves, crushed
- ¼ teaspoon lemon pepper
- 1 can (12 ounces) evaporated skim milk, divided
- 2 tablespoons all-purpose flour
- 1 tablespoon cornstarch
- ⅛ teaspoon black pepper
  Fresh basil and/or thyme sprigs for garnish

If using fresh corn, cut off tips of kernels with sharp knife, then scrape cobs with dull edge. Combine fresh or frozen corn, apple juice, chicken broth, mushrooms, onion, water, basil, thyme and lemon pepper in large saucepan. Bring to a boil over high heat. Reduce heat to low. Simmer, covered, 10 to 15 minutes for fresh corn (5 to 10 minutes for frozen) or until corn is tender, stirring occasionally.

Combine ¼ cup milk, flour and cornstarch in small bowl until smooth. Stir into mixture in saucepan. Stir in remaining milk. Cook and stir over medium heat until mixture boils and thickens. Cook and stir 1 minute more. Stir in black pepper; garnish with fresh herbs. ***Makes 4 servings***

✳ To defat chicken broth, skim fat from surface of broth with spoon. Or, place can of broth in refrigerator at least 2 hours ahead of time. Before using, remove fat that has hardened on surface of broth.

NUTRIENTS PER SERVING:			
Calories	210.9	Manganese	0.32 mg
Protein	10.71 g	Niacin (B3)	2.79 mg
Carbohydrate	42.8 g	Riboflavin (B2)	0.44 mg
Dietary Fiber	2.14 g	Sodium	188.8 mg
Fat	1.21 g	Thiamin (B1)	0.23 mg
Saturated Fat	0.22 g	Vitamin A	117.5 RE
Poly Fat	0.32 g	Vitamin C	45.06 mg
Mono Fat	0.21 g	Zinc	1.43 mg
Cholesterol	3.4 mg		
Sugar	2.02 g	DIETARY EXCHANGES:	
Beta-Carotene	104.6 RE	Milk: 1	Fruit: 0.5
Calcium	273.4 mg	Bread: 1.5	
Cobalamin (B12)	0.22 µg		
Folate	35.53 µg	% OF CALORIES FROM:	
		PRO: 19%	CARB: 76%
		FAT: 5%	

CRANBERRIES

Cranberries are truly an American fruit, for they predate the arrival of the Pilgrims. American Indians used cranberries for food as well as medicine. They believed cranberries possessed medicinal qualities that helped draw poison out of arrow wounds. Much later, American sailors depended on the vitamin C in cranberries to keep scurvy at bay when at sea.

There are more than 100 different varieties of cranberries, but only four—Early Black, Howes, Searls, and McFarlin—make up most of the cranberries grown in this country.

Health Benefits

Cranberries seem to have a yet-to-be identified substance that helps prevent urinary tract infections by interfering with the ability of bacteria to adhere to cell membranes. There is debate over how much is needed to offer urinary tract protection. But at least one study found that drinking a four- to six-ounce glass of cranberry-juice cocktail (the only kind of cranberry juice you can buy) was enough to ward off urinary tract infections. But cranberries can't cure a urinary tract infection. You'll need to see your doctor for that. Cranberries also contain a naturally occurring compound called ellagic acid that may help prevent certain types of cancer.

NUTRIENT INFORMATION			
Cranberries		Cholesterol	0
Serving Size: ½ cup		Dietary Fiber	0.6 g
Calories	23	Sodium	0.5 mg
Protein	0.2 g		
Carbohydrate	6.0 g	Vitamin C	6.4 mg
Fat	0.1 g		
Saturated	na		

Selection and Storage

Fresh cranberries are most available during the fall harvest season, September to December. They may be stored in the refrigerator for two to four weeks, and they freeze well. To freeze, put the unwashed berries into double-wrapped plastic, or freeze them in their store-bought plastic package. They'll keep for nine months to a year. Use them frozen.

Preparation and Serving Tips

Most of the cranberries that are harvested are used for either cranberry juice or cranberry sauce. But cranberry sauce has only a fraction of the vitamin C of fresh cranberries, and it also packs more than three times the calories that you'll get from fresh cranberries.

Cranberries are far too sour to eat raw, so they are usually made into sauces, relishes, and jellies and preserves. Chopped cranberries can be mixed into stuffing, muffins, cookies, and quick breads.

Because they are so tart, cranberries work best when blended with chopped, fresh or dried, naturally sweet fruits, such as raisins, apples, prunes, or apricots.

To prepare frozen cranberries for cooking, simply sort them and rinse them in cold water. You'll get the best results if you use them while they're still frozen rather than waiting for them to thaw.

SPICED ORANGE CRANBERRY MUFFINS

- ½ cup chopped cranberries
- 3 tablespoons packed brown sugar
- 1 cup orange juice
- 1 egg white
- 2 tablespoons canola *or* vegetable oil
- 1 cup whole wheat flour
- ½ cup all-purpose flour
- 1½ teaspoons baking powder
- ½ teaspoon ground cinnamon
- ¼ teaspoon ground nutmeg

Preheat oven to 400°F. Paperline eight 2½-inch muffin cups or coat with nonstick cooking spray. Combine cranberries and sugar in small bowl; let stand 5 minutes. Stir in orange juice, egg white and oil.

Combine whole wheat flour, all-purpose flour, baking powder, cinnamon and nutmeg in medium bowl. Add cranberry mixture to flour mixture; stir just until combined.

Spoon batter into prepared muffin cups, filling ¾ full. Bake 18 to 20 minutes or until wooden toothpick inserted near center comes out clean. Immediately remove from pan; cool on wire rack.   *Makes 8 muffins*

NUTRIENTS PER SERVING:			
Calories	149.5	Folate	25.81 µg
Protein	3.55 g	Sodium	71.35 mg
Carbohydrate	26.29 g	Vitamin C	16.47 mg
Dietary Fiber	2.64 g	Vitamin K	32.82 µg
Fat	3.87 g		
Saturated Fat	0.33 g	DIETARY EXCHANGES:	
Poly Fat	1.18 g	Fruit: 0.5	Bread: 1
Mono Fat	2.06 g	Fat: 1	
Cholesterol	0 mg		
Sugar	8.24 g	% OF CALORIES FROM:	
Calcium	27.38 mg	PRO: 9%	CARB: 68%
		FAT: 23%	

DANDELION GREENS

It's hard to believe that these exceptionally nutritious greens are the same weeds of the sunflower family that most people try to banish from their lawns. But it's true. Still, there's an important difference. The dandelion greens you buy in the market have been cultivated to be more tender than the wild variety.

Health Benefits

Even more so than other greens, dandelion greens are high in vitamin A in the form of the disease-fighting nutrient beta-carotene. They are also a good source of calcium and of vitamin C. If you eat a larger serving of greens than the example listed in the nutritional information, say one cup, you also get a healthy dose of iron and the B vitamins thiamin and riboflavin.

```
NUTRIENT INFORMATION
Dandelion Greens, cooked          Sodium           23 mg
Serving Size:        ½ cup
Calories             72           Vitamin A        6,084 IU
Protein              1.0 g
Carbohydrate         3.3 g        Calcium          73 mg
Fat                  0.3 g        Iron             0.9 mg
  Saturated          0
Cholesterol          0
Dietary Fiber        0.7 g
```

Selection and Storage

Look for greens that are kept chilled in the market. They can wilt and develop a bitter taste if left at warmer temperatures. Choose the smallest leaf greens you can find. They are usually the most tender. Dandelion greens should have their roots still attached.

To store them, wrap dandelion greens in damp paper towels and put them in a plastic bag; they should keep for three to five days. However, dandelion greens may not keep as well as hardier greens such as collards.

Dandelion greens are available year-round but are usually best in the spring. Look for tender greens that have been picked before the yellow flower develops. Dandelions become bitter with age. Use the greens as quickly as possible for the best flavor.

Before you decide to pick wild dandelion leaves, be sure that they have not been treated with chemicals such as weed killers or fungicides. And be aware that they will probably not have the more delicate taste or texture of those you would buy from the market.

Preparation and Serving Tips

When you're ready to cook them or serve them up in a salad, be sure to wash them well since most greens have sand and dirt still clinging to leaves. Dry the greens well in paper towels if you're going to serve them in a salad. You can leave them damp if you're going to cook them.

The small dandelion greens are likely to require less cooking time than the larger-leaf collard greens. Steaming may be enough to cook dandelion greens tender; it can take anywhere from two to fifteen minutes. As with other greens, dandelion greens cook down a great deal. One pound of raw yields only about ½ cup cooked greens.

Dandelion greens are good in salad with warm vinaigrette dressing; they also work well in soups and stuffings.

ITALIAN TOMATO AND DANDELION GREENS SOUP

  2 **cans (14½ ounces each) no-salt-added stewed tomatoes, undrained**
  1 **cup loose-pack frozen zucchini, carrots, cauliflower, lima beans and Italian beans**
  1 **cup low sodium tomato juice**
  1 **cup water**
  1 **tablespoon onion powder**
  1 **teaspoon sugar**
  1 **teaspoon dried oregano leaves, crushed**
  ½ **teaspoon dried basil leaves, crushed**
  ¼ **teaspoon garlic powder**
  ¼ **teaspoon pepper**
  2 **cups packed torn stemmed washed dandelion greens**
  ¼ **cup grated Parmesan cheese**

Combine stewed tomatoes and juice, frozen vegetables, tomato juice, water, onion powder, sugar, oregano, basil, garlic powder and pepper in large saucepan. Bring to a boil over high heat. Reduce heat to low. Simmer, covered, 4 to 5 minutes or until vegetables are tender, stirring occasionally.

Stir in dandelion greens. Cook about 1 minute or until greens wilt. Top each serving with Parmesan cheese.

Makes 4 servings

NUTRIENTS PER SERVING:

Calories	135.3	Riboflavin (B₂)	0.25 mg
Protein	7.2 g	Sodium	178 mg
Carbohydrate	23.61 g	Thiamin (B₁)	0.26 mg
Dietary Fiber	5.88 g	Vitamin A	729.5 RE
Fat	3.1 g	Vitamin C	82.97 mg
Saturated Fat	1.37 g		
Poly Fat	0.57 g	DIETARY EXCHANGES	
Mono Fat	0.7 g	Veg: 3	Bread: 0.5
Cholesterol	4.94 mg	Fat: 0.5	
Sugar	11.24 g		
Beta-Carotene	396.5 µg	% OF CALORIES FROM:	
Calcium	179.3 mg	PRO: 19%	CARB: 63%
Folate	60.85 µg	FAT: 18%	
Iron	3 mg		

DATES

Dates are among the most ancient of fruits. There is evidence that date palms grew in Egypt along the Nile during the fifth century B.C. Most of the world's dates are still grown in the Middle East, but they are also grown here in the United States in California and Arizona.

Health Benefits

Dates are an excellent source of fiber and potassium and several important vitamins and minerals. Though they provide more calories than most fruits because of their high natural sugar content, they are fat-free.

Selection and Storage

Though dates are usually harvested only in late fall and early winter, they are generally available year-round. They are sold in both fresh and dried varieties. Fresh dates are easy to find in most supermarkets, but you may have to make a trip to the local health food store to find dried dates. Whether you buy fresh or dried dates, look for plump fruit with unbroken, smoothly wrinkled skin. Don't buy dates that smell bad or have hardened sugar crystals on the skin.

Packaged dates are available in pitted, unpitted, or chopped forms. Dried dates may keep for up to a year in the refrigerator. Fresh dates should be refrigerated in tightly sealed containers, where they will keep for up to eight months. If you keep them in the kitchen cabinet, however, they will stay fresh for only about a month.

If dates dry out during storage, they can be "plumped" by soaking them in a little warm water, fruit juice, or, for fancier dishes, your favorite liqueur. Don't store dates near strongly flavored items such as garlic or onions; the dates tend to absorb outside odors.

NUTRIENT INFORMATION			
Dates, dried		Niacin	1.8 mg
Serving Size: 10 dates		Pantothenic Acid	0.6 mg
Calories	228	Vitamin (B₆)	0.2 mg
Protein	1.6 g		
Carbohydrate	61 g	Calcium	27 mg
Fat	0.4 g	Copper	0.2 mg
Saturated	na	Iron	1.0 mg
Cholesterol	0	Magnesium	29 mg
Dietary Fiber	6.4 g	Manganese	0.2 mg
Sodium	2 mg	Potassium	541 mg

Preparation and Serving Tips

Dates are great to eat out of hand, but they can also be made extra special if you stuff them with tasty fillers. Try filling dates with whole almonds or pieces of walnuts or pecans. Or for a spicy twist, slide in a piece of crystallized ginger.

Adding dates to home-baked breads, cakes, muffins, and cookies adds a richness and nutrition to otherwise ordinary recipes. And the natural moisture of dates adds to the quality of the final product.

Dates are also great in fruit compotes, salads, and fruity desserts. Chopped or slivered dates work well when they are sprinkled on side dishes such as rice, couscous, or even your favorite vegetables.

To slice or chop dates for recipes, be sure to chill them in the refrigerator before hand. The colder they are the easier they will be to slice.

DATE GINGERBREAD

1¼ cups plus 1 teaspoon all-purpose flour, divided
¾ cup finely chopped pitted dates (about 18 whole dates)
½ cup whole wheat flour
¼ cup packed brown sugar
1 tablespoon (½ ounce) finely chopped candied ginger
½ teaspoon baking powder
½ teaspoon baking soda
½ teaspoon ground ginger
½ teaspoon ground nutmeg
½ cup water
½ cup molasses
¼ cup canola or vegetable oil
2 egg whites
   Orange slices for garnish

Preheat oven to 350°F. Coat 8-inch round baking pan with nonstick cooking spray. Dust with 1 teaspoon flour; set aside.

Combine remaining 1¼ cups all-purpose flour, dates, whole wheat flour, sugar, candied ginger, baking powder, baking soda, ground ginger and nutmeg in large bowl. Add water, molasses, oil and egg whites. Beat with electric mixer at low speed until combined. Increase speed to high; beat 2 minutes. Pour into prepared pan.

Bake 38 to 40 minutes or until wooden toothpick inserted near center comes out clean. Cool in pan on wire rack 10 minutes. Cut into wedges and serve warm. Garnish with orange slices.   ***Makes 8 servings***

NUTRIENTS PER SERVING:			
Calories	283	Magnesium	23.25 mg
Protein	4.27 g	Niacin (B₃)	2.44 mg
Carbohydrate	52.25 g	Potassium	798.2 mg
Dietary Fiber	2.95 g	Sodium	108.9 mg
Fat	7.28 g	Vitamin K	58.88 µg
Saturated Fat	0.58 g		
Poly Fat	2.2 g	DIETARY EXCHANGES:	
Mono Fat	4.07 g	Fruit: 2	Bread: 1.5
Cholesterol	0 mg	Fat: 1.5	
Sugar	17.36 g		
Calcium	161.3 mg	% OF CALORIES FROM:	
Folate	10.76 µg	PRO: 6%	CARB: 72%
Iron	4.99 mg	FAT: 22%	

FIGS

Along with dates, figs are one of our most ancient fruits, dating back to the ancient Egyptians. Today, figs are one of the sweetest fruits around. About 60 percent of the carbohydrate in figs is in the form of sugar. Most of the figs in this country are grown in California and then distributed nationally. But figs have an incredibly short shelf life. Once harvested, they will last only about one week. Black Mission figs are the most commonly seen variety, but Kadota and Calimyrna, which have greenish-yellow skins, are widely available as well. The different varieties are generally available fresh from June to September; dried figs are available year-round.

Health Benefits

A Roman author once claimed that figs "increase the strength of young people, preserve the elderly in better health and make them look younger with fewer wrinkles." Today, we know that while they are no cure-all, figs are healthy, nutritious foods. Figs, especially dried figs, are good sources of potassium, calcium, magnesium, and the B vitamin niacin. If you eat enough of them, figs can have a natural laxative effect.

NUTRIENT INFORMATION			
Figs, fresh		Sodium	2 mg
Serving Size: 2 large			
Calories	94	Niacin	0.5 mg
Protein	1.0 g		
Carbohydrate	24.6 g	Calcium	44 mg
Fat	0.4 g	Magnesium	22 mg
Saturated	0.06 g	Potassium	296 mg
Cholesterol	0		
Dietary Fiber	1.5 g		

Selection and Storage

Whatever variety you buy, look for figs that are soft, but not mushy, to the touch. Color is not the best indicator of ripeness. If a fresh fig smells bad, it is bad. Put fresh figs in the refrigerator and use them as soon as possible. If figs are not yet ripe, you can ripen them by simply leaving them out of the refrigerator away from direct heat.

When you buy dried figs, be sure the package is tightly sealed, and check for freshness by pressing slightly through the packaging. If the fig gives a little, it's fresh. Dried figs should not be rock hard. You can use dried figs straight out of the package. Once you open the package, be sure to rewrap it well. Otherwise, the figs will become dry and hard. If wrapped well, they can keep for several months.

Preparation and Serving Tips

Fresh figs are great just to peel and eat. Dried figs make welcome additions to bread, muffins, coffee cakes, and cookies. As with dates, dried figs will slice easier if you place them in the refrigerator or freezer beforehand.

Chopped, dried figs can be added to cottage cheese or light cream cheese and used as a spread for crackers or as a dip for crudités. Dried figs can be substituted in any recipe that calls for another type of dried fruit. And chopped dried figs work well sprinkled on hot cereal.

FIG PAVLOVA

2 egg whites
1 teaspoon white vinegar
½ cup sugar
1½ cups sliced fresh figs (about 8 medium)
1 cup sliced strawberries
½ cup vanilla low fat yogurt
⅓ cup thawed frozen reduced fat nondairy whipped topping
¼ teaspoon grated orange peel

For meringue shells, preheat oven to 300°F. Line baking sheet with foil. Draw six 3-inch circles on foil.

Combine egg whites and vinegar in small bowl. Beat with electric mixer on medium speed until mixture forms soft peaks. Gradually add sugar, beating on high speed until mixture is stiff and glossy. Spread over circles on foil, building up sides.

NUTRIENTS PER SERVING:

Calories	151.6	Magnesium	17.43 mg
Protein	2.66 g	Niacin (B₃)	0.35 mg
Carbohydrate	35.21 g	Potassium	249.7 mg
Dietary Fiber	4.98 g	Vitamin C	15.66 mg
Fat	1.38 g		
Saturated Fat	0.18 g	DIETARY EXCHANGES:	
Poly Fat	0.15 g	Milk: 0.5	Fruit: 2
Mono Fat	0.11 g		
Cholesterol	0.83 mg	% OF CALORIES FROM:	
Sugar	24.73 g	PRO: 6%	CARB: 86%
Calcium	57.09 mg	FAT: 8%	
Folate	10.51 µg		

Bake 35 minutes. Turn off oven; let shells dry in oven with door closed at least 1 hour. Remove from foil.

Just before serving, spoon figs and strawberries into shells. Combine yogurt, whipped topping and orange peel in small bowl. Spoon over fruit. _Makes 6 servings_

FISH

Fish makes a fabulous addition to any healthy diet. Its generally low fat content (many types of fish provide 20 percent or less of calories from fat) makes it a perfect protein substitute for fatty cuts of beef.

Health Benefits

The fat that fish does contain, known as omega-3 fatty acids, is thought to offer superb health benefits such as aiding in the prevention of heart disease and cancer, treating psoriasis and arthritis, and relieving the agony of migraine headaches.

Fortunately, you don't have to buy fresh fish to get the health benefits that omega-3 fatty acids offer. Canned fish, including tuna, sardines, and salmon, offer the same omega-3s as the fresh varieties. Fatty fish tend to have more omega-3s than do leaner fish.

But fish has also been dogged by safety questions. Pesticides, mercury, and chemicals like PCB sometimes find their way into fish, sometimes making it a not-so-healthy choice after all. Fattier fish, for example, is richer in omega-3s, but it's also more likely to have a greater amount of environmental contaminants. Still, there are precautions you can take to reduce the risk of eating contaminated fish.

• Eat fish from a variety of sources.

• Whenever possible, choose open ocean fish and farmed fish over freshwater fish; they are less likely to harbor toxins.

• Eat smaller, young fish. Older fish are more likely to have accumulated chemicals in their fat.

• Before you fish, check your own state's advisories about which waters are unsafe to fish. Try the Department of Public Health or the Department of Environment Conservation.

• Don't make a habit of eating the fish you catch for sport if you fish in the same area over and over again.

• Avoid swordfish; it may be contaminated with mercury.

NUTRIENT INFORMATION

Coho Salmon, cooked Serving Size: 3 oz		Snapper, cooked Serving Size: 3 oz	
Calories	157	Calories	109
Protein	23.3 g	Protein	22.4 g
Carbohydrate	0	Carbohydrate	0
Fat	6.4 g	Fat	1.5 g
Saturated	1.2 g	Saturated	0.3 g
Cholesterol	42 mg	Cholesterol	40 mg
Dietary Fiber	0	Dietary Fiber	0
Sodium	50 mg	Sodium	48 mg
		Magnesium	31 mg
Potassium	454 mg	Potassium	444 mg

Selection and Storage

Fish doesn't stay fresh for long. In fact, fatty fish such as bluefish, tuna, salmon, mackerel, or herring lasts only about a week after leaving the water; lean fish such as cod, haddock, or perch, about ten days—if handled properly during that time. To be sure the fish you buy is fresh, check for a "fishy" smell. If you detect one, don't buy it. Whether you buy whole fish, fish fillets, or steaks, the fish should be firm, not soft, to the touch. The scales should be shiny and clean, not slimy. Check the eyes; they should be clear, not cloudy, and should be bulging, not sunken. Fish fillets and steaks should be moist. Steer clear if they look dried or curled around the edges.

If you buy whole fish, you'll need about twice as much weight per serving as you would for fillets or steaks.

It's best to cook fresh fish the same day you buy it. (Fish generally spoils faster than beef or chicken, and whole fish generally keeps better than steaks or fillets.) But it will keep in the refrigerator overnight if you place it in a plastic bag over a bowl of ice. If you need to keep it longer, freeze it. The quality of the fish is better retained if the fish is frozen quickly, so freeze fish whole only if it weighs two pounds or less. Larger fish should be cut into pieces, steaks, or fillets. Lean fish will keep in the freezer up to six months; fatty fish, only about three months.

Preparation and Serving Tips

For the uninitiated, fish may be the most perplexing of foods to prepare. But low-fat fish preparation is simple. The key to juiciness and flavor lies in taking advantage of fish's natural fat and juices. The number one rule: Preserve moistness. In practical terms, that means avoiding direct heat, especially when preparing low-fat varieties of fish. You'll get the best results with lean fish, including flounder, monkfish, pike, and red snapper, if you use moist-heat methods such as poaching, steaming, or baking with vegetables or a sauce that holds moisture in. Dry-heat methods, such as baking, broiling, and grilling, work well for fattier fish.

Fish cooks fast. That means that it can overcook quickly. You can tell fish is done when it looks opaque and the flesh just begins to flake with the touch of a fork. If it falls apart when you touch it, it's too late; the fish is overdone. The general rule of thumb for cooking fish is to cook ten minutes per inch of thickness, measured at the fish's thickest point.

Marinades do wonders for fish. But as with poultry, keep safety in mind. Never marinate at room temperature; only in the refrigerator. And never use the marinade as a sauce for prepared fish unless you boil the marinade first.

Citrus juices work well to enhance fish's natural flavor without overwhelming them. Lemon, lime, or orange juice complement almost any kind of fish. Garnish the fish with lemon, lime, or orange wedges. Flavored vinegars with a touch of flavored oil also complement the delicate flavor of fish. Some favorite fish seasonings include dill, tarragon, basil, paprika, parsley, and thyme; season to taste.

For fish soups, stews, and chowders, use leaner fish. An oily fish will overpower the flavor of the broth.

Chunks of lean cooked fish add a new twist to pasta salads. For a colorful presentation, serve an herb-broiled fillet on a bed of Boston lettuce and radicchio. Drizzle with a warm citrus-flavored vinaigrette.

POACHED SALMON WITH TARRAGON SAUCE

- 1 **cup defatted low sodium chicken broth**✻
- ¼ **cup lemon juice**
- 1 **bay leaf**
- ⅛ **teaspoon pepper**
- 4 **fresh or thawed frozen pink salmon steaks (5 ounces each), cut ¾ inch thick**
- ⅓ **cup plain nonfat yogurt**
- ¼ **cup fat free mayonnaise**
- 2 **tablespoons thinly sliced green onion**
- 2 **tablespoons chopped parsley**
- 1 **teaspoon chopped fresh tarragon** *or* **¼ teaspoon dried tarragon leaves, crushed**

Combine chicken broth, lemon juice, bay leaf and pepper in large skillet. Bring to a boil over high heat. Carefully place salmon steaks in skillet; return to a boil. Immediately reduce heat to medium-low. Simmer, covered, 8 to 10 minutes or until salmon begins to flake when tested with a fork. Remove salmon from skillet.

Meanwhile, combine yogurt, mayonnaise, green onion, parsley and tarragon in small bowl. Refrigerate covered until ready to serve. Spoon the sauce over the salmon. Salmon may be served chilled.

Makes 4 servings

* To defat chicken broth, skim fat from surface of broth with spoon. Or, place can of broth in refrigerator at least 2 hours ahead of time. Before using, remove fat that has hardened on surface of broth.

NUTRIENTS PER SERVING:

Calories	232.7	Copper	0.34 mg
Protein	24.84 g	Folate	17.63 µg
Carbohydrate	19.52 g	Iron	64.35 mg
Dietary Fiber	0.12 g	Potassium	359.5 mg
Fat	5.94 g	Sodium	526.7 mg
Saturated Fat	1.22 g		
Poly Fat	1.28 g	DIETARY EXCHANGES:	
Mono Fat	2.56 g	Bread: 1.5	Meat: 3
Cholesterol	25.75 mg		
Sugar	1.41 g	% OF CALORIES FROM:	
Calcium	76.56 mg	PRO: 43%	CARB: 34%
Cobalamin (B$_{12}$)	3.72 µg	FAT: 23%	

GAME

The spoils of hunting, such as deer, quail, or rabbit, are usually referred to as game. Today, you're likely to find a huge selection of game—more than 400 varieties—in specialty and gourmet shops and even in a growing number of adventurous restaurants. If you hunt it yourself, the availability is, of course, seasonal. But if you purchase it from a store or order it in a restaurant, it is usually available year-round. You can choose from alligator, antelope, bison, elk, bear, boar, and buffalo, just to name a few. Some shops even offer mail-order game so you don't even have to step outdoors to try it.

Game meat can taste, well, gamey. So it may be an acquired taste for you. But because most of it is considerably lower in fat than beef or pork, you might want to give it a try. Just keep in mind that game usually carries a premium price tag.

Health Benefits

Game meat's remarkably low fat content is its chief health benefit. While lean cuts of beef usually provide about 30 percent of calories from fat, most game meats provide less than 15 percent of calories from fat.

NUTRIENT INFORMATION			
Deer, roasted			
Serving Size: 3 oz		Niacin	5.7 mg
Calories	134	Riboflavin	0.5 mg
Protein	25.7 g	Thiamin	0.2 mg
Carbohydrate	0		
Fat	2.7 g	Iron	3.8 mg
Saturated	1.1 g	Magnesium	20 mg
Cholesterol	95 mg		
Dietary Fiber	0 g	Phosphorus	192 mg
Sodium	46 mg	Potassium	285 mg
		Zinc	2.3 mg

Selection and Storage

Basically, the same rules apply for game meats as they do for beef and pork. Chances are, the game you buy will be frozen. Freshness is key. If it looks freezer burned or has frozen liquid in the package, don't accept it. It is either old or has been thawed and refrozen.

As with other meats, keep game meat frozen at zero degrees Fahrenheit. Fresh game will keep in the refrigerator for one or two days.

Preparation and Serving Tips

Before you prepare your game, be sure to cut away any visible fat. Besides lowering the fat content further, it will decrease the meat's "gamey" flavor.

Game meats need a little extra care in preparation because they are so lean. If you bring home your own game from the woods, it will be leaner and probably a bit tougher than if you buy game that is farm raised—what you'll most likely find in markets that sell game. But farm-raised game is still lower in fat than most lean beef.

Game meats dry out quickly during cooking and they tend to be chewy even when prepared properly, so moist-heat methods such as braising tend to work best. Marinades will also help keep game meats tender. Game fits especially well in stews and chilis, but it can be substituted for beef, pork, and poultry in an endless number of recipes.

VENISON STEAKS WITH BLUEBERRY SAUCE

12 ounces lean boneless sirloin-cut venison steaks
 1 cup onion slices
 ½ cup carrot slices
 2 shallots, chopped
 ¼ cup defatted low sodium beef broth✻
 ¼ cup red wine vinegar
 1 tablespoon olive oil
 1 teaspoon rubbed sage
 ½ teaspoon coarsely ground black pepper
   Savory Blueberry Sauce (recipe follows)

Place venison, onion, carrots and shallots in medium bowl. Combine beef broth, vinegar, oil, sage and pepper in small bowl; pour over steaks and vegetables. Refrigerate, covered, 8 hours or overnight.

Drain steaks; reserve marinade for sauce. Prepare Savory Blueberry Sauce.

Broil or grill steaks to desired degree of doneness. Serve with Savory Blueberry Sauce. *Makes 4 servings*

✻ To defat beef broth, skim fat from surface of broth with spoon. Or, place can of broth in refrigerator at least 2 hours ahead of time. Before using, remove fat that has hardened on surface of broth.

SAVORY BLUEBERRY SAUCE

½ cup reserved marinade from venison steaks
2 cups fresh *or* frozen blueberries
2 tablespoons packed brown sugar
¼ teaspoon rubbed sage
2 tablespoons red wine vinegar
   Dash pepper

Bring marinade to a boil in medium skillet over medium-high heat. Reduce heat to low. Simmer, uncovered, 10 minutes. Strain liquid; discard solids. Return liquid to skillet; bring to a boil over medium heat. Boil until liquid is reduced by half.

Stir in blueberries, sugar and sage; simmer 5 minutes or until heated through. (Blueberries will retain their shape.) Stir in vinegar and pepper. ***Makes 1½ cups***

NUTRIENTS PER SERVING:			
Calories	223.4	Niacin (B₃)	5.33 mg
Protein	20.07 g	Potassium	482.6 mg
Carbohydrate	25.54 g	Riboflavin (B₂)	0.24 mg
Dietary Fiber	3.26 g	Sodium	62.63 mg
Fat	5.27 g	Thiamin (B₁)	0.32 mg
Saturated Fat	2.37 g	Vitamin C	15.36 mg
Poly Fat	2.11 g	Zinc	4.11 mg
Mono Fat	3.54 g		
Cholesterol	69.93 mg	DIETARY EXCHANGES:	
Sugar	14.51 g	Veg: 2	Fruit: 1
Beta-Carotene	5,066 RE	Meat: 2	
Calcium	46.3 mg		
Iron	3.14 mg	% OF CALORIES FROM:	
Magnesium	33.88 mg	PRO: 35%	CARB: 44%
		FAT: 21%	

GARLIC

Through the centuries, garlic has been both reviled and revered for its flavor and medicinal qualities. Today, the gossip about garlic, focusing on its apparent disease-preventing qualities, has reached a fevered pitch. For garlic lovers, that's good news. For those who can do without the pungent odor garlic leaves behind, there are some things you can do to lessen its aromatic effect while still getting the many health benefits of this cloven wonder.

Health Benefits

The list just seems to grow and grow. From preventing heart disease and cancer to fighting off infections, researchers are finding encouraging results with garlic. Behind all the grandiose claims for garlic are the compounds that give it its biting flavor. The chief health-promoting chemical is allicin, a sulphur-containing compound. The biggest question surrounding allicin is whether its purported disease-preventing abilities remain intact once it is cooked. No one really knows for sure. But it's believed that at least some of the health benefits linger after cooking.

Garlic has been found to lower levels of low-density lipoproteins (LDLs), the "bad" cholesterol, and raise high-density lipoproteins (HDLs), the "good" cholesterol. It may also help to dissolve clots that sometimes get stuck in narrowed arteries, triggering heart attacks and strokes.

Garlic has also been found to inhibit the growth of or kill several kinds of bacteria, including *staphylococcus* and *salmonella*, and many fungi and yeast.

Studies in animals have found that garlic helps prevent colon, lung, and esophageal cancers. How much is enough? No one knows. In many studies, garlic extracts have been used, making it impossible to translate that into a garlic prescription for better health.

What about garlic supplements? Most experts say that such supplements are an unnecessary expense. It's not even known for sure if the healthy compounds fresh garlic contains remain intact in the pill form.

```
NUTRIENT INFORMATION
Garlic                           Cholesterol      0
Serving Size: 3 cloves           Dietary Fiber    0.14 g
Calories           13            Sodium           2 mg
Protein            0.6 g
Carbohydrate       3.0 g
Fat                0.1 g
   Saturated       0
```

Selection and Storage

There's really little difference among varieties of garlic. Most varieties of garlic have the same characteristic pungent odor and bite. But generally, pink-skinned garlic tastes a little sweeter and keeps longer than white garlic. Elephant garlic, a large-clove garlic, is milder in flavor than regular white garlic. Most varieties can be used interchangeably in recipes.

You can find garlic that's sold loose or in cellophane-wrapped boxes. Opt for loose garlic if you can. It's easier to know the quality of the garlic you're getting. Look for garlic that is firm to the touch and has no visible damp or brown spots. Garlic that gives when you touch it has probably turned to dust.

Don't expect the same flavor from garlic powders and salts that you get from fresh garlic. Much of the flavor has been processed out. And garlic salt contains large amounts of sodium—as much as 900 milligrams per teaspoon.

Garlic may keep anywhere from a few weeks to a few months, depending on its age and how you store it once you get it home. Try keeping it in a cool, dark, dry spot. You can find special terra cotta garlic holders at gourmet shops, but you can do just as well storing it under a small overturned clay pot.

If you don't use garlic regularly, check on your stored garlic occasionally to make sure it's still in good shape. If one or two cloves have gone bad, remove them, being careful not to nick the remaining cloves. Any cuts into the skin will hasten the demise of the garlic that's left. If it begins to sprout, it's OK to use, but the garlic may have a milder flavor.

Garlic-in-oil blends taste great—but beware. When you drop cloves of garlic into a bottle of oil, you're creating the perfect environment for the deadly *clostridium botulinum* bacteria to flourish. Garlic sometimes carries the bacterial spores from the soil. If you then bottle garlic in oil, an oxygen-free environment, you've created the right conditions for the bacteria to multiply. Either buy commercial garlic-in-oil preparations that contain antibacterial agents such as citric or phosphoric acids or make your own fresh for each use.

Preparation and Serving Tips

There are a few rules of thumb to follow for managing garlic's flavor: Garlic pressed through a garlic press is as much as ten times stronger in flavor than garlic minced with a knife, so use pressed garlic when you want the garlic flavor to come through full force; use minced when you want to curtail it; and use whole cloves cooked slowly for a hint of garlic flavor. The longer garlic is cooked, the more flavor it will lose. So add garlic early for more flavor; later for less flavor.

For a hint of garlic in salads, rub the salad bowl with a cut clove or crushed cloves before adding salad. For even more flavor, add a few sprinkles of freshly crushed garlic.

You can make your own fat-free garlic bread by warming a loaf of bread, slicing it, then spreading the inside with a fresh cut clove of garlic. Toast the loaf under the broiler. You'll get a teaser of garlic without all the fat of traditional garlic bread.

To deal with the aftereffects of garlic, try chewing on fresh parsley, fresh mint, or citrus peel to help mask the aroma. This doesn't work for everybody, but it just might help you.

GRAPEFRUIT

Just thinking about biting into a grapefruit can get your salivary glands working overtime. Grapefruit is a tart-tasting fruit that not everyone enjoys. But for those who do, grapefruit offers a lot of good nutrition for very few calories. It's traditionally thought of as a breakfast food, but it can just as easily be eaten out of hand, anytime of the day.

Health Benefits

Grapefruit is an excellent source of vitamin C. Pink and red grapefruit are good sources of disease-fighting beta-carotene and its lesser-known carotenoid cousins. And if you peel and eat a grapefruit like you would an orange, you get a good dose of cholesterol-lowering pectin. As a member of the citrus family, it is also a storehouse of phytochemicals such as flavonoids, terpenes, and limonoids. These naturally occurring chemicals are believed to have cancer-preventing properties.

Despite its reputation as a "fat-burner," grapefruit has no special ability to burn away excess fat. Its only role in weight reduction is that it can fill you up and provide nutrients for only a few calories.

NUTRIENT INFORMATION			
Grapefruit, pink or red		Sodium	0
Serving Size: ½ fruit			
Calories	37	Vitamin A	318 IU
Protein	0.7 g	Niacin	0.2 mg
Carbohydrate	9.5 g	Vitamin C	46.8 mg
Fat	0.1 g		
Saturated	0	Potassium	158 mg
Cholesterol	0 mg		
Dietary Fiber	1.6 g		

Selection and Storage

You don't have to worry about whether the grapefruit you buy is ripe, because grapefruit isn't picked unless it's fully ripe. However, you should look for ones that are heavy for their size; they're the juiciest. Avoid those that are soft or mushy or those that are oblong, rather than round. They are generally of poorer quality, possibly pithy and less sweet. Though the peak season for grapefruit is considered to be January through June, it is available throughout the year.

There is no difference in taste among white, red, and pink varieties of grapefruit. They are equally sweet (and equally tart).

Unlike other foods that are best kept in the coldest part of the refrigerator, grapefruit keeps best in the warmest part of your refrigerator, usually the vegetable crisper. Here, they should keep for up to two months.

Preparation and Serving Tips

Wash grapefruit before you cut it to prevent bacteria on the outside from being introduced inside. Try bringing grapefruit to room temperature before you juice or slice it.

If you peel and separate into segments, try dipping the segments into something sweet like honey or yogurt. Or for something a little different, try sprinkling a little brown sugar on a grapefruit half and sticking it under the broiler until it bubbles. Try substituting grapefruit juice for orange or lemon in a citrus vinaigrette dressing recipe.

SPICY GRAPEFRUIT SALAD WITH RASPBERRY DRESSING

- 2 **cups washed watercress**
- 2 **cups washed mixed salad greens**
- 3 **medium grapefruit, peeled, sectioned, seeded**
- ½ **pound jícama, cut into julienne strips**
- 1 **cup fresh *or* frozen thawed raspberries**
- 2 **tablespoons chopped green onion**
- 1 **teaspoon balsamic vinegar**
- 1 **tablespoon honey**
- ½ **to ¾ teaspoon dry mustard**

Combine watercress and salad greens; divide between 4 salad plates. Arrange grapefruit and jícama on top of greens.

Reserve 12 raspberries for garnish. For dressing, combine remaining raspberries, green onion, vinegar, honey and mustard in food processor or blender; process until smooth. Drizzle dressing over salads; garnish with reserved raspberries.

Makes 4 servings

NUTRIENTS PER SERVING:			
Calories	113.2	Iron	1.58 mg
Protein	3 g	Magnesium	36.4 mg
Carbohydrate	26.45 g	Potassium	541.1 mg
Dietary Fiber	5.07 g	Sodium	15.79 mg
Fat	0.65 g	Vitamin C	99.31 mg
Saturated Fat	0.05 g	Vitamin K	91.85 µg
Poly Fat	0.22 g	Zinc	0.48 mg
Mono Fat	0.05 g		
Cholesterol	0	DIETARY EXCHANGES:	
Sugar	18.63 g	Veg: 1	Fruit: 1.5
Beta-Carotene	963.9 RE		
Calcium	76.71 mg	% OF CALORIES FROM:	
Folate	85.37 µg	PRO: 10%	CARB: 86%
		FAT: 5%	

GRAPES

Grapes are one of the oldest cultivated fruits in existence today, dating back as far as 4000 B.C. They are unique in that they grow on vines that sprawl along the ground for a distance of up to fifty feet. Most of the grapes in this country come from California. This small fruit is especially popular among kids (but be sure to peel and/or slice them for young children to avoid choking).

Health Benefits

Grapes may not be packed with the nutrients you're most familiar with, but they do contain a collection of phytochemicals that researchers are just beginning to realize the importance of. Among them is ellagic acid, a chemical also found in strawberries, which is thought to possess cancer-preventing properties. Grapes also contain boron, a mineral that is believed to play a role—along with calcium, magnesium, and phosphorus—in preventing the bone-destroying disease, osteoporosis.

Selection and Storage

Though the peak season for the most popular variety, Thompson seedless, is June through November, there is some variety of grape available twelve months of the year. Grapes become sweet as they ripen on the vine, but once harvested, they will not ripen further. When you choose grapes, look for clusters with plump, well-colored fruit attached to pliable, green stems. Soft or wrinkled grapes or those with bleached areas around the stem are past their prime.

There are basically three categories of grapes: the greens, the reds, and the blue/blacks. Good color is the key to good flavor. The sweetest green grapes are yellow-green in color; red varieties that are predominantly crimson/red will have the best flavor; and blue/black varieties taste best if their color is deep and rich, almost black. If you object to seeds, then look for one of the seedless varieties.

Store unwashed grapes in the refrigerator. They can keep for up to a week.

NUTRIENT INFORMATION
Grapes, American
Serving Size: 20 grapes

Calories	30	Sodium	0
Protein	0.3 g	Vitamin B$_6$	1.8 mg
Carbohydrate	8.2 g		
Fat	0.2 g	Manganese	0.3 mg
Saturated	0	Potassium	92 mg
Cholesterol	0		
Dietary Fiber	0.36 g		

Preparation and Serving Tips

Just before you serve, rinse grape clusters and drain or pat them dry. Slight chilling enhances the flavor and texture of table grapes. In addition to eating grapes as a chilled snack straight from the bunch, you can also try fruit kabobs. Skewer grapes, banana slices (dipped in lemon), apple chunks, and pineapple cubes or any of your favorite fruit. Brush with a combination of honey, lemon, and ground nutmeg. Broil until warm.

Cold, sliced grapes taste great blended in with a low-fat yogurt. Or try frozen grapes for a change of pace. Experiment with recipes that call for grapes with poultry or fish. Or use grapes as a tasty garnish in place of parsley.

SAVORY GRAPE PILAF

    1 teaspoon olive oil
   ¼ cup vermicelli, broken into small pieces
  2¼ cups defatted low sodium chicken broth✻
    1 cup uncooked brown rice
   ¼ cup water
   ½ teaspoon dried oregano leaves, crushed
   ⅛ teaspoon pepper
    1 cup seedless grapes, cut into halves
    2 tablespoons minced green onion

Heat oil in medium nonstick saucepan over medium heat. Add vermicelli; cook and stir until browned. Add broth, rice, water, oregano and pepper; bring to a boil. Reduce heat to low. Simmer, covered, 30 to 40 minutes or until rice is tender.

NUTRIENTS PER SERVING:			
Calories	150.7	Magnesium	47.26 mg
Protein	3.4 g	Manganese	1.27 mg
Carbohydrate	30.1 g	Potassium	107.7 mg
Dietary Fiber	2.08 g	Sodium	96.18 mg
Fat	1.86 g		
Saturated Fat	0.31 g	DIETARY EXCHANGES:	
Poly Fat	0.41 g	Fruit: 0.5	Bread: 1.5
Mono Fat	0.88 g		
Cholesterol	0.01 mg	% OF CALORIES FROM:	
Sugar	2.67 g	PRO: 9%	CARB: 80%
Beta-Carotene	64.42 RE	FAT: 11%	
Calcium	16.56 mg		

Stir in grapes and green onion. Cover; let stand 5 minutes before serving.   *Makes 6 servings*

✻ To defat chicken broth, skim fat from surface of broth with spoon. Or, place can of broth in refrigerator at least 2 hours ahead of time. Before using, remove fat that has hardened on surface of broth.

HERBS AND SPICES

This is a broad category that is hard to nail down. There are dozens upon dozens of herbs and spices available, from the more pedestrian black pepper to the more exotic turmeric or cardamom. But there is one uniting factor; they all add flavor and aroma to the food you prepare. Using the right blend of these taste enhancers can literally make or break a dish. That's especially true for low-fat dishes, where flavor can sometimes be lacking.

The best advice about herbs and spices is simple: Use them. Too often, they are permanently relegated to attractively labeled bottles on kitchen spice racks. That's too bad, because by knowing just a little bit about spices, you can become a superior cook.

Health Benefits

Some herbs and spices are pretty good sources of nutrients such as vitamins A and C, and they're low in calories; none provide more than 15 calories per teaspoon, dried. Paprika, for example, is an excellent source of vitamin A, parsley is rich in vitamin C, cumin is a surprising source of iron, and caraway seeds even contribute a little calcium to your diet. But new research findings suggest that several herbs are also rich sources of antioxidants that possibly prevent the growth of cancer cells and protect delicate arteries from buildup of plaque. Among them: allspice, basil, clove, coriander, dill, fennel leaves, mint, nutmeg, parsley, rosemary, and sage.

Aside from their nutrient and antioxidant contents, there are any number of health claims made for individual herbs. Here are but a few: Mint relieves gas and nausea; cinnamon enhances insulin's activity; oregano has antiseptic properties; sage contains compounds that act as antibiotics; and thyme is said to relieve cramps.

Selection and Storage

In our opinion, fresh is best. But it's not always easy to find sources of fresh herbs and spices such as basil, tarragon, or oregano. You can sometimes find them through mail order, or you can grow your own herb garden. But when fresh isn't available, almost every supermarket has a spice section brimming with a wide assortment of herbs and spices for every possible need.

Buy fresh herbs only as you need them. When you get them home, wrap them in damp paper towels, place them in a plastic bag, and refrigerate them. They should last a few days in the refrigerator.

If you decide on dried herbs and spices, beware of some spice blends, such as lemon peppers; they are sometimes deceivingly high in sodium—a far cry from pure herbs and spices, which are virtually sodium-free. Store dried herbs in airtight containers, and they will keep for up to one year. Whole spices such as cloves or cinnamon will keep much longer. Bear in mind that the flavor of dried herbs tends to fade faster than that of dried spices.

Try making and storing your own favorite blends of herbs and spices, so you'll always have them on hand. A popular French combo of bay leaf, parsley, and thyme, for example, can be ground with mortar and pestle and put away. Or try an Italian blend of basil, marjoram, oregano, rosemary, savory, and thyme.

Preparation and Serving Tips

Becoming acquainted with herbs and spices is almost a must when you're committed to low-fat or low-sodium cooking. When you remove the fat and sodium, a lot of the flavor can go with them. That flavor can be replaced with herbs.

There are a few herbs that seem to work best as flavor replacers for salt. Among them: anise seed, basil, celery seed, clove, cumin, garlic, lemon peel, oregano, pepper, sage, and tarragon.

The "proper" seasoning of a dish really doesn't exist. Taste is a personal matter. Forget what anyone else says. If it tastes good to you, it is good. What burns the taste buds of one person may seem a tad bland to another. If you're a novice at using herbs and spices, start off using only one or two herbs per dish. If you're using fresh herbs, don't be shy. The flavors are often subtle, and it often takes more than you think to get a rich flavor.

With dried herbs and spices, however, a little often goes a long way, so use them judiciously. Start with only about ¼ to ⅓ teaspoon until you get a better "feel" for the amount you like in dishes. It usually takes about three times as much fresh herb as dried to get the same degree of flavor. To bring out the full flavor of dried herbs, try marinating them in oil, or heat them in a little oil before you add them to a recipe.

If you're cooking with fresh herbs, wait until the end of the cooking time to add them so they'll retain their delicate flavor. Dried herbs and spices, on the other hand, hold their flavor well even under intense heat.

Here are a few seasoning suggestions to get you started:

Beef: bay, chives, garlic, marjoram

Fruits: caraway, cinnamon, cloves, ginger, mint, parsley, tarragon

Lamb: garlic, marjoram, mint, oregano, paprika, rosemary, savory, sage

Pasta: basil, fennel, garlic, paprika, parsley, sage

Pork: coriander, cumin, ginger, sage, thyme

Potatoes: chives, garlic, paprika, parsley, rosemary

Poultry: garlic, oregano, rosemary, sage

Rice: cumin, marjoram, parsley, saffron, tarragon, thyme, turmeric

Salads: basil, chervil, chives, dillweed, marjoram, mint, parsley, tarragon

Seafood: chervil, dill, fennel, tarragon, parsley

Vegetables: basil, caraway, chives, dillweed, marjoram, mint, nutmeg, oregano, paprika, rosemary, savory, tarragon, thyme

KALE

Kale is one of the greens of the cruciferous vegetable family—and what a family it is! Brussels sprouts, cabbage, cauliflower, and collard greens are also members of this clan, which many researchers say can help ward off cancer if you eat a lot of them. Add to that kale's other nutritional attributes, and you have a nutrition standout.

Health Benefits

Though greens in general are nutritious foods, kale stands a head above the rest. Not only is it one of the best sources of vitamin A in the form of beta-carotene, that dynamic disease-fighter we keep talking about, it also provides several other important nutrients that you seldom find together in one nice, neat food package.

NUTRIENT INFORMATION			
Kale, cooked		Vitamin A	4,810 IU
Serving Size: ½ cup		Folic Acid	8.6 µg
Calories	21	Vitamin C	26.7 mg
Protein	1.2 g		
Carbohydrate	3.7 g	Calcium	47.0 mg
Fat	0.3 g	Magnesium	15.0 mg
Saturated	0	Potassium	148.0 mg
Cholesterol	0		
Sodium	15.0 mg		

Selection and Storage

If you're having a hard time distinguishing one green from another, kale is the one that looks like collards but is frilly around the edges, and it tends to be a darker color green (a hint as to why it's so high in vitamin A). It also has a stronger flavor and a somewhat coarser texture. The peak season for kale is generally January through April.

Kale's flavor also tends to become stronger the longer it is stored. So, unless you actually prefer the strong taste, you should use kale within a day or two of buying it. Wrap fresh kale in damp paper towels, and put it in a plastic bag until you're ready to use it.

As with other greens, kale keeps best when it's on ice. And the smaller the leaf, the more tender it is likely to be and the milder the flavor. Be sure to pick kale that is a vivid green color; avoid kale that is discolored or wilted.

Preparation and Serving Tips

Like all other greens, kale should be washed thoroughly before cooking. It's not uncommon for greens to still have dirt and sand in them when you bring them home from the market. You may have to repeat the rinsing process a few times to remove all of the grit.

Kale is a hearty variety of greens that stands up well during cooking. Just about any cooking method will do, but keep cooking time to a minimum to preserve nutrients and keep kale's strong odor from permeating the kitchen.

Try simmering the greens in a well-seasoned stock or broth, covered for 10 to 30 minutes, or until tender. Don't forget that most greens cook down a great deal. One pound of raw will probably yield only about ½ cup, cooked.

KALE SOUP

   4 cups defatted low sodium chicken broth✳
   4 cups chopped kale
   1 cup julienned fennel
   1 cup juiienned carrots
   ½ cup chopped onion
   ½ teaspoon thyme leaves, crushed
   ⅛ teaspoon pepper

Combine the defatted chicken broth, kale, fennel, carrots, onion, thyme and pepper in a stockpot; bring to a boil over

NUTRIENTS PER SERVING:			
Calories	64.35	Magnesium	22.82 mg
Protein	3.69 g	Potassium	327.2 mg
Carbohydrate	11.21 g	Sodium	89.79 mg
Dietary Fiber	4.19 g	Vitamin C	40.81 mg
Fat	0.89 g	Vitamin K	251.5 µg
Saturated Fat	0.07 g		
Poly Fat	0.21 g	DIETARY EXCHANGES:	
Mono Fat	0.04 g	Veg: 2.5	
Cholesterol	0 mg		
Sugar	4.32 g	% OF CALORIES FROM:	
Beta-Carotene	5,305 RE	PRO: 22%	CARB: 66%
Calcium	87.34 mg	FAT: 12%	
Folate	19.64 µg		

high heat. Reduce heat to low. Simmer, uncovered, for 10 minutes.

Makes 4 servings

＊ To defat chicken broth, skim fat from surface of broth with spoon. Or, place can of broth in refrigerator at least 2 hours ahead of time. Before using, remove fat that has hardened on surface of broth.

KIWIFRUIT

The funny-looking fruit in the fuzzy brown packaging hit this country by storm a few years back. Now it is almost as commonly seen in supermarkets as are apples and bananas. The kiwifruit is an import from New Zealand, though it's originally a native of China. Today it is grown in California.

Health Benefits

Kiwis carry a lot of nutrition in a small package. They're packed with vitamin C, potassium, and fiber, and they're a good source of magnesium as well.

Selection and Storage

Because New Zealand and California have opposite seasons, that means opposite harvest times. That translates into kiwis being available all year. Choose kiwis that are fairly firm but that give under slight pressure. Allow firm kiwis about a week to ripen at room temperature. Unripe kiwifruit can have a strong sour taste. Kiwis can keep for one to two weeks in the refrigerator. As with several other fruits, you can hasten the ripening process by placing kiwis in a paper bag. Try adding an apple or banana to the bag; ripening apples and bananas emit a gas that speeds up the ripening process of kiwis and other fruit.

Avoid kiwi that are soft or have dark areas of skin. That usually means they've been bruised or they are overripe.

NUTRIENT INFORMATION			
Kiwifruit		Vitamin C	74.6 mg
Serving Size: 1 medium			
Calories	46	Calcium	20.0 mg
Protein	0.8 g	Magnesium	23.0 mg
Carbohydrate	11.3 g	Potassium	252.0 mg
Fat	0.3 g		
Saturated	0		
Cholesterol	0		
Dietary Fiber	2.6 g		
Sodium	4.0 mg		

Preparation and Serving Tips

Kiwis are great for garnishes because they don't discolor when they are exposed to air. That's because they contain so much vitamin C; its antioxidant properties prevent oxygen from doing damage and turning the fruit brown. With its brilliant green color and its inner circle of tiny black seeds, sliced kiwi truly adds a finishing touch to salads, entrees, vegetables, and desserts such as cakes, puddings, and souffles. The delicate flavor of kiwi gets lost with cooking, however, so it's best used only as a topper for cooked dishes.

Kiwifruit go especially well with tropical fruits such as mangoes. But they work well in any fruit salad.

Kiwifruit contain an enzyme that makes a great meat tenderizer. You can cut a kiwi in half and rub it over meat, and it won't alter the flavor of the meat. However, this same enzyme makes it impossible for gelatin to set if you add kiwi to it (unless you first briefly heat the kiwi to destroy the enzyme).

If you prefer your kiwi whole, the skin is edible if you rub off the brown fuzz. But most people prefer to peel kiwifruit before eating. You can slice it or simply peel it and eat it whole. If it's ripe, the core is edible, too.

KIWIFRUIT ANGEL SHORTCAKE

- 4 kiwifruit
- 2 tablespoons honey
- 1 teaspoon grated orange peel
- 1 cup lemon nonfat yogurt
- ½ cup thawed frozen reduced fat nondairy whipped topping
- 4 slices angel food cake, cut 1 inch thick

Peel kiwifruit; cut into ¼-inch-thick slices. Combine kiwifruit, honey and orange peel; set aside. Combine yogurt and whipped topping until well blended. Place angel food cake on 4 dessert plates; top each slice with yogurt mixture and kiwifruit mixture. Serve immediately. *Makes 4 servings*

NUTRIENTS PER SERVING:			
Calories	289.4	Magnesium	29.03 mg
Protein	7.29 g	Potassium	448.6 mg
Carbohydrate	63.76 g	Sodium	184 mg
Dietary Fiber	2.66 g	Vitamin C	75.18 mg
Fat	2.46 g		
Saturated Fat	0	DIETARY EXCHANGES:	
Poly Fat	0	Fruit: 2	Bread: 2
Mono Fat	0	Fat: 0.5	
Cholesterol	1.87 mg		
Sugar	17.98 g	% OF CALORIES FROM:	
Calcium	160.5 mg	PRO: 10%	CARB: 83%
		FAT: 7%	

KOHLRABI

This member of the cabbage family may not be a household name, but it should be. A cross between a turnip and a cabbage, it is rich in some important nutrients, and its unique flavor makes it a great addition to traditional dishes. Unlike some other similar vegetables, it's the bulb, rather than the leaves, of kohlrabi that are usually prepared. The leaves can, however, be cooked and eaten as a cooking green.

While kohlrabi offers the same good nutrition as some other members of the cruciferous family, it tends to have a milder flavor. That's good news if you're not a fan of the hearty flavors (or smells) of cabbage, broccoli, or cauliflower.

Health Benefits

An often-untapped source of vitamin C, kohlrabi carries a double nutrition bonus because it's also a member of the cruciferous family of vegetables. Cancer researchers long ago discovered that people who regularly include cruciferous vegetables in their diets are less likely to suffer cancer than people who seldom have them at the table.

NUTRIENT INFORMATION			
Kohlrabi, cooked		Niacin	0.3 mg
Serving Size: ½ cup		Vitamin C	44.3 mg
Calories	24		
Protein	2.5 g	Calcium	20 mg
Carbohydrate	5.5 g	Potassium	279 mg
Fat	0.1 g		
Saturated	0		
Cholesterol	0		
Dietary Fiber	0.8 g		
Sodium	17 mg		

Selection and Storage

Kohlrabi is available mainly through the summer months. Look for smaller bulbs. Larger bulbs mean the kohlrabi is older and probably tougher. Remove the leaves and stems before you store it in a cold spot in the refrigerator.

If you plan on cooking the leaves as well, look for kohlrabi with small, fresh-looking leaves. Avoid them if they are wilted or discolored. When you remove them from the bulb, treat them as you would any other cooking green. Wash them well, wrap them in damp paper towels, place them in a plastic bag, and refrigerate. They should keep for four or five days.

Preparation and Serving Tips

The leaves should be attached when you buy kohlrabi, but you should cut off the leaves and stems and peel the bulb before you cook it or eat it raw. Sliced kohlrabi tastes great with a low-fat dip. And it is terrific in stir-fry dishes. Toss slices in the wok with snow peas, sprouts, onions, and mushrooms to really round out the meal.

If you want to try it alone, steam it. Steaming will help preserve the fragile vitamin C it contains. Though it releases the same familiar cabbage-like smell that other cruciferous vegetables do, it's not nearly as strong.

Kohlrabi is also perfect, sliced or cubed, in hearty vegetable soups or stews.

KOHLRABI WITH RED PEPPERS

    3 tablespoons cider vinegar
    3 tablespoons water
    2 teaspoons olive *or* canola oil
    1 tablespoon sugar
    1 clove garlic, minced
    ½ teaspoon dried tarragon leaves, crushed
    ⅛ teaspoon black pepper
    2 pounds kohlrabies, peeled, sliced
    ¾ cup sliced red bell pepper
    ½ cup sliced onion

Bring vinegar, water, oil, sugar, garlic, tarragon and black pepper to a boil in large skillet over high heat. Add kohlrabies, bell pepper and onion; reduce heat to low. Simmer, covered, about 20 minutes or until kohlrabies are crisp-tender, stirring occasionally. *Makes 4 servings*

NUTRIENTS PER SERVING:

Calories	76.25	Sodium	24.05 mg
Protein	2.43 g	Vitamin C	88.43 mg
Carbohydrate	14.09 g		
Dietary Fiber	2.71 g	DIETARY EXCHANGES:	
Fat	2.45 g	Veg: 2	Fat: 0.5
Saturated Fat	0.35 g		
Poly Fat	0.28 g	% OF CALORIES FROM:	
Mono Fat	1.67 g	PRO: 11%	CARB: 64%
Cholesterol	0 mg	FAT: 25%	
Sugar	8.75 g		
Beta-Carotene	42.08 RE		
Calcium	37.52 mg		
Folate	26.13 µg		
Potassium	482.1 mg		

LEMONS AND LIMES

Probably the most tart of fruits, lemons and limes are rarely eaten alone. But their tart juice adds life to everything from salads to pies. These tropical plants are native to Southeast Asia and are thought to have been first cultivated in China, India, and Japan. Today, they are grown in southern Florida and southern California.

Health Benefits

Both lemons and limes are excellent sources of vitamin C, that all-important antioxidant nutrient that helps fight several diseases, including heart disease and cancer. They are also a good source of potassium, which can be good news for your blood pressure. Lemons and limes also contain phytochemicals (naturally occurring chemicals found in plants) such as terpenes and limonenes. If you remember from previous sections of this book, phytochemicals are thought to play a role in preventing some cancers.

NUTRIENT INFORMATION

Lemon Serving Size: 1 medium		Lime Serving Size: 1 medium	
Calories	17	Calories	20
Protein	0.6 g	Protein	0.5 g
Carbohydrate	5.4 g	Carbohydrate	7.1 g
Fat	0.2 g	Fat	0.1 g
Saturated	0	Saturated	0
Cholesterol	0 mg	Cholesterol	0 mg
Dietary Fiber	3 g	Dietary Fiber	2.0 g
Sodium	1 mg	Sodium	1 mg
Folic Acid	6.2 µg	Folic Acid	5.6 µg
Vitamin C	30.7 mg	Vitamin C	19.5 mg
Calcium	15 mg	Calcium	22 mg
Potassium	80 mg	Potassium	68 mg

Selection and Storage

Look for firm, unblemished lemons and limes that are heavy for their size. That indicates a lot of juice. Thin-skinned fruit will yield the most juice. Lemons and limes contain little starch, so they are pretty much as ripe as they're going to get when you bring them home from the market.

Put them in the refrigerator whole and they will keep for a month or two. Lemons are somewhat sturdier, and will keep for a week or two at room temperature, but limes should be refrigerated immediately.

There are several varieties of lemons that vary only in the amount of juice they produce, the number of seeds they contain, and the thickness of their skin. However, one variety of lime, the Key lime, is more flavorful because of its greater acidity. The Key lime is small and round whereas other varieties of lime look more like green lemons. Limes take on a yellowish color as they ripen, but it's the very green limes that have the best flavor.

Preparation and Serving Tips

The juice of both lemons and limes is used to tenderize meats and to add flavor to a variety of dishes. You can marinate any cut of beef, poultry, or pork with the juice of these fruits to make it more tender.

You'll get more juice from the fruit if you first bring it to room temperature and roll it back and forth on a table or countertop under the palm of your hand before you cut and squeeze it.

Perhaps the most flavorful part of the lemon or lime is its "zest." That's the term used to describe the colorful skin of either fruit. You can scrape it off with a grater, a vegetable peeler, or a paring knife and use it in desserts, fruit salads, and veal and poultry dishes. It can really add life to an otherwise ordinary dish.

LENTILS

Lentils haven't yet attained superstar nutrition status, but they are slowly gaining the recognition they deserve as being an unbelievably nutritious food. This generation is far from being the first to discover the wonders of lentils. Archeologists have dug up remnants of lentils from ancient Egyptian tombs, and lentils are mentioned in the bible as Esau traded his birthright to Jacob for "a potage of lentils." Why the Egyptians thought lentils were worthy of the tombs of the pharaohs is anyone's guess. But modern man is impressed with their nutritional value.

Health Benefits

Lentils belong to the legume family and boast a bevy of nutrients—from folic acid and niacin to potassium and zinc. It's unusual to find so many different nutrients wrapped up in one hearty food package. Its high fiber content is a boon to health because the fiber is mostly soluble, the kind that lowers blood cholesterol. And it's exceptionally high in folic acid, a sometimes hard-to-get nutrient that researchers have just recently discovered can help prevent certain types of birth defects. Lentils are also an important source of iron for vegetarians.

NUTRIENT INFORMATION			
Lentils, cooked		Thiamin	0.2 mg
Serving Size: ½ cup		Vitamin B$_6$	0.2 mg
Calories	115		
Protein	8.9 g	Calcium	19.0 mg
Carbohydrate	19.9 g	Copper	0.3 mg
Fat	0.4 g	Iron	3.3 mg
Saturated	0	Magnesium	35 mg
Cholesterol	0	Manganese	0.5 mg
Dietary Fiber	5.2 g	Phosphorus	178 mg
Sodium	2 mg	Potassium	366 mg
		Zinc	1.3 mg
Folic Acid	178.9 µg		
Niacin	1.0 mg		

Selection and Storage

Though a large variety of lentils are grown around the world, brown, green, and red are most common in the United States. In the supermarket, you'll probably find them prepackaged. But in health food stores and gourmet markets, they're more likely to be sold loose in bins.

If you buy them prepackaged, look for well-sealed bags or boxes of uniformly sized, brightly colored, disk-shaped lentils. If you buy in bulk, check for insects. Evidence that the bin is infested may show up as pinholes in the tiny legumes. Also make sure the lentils are not cracked or broken.

When you get them home, they should keep for up to a year if you keep them in a well-sealed container at a cool temperature.

Preparation and Serving Tips

Red lentils cook quickly and tend to become mushy. They work best in soup, purées, or dips, where the lentils need to be soft. Brown or green lentils, on the other hand, retain their shape if they're not overcooked and can be used in salads or any dish in which you don't want the lentils reduced to mush. Most varieties of lentils cook in 30 to 45 minutes or less, and none require soaking, as dried beans do. Some red varieties cook in only ten minutes.

Lentils tend to take on the flavors of the foods around them, so they are willing recipients of flavorful herbs and spices. They are a favorite in Indian, Middle Eastern, and African recipes.

LENTIL BURGERS

  1 **can (about 14 ounces) defatted low sodium chicken broth**∗

  1 **cup dried lentils**

  1 **small carrot, grated**

 ¼ **cup coarsely chopped mushrooms**

  1 **egg**

 ¼ **cup dry unseasoned bread crumbs**

  3 **tablespoons finely chopped onion**

  2 **to 4 cloves garlic, minced**

  1 **teaspoon dried thyme leaves, crushed**

     Nonstick cooking spray

 ¼ **cup plain nonfat yogurt**

 ¼ **cup chopped seeded cucumber**

 ¼ **teaspoon dried dill weed, crushed**

 ½ **teaspoon dried mint leaves, crushed**

 ¼ **teaspoon black pepper**

 ⅛ **teaspoon salt**

     Dash hot pepper sauce

Bring chicken broth to a boil in medium saucepan over high heat. Stir in lentils; reduce heat to low. Simmer, covered, about 30 minutes or until lentils are tender and liquid is absorbed. Let cool to room temperature.

Place lentils, carrot and mushrooms in food processor or blender; process until finely chopped but not smooth. (Some whole lentils should still be visible.) Stir in egg, bread crumbs, onion, garlic and thyme. Refrigerate, covered, 2 to 3 hours.

Shape lentil mixture into four ½-inch-thick patties. Coat large skillet with cooking spray; heat over medium heat. Cook patties over medium-low heat about 10 minutes or until browned on each side.

For sauce, combine yogurt, cucumber, dill, mint, black pepper, salt and hot pepper sauce in small bowl. Serve sauce over burgers. **_Makes 4 servings_**

* To defat chicken broth, skim fat from surface of broth with spoon. Or, place can of broth in refrigerator at least 2 hours ahead of time. Before using, remove fat that has hardened on surface of broth.

NUTRIENTS PER SERVING:			
Calories	124.1	Folate	47.5 µg
Protein	8.76 g	Iron	2.84 mg
Carbohydrate	20.69 g	Magnesium	30.17 mg
Dietary Fiber	0.93 g	Potassium	313.8 mg
Fat	2.11 g	Sodium	166.4 mg
Saturated Fat	0.52 g	Vitamin C	10.07 mg
Poly Fat	0.4 g		
Mono Fat	0.64 g	DIETARY EXCHANGES:	
Cholesterol	53.5 mg	Veg: 2.5	Bread: 0.5
Sugar	2.51 g	Meat: 0.5	
Beta-Carotene	512.7 RE		
Calcium	71.8 mg	% OF CALORIES FROM:	
		PRO: 26%	CARB: 61%
		FAT: 14%	

LETTUCE

Iceberg lettuce is one of the most popular vegetables in the United States. But it's not the most nutritious. You have to look to the darker green varieties, like Romaine, to get a real nutrient contribution to your diet. Whether you eat a salad before the meal (as is the custom in this country) or after a meal (like the French) or just like to munch on greenery during the day to stave off hunger, you have a wide choice of nutrient-dense leaves to choose from.

Health Benefits

Generally, the darker the lettuce leaf, the greater the nutrition. That's why the pale leaves from a head of iceberg lettuce offer few nutrients compared to the darker, heartier leaves of Romaine or red leaf lettuce. Romaine's dark-green hue is your clue that it's an excellent source of beta-carotene.

NUTRIENT INFORMATION			
Lettuce, Romaine		Calcium	10 mg
Serving Size: ½ cup, shredded		Potassium	81 mg
Calories	4		
Protein	0.5 g	Vitamin A	728 IU
Carbohydrate	0.7 g	Folic Acid	38 µg
Fat	0.1 g	Vitamin C	6.7 mg
Saturated	0 g		
Cholesterol	0 mg		
Dietary Fiber	0.2 g		
Sodium	2 mg		

Selection and Storage

Though lettuce comes in an array of shapes, sizes, and shades of green, there are three basic types: cabbage, or butterhead; cos, or romaine; and loose leaf. Cabbage lettuce has a round head and tightly bound leaves. Cos lettuce is a crisp, long-leaved lettuce with its leaves growing out from a stem rather than from a core. Loose leaf is an umbrella term used to include several varieties that possess short, curly leaves that grow from a stem.

Most varieties are available year-round, though varieties other than iceberg tend to become a little more scarce and expensive during winter months.

Look for well-proportioned heads. Lettuce that is uncharacteristically pale is probably past its prime. Avoid lettuce that is beginning to wilt or has brown-edged or slimy leaves. It's definitely not long for this world. Look for lettuce with attractive, dark-green outer leaves. This darker growth is the most nutritious, so you don't want to have to throw it out once you get home. Though you won't always find it, look for lettuce that is stored on ice, or at least in a cold spot in the market.

Lettuce tends to be gritty, especially long and loose-leaved varieties, and needs a thorough washing once you get it home. Wash the leaves in cold water, dry them, and store them in a plastic or paper bag in the refrigerator. It's not necessary to wash the interior leaves of iceberg lettuce.

The varieties you are likely to encounter at the market are:

Iceberg: Though it's the least nutritious and the least flavorful, it's the best-seller in the United States. It holds up well in the refrigerator for relatively long periods—up to two weeks—and its super-crispy texture is a plus when topping foods such as tacos. If you buy it already wrapped in cellophane, refrigerate it with the wrap still in place.

Romaine: Also known as cos, romaine lettuce comes in bunches with fluted leaves 6 to 12 inches long. Each leaf has a thick midrib, is crispy, and has an oh-so-slight bitter taste. Romaine is a hearty lettuce and holds up fairly well in storage for up to ten days.

Boston and Bibb: Referred to as butterheads, these small, loosely clustered, somewhat crinkled leaves are light green in color and have a smooth, almost waxy feel. Butterheads will keep only about three or four days, refrigerated.

Leaf Lettuce: This is actually a catch-all term used to describe a class of loose-leaf lettuces. Colors range from light to dark green; some have red-tinged leaves. These lettuces are somewhat fragile and bruise easily. Like Boston varieties, they will keep only a few days in the refrigerator. But they are best used in a day or two.

Preparation and Serving Tips

After you wash and dry lettuce leaves, you can either tear or cut lettuce leaves for a salad. Even culinary experts disagree as to which method is best. Do whatever works for you. Washed and dried lettuce leaves should also be "crisped" before you serve them. To do that, simply place them, loosely packed, in a plastic bag and return them to the refrigerator for an hour or two before you add the dressing.

For the dressing, most cooks recommend making your own and using only high-quality walnut or olive oil. They're expensive, but they impart a deep, rich flavor to dressings that you won't get from other vegetable oils. You can also make your own herb vinegar, by adding a sprig of fresh tarragon or basil to a bottle of vinegar and letting it "age." Wait until you're almost ready to serve to make your dressing.

Though salads are by far the number one way to serve up lettuce, it can also be braised and served as a side dish or heated and served "wilted" with green peas. All are excellent ways to use up leftover lettuce before it goes bad.

TAOS TOSSED SALAD

Baked Tortilla Strips (recipe follows)
¼ cup orange juice
1 tablespoon white wine vinegar
1 teaspoon olive *or* canola oil
2 cloves garlic, minced
¼ teaspoon ground cumin
¼ teaspoon pepper
3 cups torn washed romaine leaves
1 cup torn washed Boston lettuce
1 cup julienned jícama
2 medium oranges, cut into segments

1 medium tomato, cut into wedges
¼ cup thinly sliced red onion

Prepare Baked Tortilla Strips; set aside.

For dressing, combine orange juice, vinegar, oil, garlic, cumin and pepper in small jar with tight-fitting lid; shake well. Refrigerate until ready to use.

Combine romaine, Boston lettuce, jícama, oranges, tomato and onion in large bowl. Shake dressing; pour over salad and toss gently to coat. Sprinkle with tortilla strips. Serve immediately. **Makes 6 servings**

BAKED TORTILLA STRIPS

2 (6-inch) flour tortillas
Nonstick cooking spray
Dash paprika

Preheat oven to 375°F. Cut tortillas into halves; cut halves into ¼-inch-wide strips. Arrange tortilla strips on cookie sheet. Spray lightly with cooking spray; toss to coat. Sprinkle with paprika.

Bake about 10 minutes or until browned, stirring occasionally. Let cool to room temperature.

Makes about 1½ cups.

NUTRIENTS PER SERVING:			
Calories	93.4	Folate	67.2 µg
Protein	2.77 g	Iron	1.19 mg
Carbohydrate	17.44 g	Potassium	321 mg
Dietary Fiber	2.31 g	Sodium	61.62 mg
Fat	1.85 g		
Saturated Fat	0.26 g	DIETARY EXCHANGES:	
Poly Fat	0.48 g	Veg: 2	Fruit: 0.5
Mono Fat	0.92 g	Fat: 0.5	
Cholesterol	0 mg		
Sugar	6.46 g	% OF CALORIES FROM:	
Beta-Carotene	35.48 RE	PRO: 11%	CARB: 72%
Calcium	56.63 mg	FAT: 17%	

MANGOES

This "fruit of India," as it is sometimes called, is unique in its richness of flavor and wealth of nutrients. The pungent flavor may be an acquired taste for some, but the one-two nutrition punch it delivers is worth the acquisition.

Health Benefits

Mangoes are a superior source of vitamin A in the form of beta-carotene. In fact, mangoes are one of the top beta-carotene providers in this book. One mango also provides almost a whole day's recommended intake of vitamin C. And unlike many other fruits, it contributes several B vitamins, in addition to the minerals calcium and magnesium.

NUTRIENT INFORMATION			
Mangoes		Vitamin A	8,060 IU
Serving Size: 1 mango		Niacin	1.2 mg
Calories	135	Riboflavin	0.1 mg
Protein	1.1 g	Thiamin	0.1 mg
Carbohydrate	35.2 g	Vitamin B$_6$	0.3 mg
Fat	0.6 g	Vitamin C	57.3 mg
Saturated	0.1 g		
Cholesterol	0 mg	Calcium	21 mg
Dietary Fiber	5.8 g	Magnesium	18 mg
Sodium	4 mg	Potassium	322 mg

Selection and Storage

There are literally hundreds of varieties of mangoes and they come in a wide range of shapes, sizes, and colors. But most of the mangoes that are available in the United States are round, oval, or kidney-shaped and are about the size of a large California avocado. The color of a mango can range from gold or yellow to red. The color of the mango deepens as the fruit ripens, though patches of green may remain even in perfectly ripened fruits.

The mango's peak season is in the warm summer months from May through August, though the best month for mangoes is June.

When ripe, a mango has a sweet, perfumey smell. If it has a fermented aroma, the fruit is past its prime. Choose mangoes that feel firm but yield to slight pressure. The skin should be unbroken and the color should have begun to change from green to yellow, orange, or red. Though it's normal for mangoes to have some black spots, avoid those that are mottled with too many. It's a sign that the fruit is overripe. The same thing goes for loose or shriveled skin.

If you bring home a mango that is not yet ripe, you can speed the process by placing it in a paper bag with a ripe mango. Check them daily to be sure they are not becoming overripe.

Preparation and Serving Tips

Chilled mangoes are great to eat sliced as a dessert or as a breakfast fruit. Just sprinkle a little lime juice on them for a real taste treat. Because mangoes are so juicy, they can be a real mess to cut and serve. You can peel the fruit and eat it as you would a peach or a plum, just be sure to have plenty of napkins or paper towels on hand to sop up the juice that runs down your chin. Mangoes are also an indispensable ingredient in sauces and chutneys.

SMOOTH MANGO SHAKE

1½ **cups skim milk**
  2 **medium very ripe mangoes,* peeled, pitted, sliced**
  1 **cup vanilla nonfat sugar-free ice cream or frozen yogurt**
  3 **to 4 teaspoons lime juice**
¼ **teaspoon ground mace**
     Mint sprigs for garnish

Combine milk and mangoes in food processor or blender; process until smooth. Add ice cream, lime juice and mace; process until smooth. Pour into tall glasses; garnish with mint sprigs. ***Makes 4 servings***

* Very ripe mangoes are essential for the flavor of the shake.

NUTRIENTS PER SERVING:			
Calories	151.3	Calcium	124.3 mg
Protein	4.69 g	Folate	19.69 µg
Carbohydrate	33.96 g	Magnesium	19.92 mg
Dietary Fiber	2.38 g	Potassium	317.9 mg
Fat	0.49 g	Sodium	74.37 mg
Saturated Fat	0.19 g	Vitamin A	459.4 RE
Poly Fat	0.06 g	Vitamin C	30.68 mg
Mono Fat	0.16 g		
Cholesterol	1.5 mg	DIETARY EXCHANGES:	
Sugar	18.87 g	Milk: 0.5	Fruit: 2
Beta-Carotene	403.3 RE		
		% OF CALORIES FROM:	
		PRO: 12%	CARB: 85%
		FAT: 3%	

MELONS

It's believed that this succulent fruit was first cultivated in ancient Egypt and reached Europe only as recently as the Renaissance. Today, it is grown in countries all over the world, from the United States to Israel. California is the top melon-producing state in this country. Though melons come in different shapes, sizes, and colors, they all have one thing in common: a pulp that is soft, sweet, and juicy.

Health Benefits

Melons are rich in vitamin C, one of the all-important disease-fighting antioxidant trio we've talked about so often, and in potassium, a nutrient that's believed to help control blood pressure and possibly prevent strokes. Melons, especially cantaloupe, are also major sources of vitamin A in the form of beta-carotene, another member of the antioxidant trio.

NUTRIENT INFORMATION			
Cantaloupe Serving Size: ½ melon		Watermelon Serving Size: ¹⁄₁₆ fruit	
Calories	94	Calories	152
Protein	2.3 g	Protein	2.9 g
Carbohydrate	22.3 g	Carbohydrate	34.6 g
Fat	0.7 g	Fat	2.1 g
Saturated	na	Saturated	na
Cholesterol	0	Cholesterol	0 mg
Dietary Fiber	2.9 g	Dietary Fiber	2.9 g
Sodium	23 mg	Sodium	10 mg
Vitamin A	8,608 IU	Vitamin A	1,762 IU
Folic Acid	45.6 µg	Niacin	1.0 mg
Niacin	1.5 mg	Pantothenic Acid	1.0 mg
Vitamin B₆	0.3 mg	Thiamin	0.4 mg
Vitamin C	113 mg	Vitamin B₆	0.7 mg
		Vitamin C	46.5 mg
Calcium	28 mg		
Magnesium	28 mg	Calcium	38 mg
Potassium	825 mg	Magnesium	52 mg
		Potassium	560 mg

Selection and Storage

The three most popular melons in the United States are watermelon, honeydew, and cantaloupe (that's actually not the proper name; the fruit we call cantaloupe is really muskmelon). In general, you should look for melons that are evenly shaped and have no bruises, cracks, or soft spots. And when you store melons, do not remove the seeds, even if you cut the fruit, until you're ready to serve. The seeds help keep the fruit moist.

Cantaloupes should have a prominent brown netting that stands out from the underlying smooth skin and a depressed "thumbprint" where the stem used to be. If the stem is still attached, the melon was picked too early and is not yet ripe.

Ripe cantaloupes should give off a mildly sweet fragrance. If it smells sickeningly sweet, or if there is mold where the stem used to be, it is overripe and may well be rotten. Mature melons will continue to ripen off the vine. So if you buy it at its peak, eat it as soon as possible. Select cantaloupes that are heavy for their size. They tend to be juicier than their lightweight counterparts. The peak season for cantaloupe is June through October.

Watermelons are ripe when the underside has a yellowish tint and is firm. If it is white or green, the melon is not yet mature. There are countless varieties of watermelons, some with orange or pink flesh, but the taste is pretty much the same—sweet and juicy. In fact, over 90 percent of the weight of a watermelon is water. Choosing a watermelon is a little chancier proposition than choosing other types of melons. Unless the market is willing to let you sample it, which is unlikely, there are really only a few outward signs that indicate the ripeness of a watermelon.

As watermelons ripen on the vine, they develop a creamy yellow underbelly. This is probably the single most reliable indicator that a melon is ripe. Watermelons don't ripen much after they are picked, so what you see is basically what you get. A whole watermelon will keep in your refrigerator for up to a week. But a cut watermelon should be eaten as soon as possible. The flesh tends to deteriorate rapidly and takes on an unappetizing slimy texture. Peak season runs from mid-June to late August.

When picking a honeydew, look for one that is off-white to yellowish white on the outside. A yellowish-white pigment is your clue that the honeydew has ripened. Avoid honeydews that are dead-white or greenish white. If it's green, it will never ripen. If the skin of a honeydew is smooth, that also generally means that the melon was picked prematurely. The skin should have a very slight wrinkled feel. Ripe honeydew are the sweetest of the melons, and larger ones are generally the best tasting. Honeydew has the advantage of being available through the winter months, but August and September are really the peak months.

Honeydews generally keep longer than cantaloupes, but they should still be refrigerated. Try not to leave the whole fruit in the refrigerator for more than four or five days.

Preparation and Serving Tips

Though all melons taste best when chilled, watermelons taste best icy cold. Melon cutters can be used with any variety of melon to make melon balls, an attractive addition to fruit salads. A multicolored melon-ball salad topped with fresh, chopped mint makes a refreshing dish. Cantaloupe wedges wrapped in prosciutto make an attractive appetizer with contrasting sweet and salty flavors. Chilled melon soup is a refreshing cool change in hot weather. And the natural cavity left in a cantaloupe after removing the seeds is a perfect place for fillers like cottage cheese, yogurt, frozen desserts, or fruit salad.

SPINACH-MELON SALAD

    6 cups torn stemmed washed spinach
    4 cups mixed melon balls, such as cantaloupe, honeydew
         and/or watermelon
    1 cup sliced zucchini
   ½ cup sliced red bell pepper
   ¼ cup thinly sliced red onion
   ¼ cup red wine vinegar
    2 tablespoons honey
    2 teaspoons olive oil
    2 teaspoons lime juice
    1 teaspoon poppy seeds
    1 teaspoon dried mint leaves, crushed

Combine spinach, melon balls, zucchini, bell pepper and onion in large bowl.

For dressing, combine vinegar, honey, oil, lime juice, poppy seeds and mint in small jar with tight-fitting lid; shake well. Pour over salad; toss gently to coat. **Makes 6 servings**

NUTRIENTS PER SERVING:			
Calories	99.19	Potassium	673.9 mg
Protein	2.9 g	Sodium	53.67 mg
Carbohydrate	19.82 g	Vitamin A	525.9 RE
Dietary Fiber	3.04 g	Vitamin C	63.51 mg
Fat	2.28 g	Vitamin K	150.8 µg
Saturated Fat	0.28 g		
Poly Fat	0.39 g	Dietary Exchanges:	
Mono Fat	1.15 g	Veg: 0.5	Fruit: 1
Cholesterol	0 mg	Fat: 0.5	
Sugar	14.52 g	% of Calories from:	
Beta-Carotene	3,093 RE	PRO: 10%	CARB: 71%
Calcium	79.17 mg	FAT: 18%	
Folate	125.2 µg		
Iron	2.03 mg		
Magnesium	63.79 mg		

MILK, SKIM

Milk was long ago dubbed "nature's most perfect food." While it's not truly perfect, skim milk certainly comes close with its high protein and B_{12} contents, exceptional calcium counts, and bevy of B vitamins. All this for only 86 calories in an eight-ounce glass. However, not everyone can enjoy milk without gastrointestinal distress. A large percentage of the world's population suffers lactose intolerance, the inability to digest lactose, the natural sugar in milk. If you are one of them, try lactose-free and lactose-reduced milks. They come in several varieties, including low fat and skim.

Though milk is often thought of as being a highly allergenic food, only a small fraction of the two percent of people who suffer food allergies are allergic to milk. Any side effects of drinking milk are likely the result of some degree of lactose intolerance, a much more common problem.

Health Benefits

Like full-fat milk, skim milk is an excellent source of calcium. In fact, eight ounces provides about 30 percent of the U.S. Recommended Daily Allowance for the mineral, which plays a critical role in preventing the bone-destroying disease, osteoporosis. Women are most at risk for developing osteoporosis later in life, and few get nearly enough calcium. Getting two to three servings of milk and other dairy products each day, coupled with the lesser amounts of calcium found in countless other foods, ensures you of getting the calcium your body needs. And the calcium from milk may be absorbed better than calcium from supplements because of the milk's lactose content. This natural sugar found in milk appears to aid in the absorption of calcium.

Milk in this country is fortified with vitamins A and D (too little vitamin D can interfere with your body's absorption of calcium). Milk also provides riboflavin and other B vitamins, magnesium, and phosphorus (phosphorus works in tandem with calcium to help build bone).

NUTRIENT INFORMATION			
Milk, Skim		Vitamin B12	0.9 µg
Serving Size: 8 oz		Niacin	0.2 mg
Calories	86	Pantothenic Acid	0.8 mg
Protein	8.4 g	Riboflavin	0.3 mg
Carbohydrate	11.9 g	Vitamin D	2.5 µg
Fat	0.4 g		
Saturated	0.3g	Calcium	302 mg
Cholesterol	4.0 mg	Phosphorus	247 mg
Dietary Fiber	0	Potassium	406 mg
Sodium	126 mg		
Vitamin A	500 IU		

Selection and Storage

Obviously, you're better off nutritionally if you choose skim, or at least one-percent, milk to keep fat to a minimum.

The good news is that all other nutrients in milk remain the same regardless of the fat content.

However, if you have children under the age of two, give them whole milk. Young, rapidly growing children need the calories and fat that whole milk provides.

You might also want to give buttermilk a try. With its distinctively tart, sour taste, it's not for everyone, but many people prefer its flavor. Buttermilk is not as fattening as it sounds. Though originally a by-product of butter, today buttermilk is made by adding bacterial culture to skim or low-fat milk. Be sure to read the carton carefully to be sure you're getting the skim variety. Buttermilk tends to be saltier than regular milk, and it may not be fortified with vitamins A and D.

All milk should have a "sell-by" date stamped on the carton. Buy only as much milk as you think you will need and don't depend on milk to stay fresh much longer than the date on the carton. Milk lasts longer in the refrigerator if it hasn't been opened.

Milk in plastic jugs is more susceptible to considerable losses of riboflavin and vitamin A than milk in paperboard cartons. That's because light, even the fluorescent lights in supermarkets, destroy these two light-sensitive nutrients.

Today, you may also find milk not in the refrigerator section, but out on the shelf with packaged goods. This is called UHT or ultra-high temperature milk, referring to the processing technique. Though it must be refrigerated once you open it, unopened UHT milk will keep at room temperature for up to six months. UHT milk is just as nutritious as the milk you buy in the refrigerated section.

Whatever you do, don't buy raw milk or products that are made with raw milk, such as some cheeses. Raw milk has not been pasteurized and it often carries bacteria that can make you sick. Pasteurization is the heat process used on 99 percent of milk sold; it destroys disease-causing bacteria that milk straight from the cow can harbor. It's especially dangerous to give raw milk to children, the elderly, or people with impaired immune systems. Both the Centers for Disease Control and Prevention and the Food and Drug Administration consider raw milk to be unsafe for human consumption because of these risks.

Preparation and Serving Tips

Milk tastes great when you drink it straight from the glass. But it tastes best if it's icy cold. Skim and one-percent milk can be substituted in most instances for whole milk. There are, of course, some recipes that just won't work well with skim milk, but most do just fine. When you need to heat any kind of milk, don't allow it to come to a boil. Boiling milk forms a film on the surface that won't dissolve. Your best bet is to heat milk over a very low heat and stir it with a whisk to keep it from scorching.

MILLET

In the United States, millet is used mainly for fodder and birdseed, but this nutritious grain is a staple in the diets of a large portion of the world's population, including Africa and Asia. It has been cultivated for about 6,000 years. There are several varieties of millet available throughout the world. In Ethiopia, it is used to make porridge; in India, to make roti (a traditional bread); and in the Caribbean, it is cooked with peas and beans.

Health Benefits

Millet is a remarkable source of protein, making it perfect for vegetarian diets. It is also a good source of niacin, copper, and manganese. You may want to give millet a try if you are allergic to wheat. Chances are, you'll be able to eat it without having an allergic reaction.

NUTRIENT INFORMATION			
Millet			
Serving Size: ½ cup			
Calories	143	Niacin	1.6 mg
Protein	4.2 g		
Carbohydrate	28.4 g	Copper	0.2 mg
Fat	1.2 g	Magnesium	52 mg
Saturated	0.2 g	Manganese	0.3 mg
Cholesterol	0 mg		
Dietary Fiber	4.3 g		
Sodium	2 mg		

Selection and Storage

Look for this slightly bland-flavored grain in health food stores, Asian markets, and gourmet food shops. Millet is a tiny, pale-yellow bead. Store it in an airtight container in a cool, dry place, and it should keep for up to a month. It will keep up to a year in the freezer.

You may occasionally see cracked millet sold as couscous. But couscous is most often made from semolina.

Preparation and Serving Tips

Millet has no characteristic flavor of its own, and it tends to take on the flavor of the foods it is prepared with. To cook millet, add one cup of whole millet and a teaspoon of margarine or oil to two cups of boiling water. Simmer, covered, for 25 to 30 minutes. It should double in volume once all the water is absorbed. Keep it covered and undisturbed while it cooks, and you'll produce a millet that is fluffy; stir it often and it will have a creamy consistency, like a cooked cereal.

For a change from the same old thing, try millet on its own as a hot breakfast cereal. You can cook it with apple juice, instead of water, and top it off with raisins, brown sugar, or nuts.

Cooked millet can also be combined with cooked beans or peas to make vegetarian "burgers." Simply combine the two (they should be moist enough to hold together), and shape into patties.

Millet also works well in soups and stews. Simply rinse the millet in a strainer or colander and add to the mix. It should take about 20 to 30 minutes for the millet to absorb the liquid and become tender.

ITALIAN EGGPLANT WITH MILLET AND PEPPERS STUFFING

- ¼ **cup uncooked millet**
- 2 **small eggplants (about ¾ pound total)**
- ¼ **cup chopped red bell pepper, divided**
- ¼ **cup chopped green bell pepper, divided**
- 1 **teaspoon olive oil**
- 1 **clove garlic, minced**
- ⅔ **cup defatted low sodium chicken broth✻**
- ½ **teaspoon ground cumin**
- ½ **teaspoon dried oregano leaves, crushed**
- ⅛ **teaspoon crushed red pepper**

Stir the millet in a large, heavy skillet over medium heat for 5 minutes or until golden in color. Transfer the millet to a small bowl; set aside.

Cut eggplants lengthwise into halves. Scoop out flesh, leaving shell about ¼-inch thick. Reserve shells; chop eggplant flesh. Combine 1 teaspoon red bell pepper and 1 teaspoon green bell pepper in small bowl; set aside.

Heat oil in same skillet over medium heat. Add chopped eggplant, remaining red bell pepper, remaining green bell pepper and garlic; cook and stir about 8 minutes or until eggplant is tender.

Stir in toasted millet, chicken broth, cumin, oregano and crushed red pepper. Bring to a boil over high heat. Reduce heat to medium-low. Cook, covered, 20 minutes or until all liquid has been absorbed and millet is tender. Remove from heat; let stand, covered, 10 minutes. Preheat oven to 350°F. Pour 1 cup water into 8-inch square baking pan.

Fill reserved eggplant shells with eggplant-millet mixture. Sprinkle shells with reserved chopped bell peppers, pressing in lightly. Carefully place filled shells in prepared pan. Bake 15 minutes or until heated through.   ***Makes 4 servings***

* To defat chicken broth, skim fat from surface of broth with spoon. Or, place can of broth in refrigerator at least 2 hours ahead of time. Before using, remove fat that has hardened on surface of broth.

NUTRIENTS PER SERVING:			
Calories	88.96	Copper	0.19 mg
Protein	2.51 g	Magnesium	27.75 mg
Carbohydrate	16.16 g	Manganese	0.36 mg
Dietary Fiber	4.5 g	Niacin (B$_3$)	1.37 mg
Fat	2.02 g		
Saturated Fat	0.3 g	DIETARY EXCHANGES:	
Poly Fat	0.47 g	Veg: 1	Bread: 0.5
Mono Fat	0.95 g	Fat: 0.5	
Cholesterol	0 mg		
Sugar	0.01 g	% OF CALORIES FROM:	
Calcium	15.95 mg	PRO: 11%	CARB: 70%
		FAT: 20%	

MUSHROOMS

Mushrooms may be standard fare in Asian cultures, but Americans are only beginning to appreciate them. It takes a while to get used to the idea of eating a fungus, which is what a mushroom is. But besides lending wonderful flavor to foods, they contribute more nutrition than you might think.

Health Benefits

Mushrooms provide an unusual array of nutrients, not unlike those in meat. It is, then, a particularly appropriate food for vegetarians to embrace. Cooked mushrooms provide a surprising amount of protein, which, even though it's incomplete, can easily be complemented by grains.

You may not think of mushrooms as a source of iron, riboflavin, and niacin, but a half-cup provides over ten percent ofdaily recommended levels. Potassium and zinc are present in substantial amounts, too, as is fiber.

You're better off with cooked mushrooms than with raw. For the same volume, you get two, three, even four times the nutrients when cooked as when raw. That's because cooking, like drying, removes the high water content of mushrooms, concentrating nutrients and flavor. It also breaks down cell walls that can hinder nutrient availability when raw (chewing raw mushrooms well serves a similar purpose).

Moreover, hydrazines—toxic compounds found naturally in raw mushrooms—are eliminated when mushrooms are cooked or dried. Although they have been shown to produce tumors in animals, how much of a problem hydrazines are for humans is unknown. Lots of foods contain natural toxins. In this case, since cooked mushrooms are so superior in nutrition and flavor, the choice seems obvious. If you add raw mushrooms to your salad once in a while, that's OK.

Ironically, some research points to cooked mushrooms as having antitumor activity by boosting the immune system. Research has focused on enoki, oyster, shiitake, pine, and straw mushrooms. Indeed, mushrooms have long enjoyed notoriety as Chinese and Japanese cure-alls. One of the more intriguing claims concerns the wood-ear mushroom, which exhibits blood-thinning properties and may help prevent the clotting that contributes to heart disease. But how much of this mushroom might help and how effective it may be is not known.

Selection and Storage

Despite the tens of thousands of varieties of mushrooms that exist, you're likely to find only one in your supermarket—the white button mushroom. It's a cultivated variety available year-round. It has a delicate flavor.

If you crave more flavor, extend your horizons and seek out specialty varieties, available in up-scale stores, specialty shops, and Oriental markets. Some of these include the Japanese shi-

NUTRIENT INFORMATION			
Button Mushrooms, fresh, cooked			
Serving Size: ½ cup, pieces		Riboflavin	0.2 mg
Calories	21	Niacin	3.5 mg
Protein	1.7 g		
Carbohydrate	4 g	Iron	1.4 mg
Fat	0.4 g	Potassium	277 mg
Saturated	0	Zinc	0.7 mg
Cholesterol	0		
Dietary Fiber	1.7 g		
Sodium	2 mg		

itake, most popular worldwide; chanterelle, which is trumpet-shaped; Japanese enoki, which comes in tiny sprout-like bunches; morel, which is a small, brown, expensive, and intensely flavored mushroom with a spongy cap; the huge oyster; portobello, an Italian mushroom with a hearty flavor; and crunchy Chinese wood ear, often sold dried. Many of these are now cultivated in this country.

As you no doubt already know, you shouldn't go picking wild mushrooms on your own. There are too many poisonous varieties that look just like nonpoisonous ones. Even experienced foragers can be fooled. Stick to cultivated varieties of wild mushrooms.

When selecting the supermarket button mushroom, look for those with caps that extend completely down to the stems, with no brown "gills" showing. If mushrooms have "opened" —meaning the gills are showing—they are older and won't last as long. They are perfectly acceptable to use, if you use them right away, but they have a stronger flavor.

The color should be creamy white or soft tan. Growers no longer add sulfites to keep them white longer—good news for those who are allergic to the additive. Avoid those that have dark-brown soft spots or long, woody stems.

Mushrooms like cool humidity, but they also need circulating air. To store mushrooms, place them in a paper bag or a ventilated container in your refrigerator, but not in the crisper drawer. Do not use a plastic bag, or the mushrooms will get slimy. Mushrooms only last a couple of days in pristine white condition, but you can still use them for flavoring even after they've turned brown.

Preparation and Serving Tips

Don't wash mushrooms; they absorb water like a sponge. To remove dirt, use a mushroom brush or wipe with a barely damp cloth. Trim the stems and save them to use for flavor in soup stocks. Don't cut mushrooms until you're ready to use them; otherwise, they'll darken.

Mushrooms cook quickly. Overcooking is what makes them rubbery and tough. If you are sautéing them, be careful how much butter or margarine you add to the pan, because the mushrooms will absorb it like water. And you'll suffer the consequences of all that added fat. Try adding a bit of wine to the pan instead.

Adding mushrooms to any dish will heighten its flavor, probably because mushrooms contain glutamic acid—the same chemical in MSG (monosodium glutamate)—without the sodium. Add fresh mushrooms to any casserole, stir-fry, soup, or stew. Remember, their water content will add liquid.

Mushrooms and grains complement each other nutritionally. And the mushroom flavor gives punch to the blander grain without overpowering it.

Stuffed mushrooms are delicious but often fat-laden. You can avoid this by stuffing them with seasoned bread crumbs and chopped onion, then only lightly drizzling with olive oil before baking.

QUICK AND EASY STUFFED MUSHROOMS

    1   slice whole wheat bread
   16   large mushrooms*
    1   clove garlic
   ½   cup sliced celery

½ **cup sliced onion**
1 **teaspoon Worcestershire sauce**
½ **teaspoon marjoram leaves, crushed**
⅛ **teaspoon ground red pepper**
 Dash paprika

Tear bread into pieces; place in food processor. Process 30 seconds or until crumbs form. Transfer to small bowl; set aside.

Remove stems from mushrooms; reserve caps. Place mushroom stems, garlic, celery and onion in food processor. Process with on/off pulses until vegetables are finely chopped.

Preheat oven to 350°F. Coat nonstick skillet with cooking spray. Add mushroom mixture; cook and stir over medium heat 5 minutes or until onion is tender. Turn into bowl. Stir in bread crumbs, Worcestershire sauce, marjoram and ground red pepper.

Fill mushroom caps with mixture, pressing down firmly. Place filled caps in shallow baking pan about ½ inch apart. Spray lightly with nonstick cooking spray. Sprinkle with paprika. Bake 15 minutes or until hot. *Makes 8 servings*

✴ Mushrooms may be stuffed up to 1 day ahead. Refrigerate filled mushroom caps, covered, until ready to serve. Bake in preheated 300°F oven 20 minutes or until hot.

NUTRIENTS PER SERVING:			
Calories	19.62	Niacin (B₃)	1.22 mg
Protein	1 g	Potassium	121.4 mg
Carbohydrate	3.88 g	Riboflavin (B₂)	0.08 mg
Dietary Fiber	1.09 g	Sodium	29.06 mg
Fat	0.28 g	Zinc	0.29 mg
Saturated Fat	0.03 g		
Poly Fat	0.09 g	DIETARY EXCHANGES:	
Mono Fat	0.03 g	Veg: 1	
Cholesterol	0 mg		
Sugar	0.78 g	% OF CALORIES FROM:	
Calcium	8.79 mg	PRO: 18%	CARB: 70%
Iron	0.63 mg	FAT: 11%	

MUSTARD GREENS

Mustard greens, like collards, are a traditional food used in Southern cooking. But even if you don't hail from the South, there's no reason to ignore this nutritious plant.

Health Benefits

As a member of the cruciferous vegetable family, mustard greens share the health treasures of broccoli, cabbage, cauliflower, and kale. That is, they have cancer-preventive properties that no one understands yet but that seem real. As a bonus, mustard greens are rich in beta-carotene, an antioxidant that may reduce the risk of certain cancers, as well as heart disease and cataracts. Ditto for its supply of vitamin C, another antioxidant.

Women would do well to include greens in their diets, since greens provide specific nutrients that many women do not get enough of. For example, mustard greens are a little-appreciated source of calcium. Like kale, the calcium in mustard greens is much better absorbed than scientists used to think. It makes a serious contribution to calcium intake for both dairy and nondairy users. Even the iron content of mustard greens is significant, considering what a difficult nutrient this is to obtain.

NUTRIENT INFORMATION			
Mustard Greens, fresh, cooked			
Serving Size: ½ cup, chopped			
Calories	11	Vitamin A	2,122 IU
Protein	1.6 g	Vitamin C	17.7 mg
Carbohydrate	1.5 g		
Fat	0.2 g	Calcium	52 mg
Saturated	0		
Cholesterol	0		
Dietary Fiber	0.8 g		
Sodium	11 mg		

Selection and Storage

Mustard greens are a winter vegetable, perfect for when other vegetables are not in season. It looks a bit like kale but is lighter green in color and more delicate, even feathery. The taste is very pungent—typical of the cabbage family. If you desire a milder flavor, try Chinese mustard greens, somewhat similar to cabbage or bok choy in texture and taste, but darker green in color.

Choose mustard greens with leaves that are green and crisp-looking; yellow or wilted leaves are a sign of aging. Select leaves that are small; the larger they are, the less tender and more pungent they are. Avoid those with seeds attached; they are overmature. The stems should be firm, not flabby.

Store greens in a plastic bag in the crisper drawer. They'll keep for three days or more, especially if wrapped in damp paper towels. But the flavor may intensify the longer you keep them.

Preparation and Serving Tips

Wash the greens well and trim the stems just before cooking. Mustard greens don't work well in salads; they're too strongly flavored for most people. But they steam up nicely. You don't need to use a steamer or add water; the water that clings to the leaves after washing is enough. Steam until just wilted.

Try to steer clear of the fattier sauces for mustard greens or the traditional bacon fat or salt pork. Try steaming with some garlic.

Mustard greens work well in stir-fries. You can braise them with broth or add them to soups and stews.

GARLICKY MUSTARD GREENS

- 2 **pounds mustard greens**
- 1 **teaspoon olive oil**
- 1 **cup chopped onion**

2 cloves garlic, minced
¾ cup chopped red bell pepper
½ cup defatted low sodium chicken broth✳
1 tablespoon cider vinegar
1 teaspoon sugar

Wash greens well; remove stems and any wilted leaves. Stack several leaves; roll up jelly-roll style. Cut crosswise into 1-inch slices. Repeat with remaining greens.

Heat oil in Dutch oven or large saucepan over medium heat. Add onion and garlic; cook and stir 5 minutes or until onion is tender. Stir in greens, bell pepper and chicken broth. Reduce heat to low. Cook, covered, 25 minutes or until greens are tender, stirring occasionally.

Stir vinegar and sugar in small cup until sugar is dissolved. Stir into cooked greens; remove from heat. Serve immediately.

Makes 4 servings

✳To defat chicken broth, skim fat from surface of broth with spoon. Or, place can of broth in refrigerator at least 2 hours ahead of time. Before using, remove fat that has hardened on surface of broth.

NUTRIENTS PER SERVING:

Calories	71.58	Folate	178.6 µg
Protein	5.99 g	Iron	1.85 mg
Carbohydrate	11.26 g	Potassium	563.7 mg
Dietary Fiber	5.28 g	Sodium	41.55 mg
Fat	1.83 g	Vitamin A	698.5 RE
Saturated Fat	0.21 g	Vitamin C	76.89 mg
Poly Fat	0.25 g		
Mono Fat	1.09 g	DIETARY EXCHANGES:	
Cholesterol	0 mg	Veg: 2.5	
Sugar	2.49 g		
Beta-Carotene	693.4 RE	% OF CALORIES FROM:	
Calcium	180.4 mg	PRO: 28%	CARB: 53%
		FAT: 19%	

NECTARINES

Many people mistakenly think a nectarine is a cross between a peach and a plum. Not true. Although nectarines and peaches are botanical cousins, they started out as distinctly different fruit, albeit from the same ancestor. Today, through cross-breeding, they are closer in looks and taste than ever. Perhaps that accounts for the confusion.

Health Benefits

A ripe nectarine can taste heavenly sweet, and it supplies beneficial nutrients to boot. Nectarines may seem like peaches without the fuzz, but nutritionally they're in a league of their own, providing twice the protein, twice the vitamin A, slightly more vitamin C, and a lot more potassium than you'll find in a peach. The nectarine falls a bit short of a peach in fiber, however, and packs almost twice the calories. Still, the extra antioxidant vitamins A and C make the nectarine a slightly better choice than a peach. But in the pursuit of variety, we'd suggest eating both.

```
NUTRIENT INFORMATION
Nectarine, fresh
Serving Size: 1 medium
Calories         67
Protein          1.3 g        Vitamin A      1,001 IU
Carbohydrate     16 g         Vitamin C      7.3 mg
Fat              0.6 g        Niacin         1.3 mg
  Saturated      0
Cholesterol      0            Potassium      288 mg
Dietary Fiber    1.8 g
Sodium           0
```

Selection and Storage

Nectarines used to be whitish to pale yellow, but they're more golden-red these days, owing to frequent cross-breeding with peaches. Their flesh has traveled the same route. They may look the same, but nectarine flesh is still firmer and less juicy than that of a peach.

Nectarines are available from late spring to early fall—best in the dead of summer. Buy them fairly ripe. They shouldn't be rock-hard, just a bit yielding to the touch along the seam. Avoid the telltale green tinge, which signals it was picked too early and won't ripen. A just-ripe nectarine has a hint of aroma. The red blush isn't a sign of ripeness, just the variety. Avoid fruit with bruises, cuts, or pinholes.

To ripen, keep at room temperature, preferably in a ventilated paper bag. They'll ripen in two or three days. If they don't, they were picked too early and will get soft but never sweet. More than likely, they'll be mealy. Once ripe, refrigerate them. But they taste best at room temperature when eaten.

Preparation and Serving Tips

Wash nectarines well under running water to rid them of dirt and pesticide residues. Don't cut them up ahead of time, or the flesh will darken. To prevent this, rub the fleshy surfaces with lemon juice.

Besides enjoying them whole, slice nectarines over cereal, waffles, yogurt, or ice milk. Try blending them with bananas, strawberries, and yogurt for a super-smooth fruit drink. Or bake them into pies and cobblers, using any recipe that calls for peaches. Cut the sugar and fat in the recipe in half; the end product won't suffer and neither will your waist.

FRESH NECTARINE PIE WITH STRAWBERRY TOPPING

    Pie Crust (recipe follows)
1½ **pounds nectarines, pitted, cut into ½-inch-thick slices**
  ½ **cup sugar, divided**
   1 **pint strawberries, hulled**
   1 **tablespoon lemon juice**
   1 **tablespoon cornstarch**

Preheat oven to 425°F. Prepare Pie Crust. Reserve 6 to 8 nectarine slices for garnish. Chop remaining nectarines; place on top of pie crust. Sprinkle evenly with 2 tablespoons sugar. Bake 30 minutes or until crust is browned and fruit is easily pierced with sharp knife. Let cool, uncovered, on wire rack 30 minutes or until room temperature.

Meanwhile, place strawberries in food processor; process until strawberries are puréed, scraping down side of bowl once or twice. Press purée through strainer, discarding seeds and pulp. Pour liquid into 1-cup measure. Add lemon juice and enough water to equal 1 cup liquid.

Combine remaining 6 tablespoons sugar with cornstarch in small saucepan. Gradually blend in strawberry mixture until sugar and cornstarch are dissolved. Bring to boil over medium heat. Cook and stir 5 minutes or until mixture boils and thickens. Remove from heat; let cool 15 minutes. Spoon mixture over pie, spreading to cover nectarines. Let cool completely.

Refrigerate at least 2 hours or up to 8 hours before serving. Cover with plastic wrap after 1 hour in refrigerator.

Makes 8 servings

Pie Crust

1¼ **cups all-purpose flour**
¼ **teaspoon baking powder**
   Dash salt
¼ **cup canola *or* vegetable oil**
3 **tablespoons skim milk, divided**

Combine flour, baking powder and salt in medium bowl. Add oil and 2 tablespoons milk; mix well. Add enough remaining milk to hold mixture together. Shape dough into a ball.

Flatten dough to 1-inch thickness on 12-inch square of waxed paper; cover with second square of waxed paper. Roll out gently to form 12-inch round crust. Mend any tears or ragged edges by pressing together with fingers. *Do not moisten.* Remove 1 layer of waxed paper from crust. Place dough, paper side up, in 9-inch pie pan. Carefully peel off remaining paper. Press pastry gently into pan and flute edge.

NUTRIENTS PER SERVING:			
Calories	227.2	Thiamin (B₁)	0.18 mg
Protein	3.09 g	Vitamin A	54.58 RE
Carbohydrate	38.92 g	Vitamin C	25.73 mg
Dietary Fiber	2.6 g		
Fat	7.47 g	DIETARY EXCHANGES:	
Saturated Fat	0.56 g	Fruit: 1.5	Bread: 1
Poly Fat	2.32 g	Fat: 1.5	
Mono Fat	4.16 g		
Cholesterol	0.09 mg	% OF CALORIES FROM:	
Sugar	19.76 g	PRO: 5%	CARB: 66%
Beta-Carotene	56.88 RE	FAT: 29%	
Calcium	20.48 mg		
Folate	14.82 µg		
Potassium	238.7 mg		
Sodium	14.14 mg		

NUTS

This category is just a little nutty. It encompasses some foods that aren't true nuts but have been given honorary status due to their similar nutrition. This includes the peanut (really a legume), the Brazil nut, and the cashew (both technically seeds).

Health Benefits

Nuts are one of those good news/bad news foods. They are high in protein and nutrients, but at a price. Their fat content, albeit mostly of the preferred monounsaturated variety, is so high, it precludes eating too many at a time (see "Watch Out for the Fat in Nuts"). Macadamia, the gourmet of nuts, is the worst culprit. Chestnuts are the only truly low-fat nut.

NUTRIENT INFORMATION

Cashews, dry-roasted Serving Size: 1 oz		Peanut Butter, smooth style Serving Size: 2 Tbsp	
Calories	163	Calories	188
Protein	4.4 gm	Protein	7.9 gm
Carbohydrate	9.3 gm	Carbohydrate	6.6 gm
Fat	13.2 gm	Fat	16 gm
Saturated	2.6 gm	Saturated	3.1 gm
Cholesterol	0	Cholesterol	0
Dietary Fiber	1.7 gm	Dietary Fiber	2 gm
Sodium	4 mg	Sodium	153 mg
Copper	0.6 mg	Niacin	4.2 mg
Iron	1.7 mg	Vitamin E	3 mg
Magnesium	74 mg		
Phosphorus	139 mg	Copper	0.2 mg
Zinc	1.6 mg	Magnesium	50 mg
		Manganese	0.5 mg
		Phosphorus	103 mg
		Potassium	231 mg
		Zinc	0.8 mg

Still, nuts have a lot to offer, especially to vegetarians. Their protein content is legendary. Peanuts, not being true nuts, provide the most complete protein. Other nuts are missing the amino acid lysine. But all are easily complemented with grains.

Nuts are chock-full of hard-to-get minerals, such as copper, iron, and zinc. They're also good sources of minerals that help to keep your bones strong, such as magnesium, manganese, and boron, though precise values are not available for the latter two.

Recent research has heartened many nut lovers. Studies at Loma Linda University in California found that eating nuts five times a week—about two ounces a day—lowered participants' blood-cholesterol levels by 12 percent. Walnuts were used, but similar results have been reported with almonds and peanuts. The results have researchers a bit puzzled, but they theorize that replacing saturated fat in the diet with the monounsaturated fat in nuts may be the key. It makes sense, then,

WATCH OUT FOR THE FAT IN NUTS

	% of Calories From Fat
Chestnuts	8
Cashews	73
Pistachios	75
Peanuts	78
Almonds	80
Walnuts, black	84
Filberts/Hazelnuts	89
Pine nuts (pignoli)	89
Brazil nuts	91
Pecans	91
Macadamia nuts	95

to eat nuts instead of other fatty foods, not just to gobble them down on top of your regular fare.

Some nuts, notably walnuts, are rich in omega-3 fatty acids, which may contribute further to the fight against heart disease and possibly even arthritis. Some nuts contain significant amounts of vitamin E. Peanuts and peanut butter are super sources of niacin. The fiber in nuts is mainly insoluble—a boon to keeping your digestive tract running smoothly.

Brazil nuts are astonishingly high in selenium—perhaps too high. While selenium plays a role in your body's antioxidant defense system, it's only desirable to get more if you are deficient in the mineral in the first place. That's because too much selenium is toxic. Just six nuts can exceed the recommended dietary level by ten times! Even this probably isn't dangerous unless you make a habit of eating them.

Selection and Storage

Most fresh nuts are available only in the fall and winter. One of the treats of visiting New York City during the winter holiday

season is buying freshly roasted chestnuts from street ven-
dors.

Shelled nuts can be purchased anytime. Look for a freshness date on the package or container. If you can, check to
be sure there aren't a lot of shriveled or discolored nuts. Be
wary if you buy nuts in bulk; they should smell fresh, not
rancid.

A caution: Aflatoxin, a known carcinogen produced by a
mold that grows naturally on peanuts, can be a problem.
Discard peanuts that are discolored, shriveled, or moldy or
that taste bad. And stick to commercial brands of peanut
butter. A survey found that best-selling brands contained
only trace amounts of aflatoxin, supermarket brands had
five times as much, while fresh-ground peanut butters—like
those sold in health-food stores—averaged more than ten
times as much.

Because of their high fat content, you must protect nuts
from rancidity. Unshelled nuts can be kept for a few months
in a cool, dry location. But once they've been shelled or the
container opened, the best way to preserve them is in the refrigerator or freezer.

Preparation and Serving Tips

To munch, nuts are pretty much a self-serve affair. For
nuts that are tough to crack, use a nutcracker or even pliers.
A nut pick is useful for walnuts. Brazil nuts open easier if
chilled first. Almonds can be peeled by boiling then dunking
in cold water.

Learn how to roast chestnuts to save fat and calories:
Slice an X in the flat end, then bake in a shallow pan, covered, at 450 degrees Fahrenheit for 30 minutes, turning
them occasionally. Or, for authenticity, roast them over an
open fire in an old-fashioned corn popper. Peel the tough
outer skin and the inner papery skin while the chestnuts are
still warm.

When you use nuts in cooking and baking, you benefit from their nutrition without overdoing the fat and calories, since a little flavor goes a long way. Nuts on cereal can boost your morning fiber intake. Peanut butter makes a great snack on apple wedges or celery or simply on a piece of hearty whole-wheat toast. Walnuts go well in Waldorf salad or with orange sections and spinach. Almonds dress up almost any vegetable when sprinkled on top. Nuts give grains extra pizzazz and crunch. Pignoli nuts add a dash of the Mediterranean when included in pasta dishes. Nuts stirred into yogurt make it a more satisfying meal. Spice cakes, quick-bread mixes, and even pancake batters are extra-special with nuts.

OATS

Whether you think of horse feed or muffins when you think oats, you're probably underestimating this truly healthful grain.

Health Benefits

Unless you've been living on the moon for the past decade, surely you witnessed the rise and fall of oat bran as a wonder food. While the media attention may have vanished, oats remain as nutritious as ever, with the same potential for reducing risk of disease as before. Fortunately, what you don't see anymore are manufacturers, driven by marketers, adding oat bran to anything and everything in sight, no matter how ridiculous.

Why the attention on oat bran in the first place? The bran of the oat grain, like wheat bran, is the outer layer of the whole-oat kernel, or groat, where much of the fiber and many nutrients reside. Whole oats—rolled, steel-cut, or whatever—contain the bran along with the rest of the oat kernel. Oat bran, by itself, is a more concentrated form of the nutrients and fiber in whole oats. So eating whole oats will give you the same benefits of oat bran; you'll just need to eat more of it to get the same effect. And because much of the considerable fiber in oats is soluble—the same beta-glucans in barley—you profit in health terms.

A recent analysis of ten different studies showed the effect of soluble fiber on blood-cholesterol levels. On average, eating three grams of soluble (not total) fiber a day—the amount in two bowls of oatmeal or one cup of cooked oat bran—reduced cholesterol by six points in three months. Participants with the highest cholesterol levels saw the best response; those whose blood-cholesterol levels were in the "high" range, or over 230 mg/dl, saw their levels drop by 16. And those who ate the most oat bran benefitted the most. Another study showed that oat bran can be as effective—and certainly much less expensive—than medication in certain individuals.

Similarly exciting results have been seen with diabetics and those with borderline blood-sugar levels. The soluble fiber in oats means slower digestion, spreading the rise in blood sugar over a longer time period. Some diabetics on a diet high in soluble fiber that includes oats and beans have been able to reduce their medication.

But oats have a lot to offer all of us. Oats are tops in protein and provide 50 percent of the recommended intake of manganese. In addition, they offer an unusual amount of iron, thiamin, and magnesium, not to mention fiber. Best of all, because the bran and germ remain, eating almost any kind of oats will provide these nutrients.

Selection and Storage

Though several types of oats are sold, the difference is mainly in cooking time and texture, not in nutrition.

Steel-cut oats, sometimes called Scotch oats or Irish oats, are whole oat groats sliced into long pieces for a coarse, chewy texture. They take about 20 minutes to cook.

Rolled oats are groats that are steamed and flattened between steel rollers. Because this exposes more surface area for the boiling water to reach, they cook more quickly—in about five minutes. You may find them easier to chew.

Quick oats are cut into smaller pieces before being rolled, so they cook even more quickly—in about a minute. But the time you save cooking quick oats rather than rolled oats may not be worth it, considering what you sacrifice in flavor and texture.

Instant oats are precooked and pressed so thin that it only takes boiling water to "reconstitute" them. Generally, they have a lot of sodium added; the flavored versions also have added sugar.

Keep oats in a dark, dry location in a well-sealed container to keep bugs out. Store the container in the refrigerator if you live in a humid locale. The oats will keep up to a year. Whole oat groats are more likely to become rancid, so be sure to refrigerate them.

NUTRIENT INFORMATION			
Rolled Oats, cooked (Oatmeal uncooked)			
Serving Size: ¾ cup (⅓ cup)			
Calories	108	Thiamin	0.2 mg
Protein	4.5 g		
Carbohydrate	18.9 g	Iron	1.2 mg
Fat	1.8 g	Magnesium	42 mg
Saturated	0.3 g	Manganese	1 mg
Cholesterol	0 mg	Phosphorus	133 mg
Dietary Fiber	2.8 g	Zinc	0.9 mg
Sodium	1 mg		

Preparation and Serving Tips

To make oatmeal, all you do is simmer rolled oats in water on the stove for five minutes (or one minute for quick oats). Do not overcook your oatmeal, however, or you'll have a thick, gummy mess. If you like, sprinkle cinnamon or cinnamon sugar on top, then pour low-fat milk over it all. Oat bran can also be served as a hot cereal—it takes about six minutes to cook—although the taste might take some getting used to.

Granola is traditionally made with oats. By making it your-self, you can avoid the fat trap that many commercial varieties fall into. Here's how: First toast the oats in a shallow pan in an oven set for 300 degrees Fahrenheit, stirring occasionally until brown. Then combine the oats with wheat germ, raisins, your favorite nuts and/or seeds (toasted), dried fruit if you like, and a little honey. Let it cool, then store it in an air-tight container in the refrigerator.

Whole oat groats can be cooked (simmer for six minutes) and combined with rice for a pilaf or mixed with vegetables and seeds for a main dish. They also make a nutritious exten-der for meat loaf.

Both oat bran and oats (rolled or quick) can be used in baking. Oats alone don't contain enough gluten to make bread, but you can try modifying your recipes to include oats as half the grain. Oatmeal chocolate-chip cookies are delicious (also add wheat germ, and cut the fat and sugar). Oats can be added to quick breads and pancake batters, too.

OAT CAKES WITH FRESH FRUIT TOPPING

- 1 pint hulled strawberries, raspberries *or* blueberries, divided
- ½ cup sugar, divided
- 2 tablespoons cornstarch
- ½ cup water
- 1 teaspoon lemon juice
- ½ cup uncooked oats
- 1 cup whole wheat flour
- 2½ teaspoons baking powder
- 1¼ cups skim milk
- ½ cup plain nonfat yogurt
  Nonstick cooking spray

Place half of strawberries in medium bowl; mash with potato masher. Slice remaining strawberries; set aside. (If using raspberries or blueberries, do not slice.)

Combine ⅓ cup sugar and cornstarch in small saucepan. Stir in water until cornstarch is dissolved. Cook and stir over medium heat until mixture comes to a boil. Add lemon juice and mashed strawberries; return to a boil. Remove from heat; let stand 15 minutes. Stir in sliced strawberries.

Stir oats in heavy skillet over medium heat 3 minutes or until slightly browned. Turn into medium bowl; cool 10 minutes. Stir in flour, baking powder and remaining sugar. Combine milk and yogurt in small bowl; stir into flour mixture just until all ingredients are moistened. (Batter will be lumpy.)

Coat nonstick griddle or heavy skillet with nonstick cooking spray. Heat over medium heat until water droplets sprinkled on griddle bounce off surface. Drop batter by scant ¼ cupfuls onto griddle; spread batter to form 4-inch round cakes. Cook 2 minutes or until bubbles appear on entire top of batter. Turn cakes; cook 2 minutes longer or until browned. Serve warm with fruit sauce.

Yield: 6 servings (2 oat cakes and ⅓ cup sauce per serving)

NUTRIENTS PER SERVING:			
Calories	209.1	Niacin (B₃)	1.51 mg
Protein	6.95 g	Potassium	322.8 mg
Carbohydrate	45.36 g	Thiamin (B₁)	0.18 mg
Dietary Fiber	4.15 g	Vitamin A	34.7 RE
Fat	1.11 g	Vitamin C	29.22 mg
Saturated Fat	0.23 g		
Poly Fat	0.41 g	DIETARY EXCHANGES:	
Mono Fat	0.24 g	Milk: 0.5	Fruit: 1
Cholesterol	1.17 mg	Bread: 1.5	
Sugar	21.48 g		
Calcium	142 mg	% OF CALORIES FROM:	
Iron	1.3 mg	PRO: 13%	CARB: 83%
Magnesium	52.16 mg	FAT: 5%	
Manganese	1.15 mg		

OIL, CANOLA

Everyone needs to use an oil now and then. And sometimes olive oil imparts too strong a flavor or is too expensive for the intended use. In its place, we suggest canola oil.

If it seems as if canola oil came out of nowhere, that's because it did—at least the name did. There is no canola plant; canola oil comes from the rapeseed plant. Canola oil derives its name from Canada, where the process to remove erucic acid from rapeseed oil was so highly developed. Its nutritional advantages have all but overshadowed corn, soybean, safflower, and sunflower oils.

Health Benefits

All oils contain saturated, polyunsaturated, and monounsaturated fatty acids, but in different proportions. (See Fat in Part I.) Canola oil stands out because it's the absolute lowest in saturated fat of all the oils—6 percent compared to 10 to 15 percent for other vegetable oils. Moreover, it is second only to olive oil in monounsaturated fatty acids—both containing far more than other vegetable oils. Why is that important? Scientists now think monounsaturates are preferable to polyunsaturates, because although both types lower "bad" LDL cholesterol levels, monounsaturates don't lower "good" HDL-cholesterol levels like polyunsaturates do.

Canola oil may have another health advantage over other oils. Ten percent of its fats are omega-3 fatty acids. Omega-3 fatty acids in fish appear to prevent blood clotting, thereby helping prevent heart attacks. They've also shown promise in the fight against arthritis. Whether or not the omega-3s from plant sources such as rapeseed have the same effect, however, is still unclear.

NUTRIENT INFORMATION		Fat	13.6 g
Canola Oil		Saturated	0.9 g
Serving Size: 1Tbsp		Cholesterol	0
Calories	120	Dietary Fiber	0
Protein	0	Sodium	0
Carbohydrate	0		

Selection and Storage

Look for an oil that is 100 percent canola oil. Many companies now sell oil blends that combine their signature oil with canola. But they offer no nutritional advantage and there's no discernable difference in taste.

As with all oils, you must keep canola oil away from light and heat. As it oxidizes, it develops undesirable compounds with off flavors. If your oil starts to smell funny, throw it out. You cannot resurrect it. When truly rancid, the odor and taste are so objectionable it can't be ignored. If you refrigerate it, however, it gets cloudy. Keeping it in a cool, dark pantry is your best bet.

Preparation and Serving Tips

Just because canola is a healthier oil doesn't mean you should use a lot of it. As with all fats and oils, use as little as possible. Canola has the same amount of fat calories as other oils.

Most recipes can survive just fine with less oil than they call for. So pay no attention to the amount in the recipe, especially when sautéing. Start off with only a little—one or two teaspoons. If you get in the habit of using nonstick pots and pans, you can sauté with practically no oil.

OIL, OLIVE

Olive trees have been cultivated for the oil their fruit produces since 6000 B.C. Olive oil is still revered as a health food and gourmet ingredient in many Mediterranean countries. And, indeed, it may be both.

Health Benefits

Olive oil is a mainstay of the Mediterranean diet, which many experts believe is the healthiest diet you can eat. People of this region suffer low rates of heart disease, despite eating a diet that's fairly high in fat. Though many factors are probably responsible for their good health, including a slower-paced lifestyle and a diet that is rich in complex carbohydrates from fruits and vegetables, the fact that the fat they eat is mostly monounsaturated olive oil is probably not coincidental.

As discussed in the profile of canola oil, monounsaturates pack a double health punch because they lower blood levels of damaging LDL cholesterol without lowering beneficial HDL cholesterol. When they are substituted for saturated fat in the diet, monounsaturates can have a protective effect in terms of heart-disease risk. A recent study demonstrated that by using a liquid oil instead of margarine, you can cut your LDL-cholesterol level an additional seven percent over the ten percent drop you get by switching from butter to margarine.

Research also suggests benefits for diabetics, although this is less clear. Some diabetics don't do well on a high-carbohydrate diet, because their blood levels of triglycerides spiral upwards. Some experts say it may prove beneficial for these individuals to lower their carbohydrate intake, allowing for a slightly higher fat intake, provided it is primarily monounsaturated. (If you are diabetic, however, do not modify your diet without first talking to your doctor or dietitian.)

Remember, you can't just add olive oil to a fatty diet and expect to be healthier. You need to replace other oils and fats in your diet with the healthier olive oil if you expect to enjoy a health advantage. Cutting down on the total amount you consume is still a priority.

NUTRIENT INFORMATION		Cholesterol	0
Olive Oil		Dietary Fiber	0
Serving Size: 1 Tbsp		Sodium	0
Calories	120		
Protein	0		
Carbohydrate	0		
Fat	13.5 g		
Saturated	1.8 g		

Selection and Storage

Olive oils reflect the olives from which they are pressed. There is no one *right* oil to buy. It depends on its use and your taste preference. Many cooks and chefs keep several types of olive oil on hand to meet different cooking needs.

The grading of olive oil is confusing to some people. But it is simply based on the acid content of the oil as defined by the International Olive Oil Council, which is made up of countries that produce olive oil. The lower the acid, the better the oil tastes. Grading has nothing to do with how much monounsaturated fat is in the oil. All types of olive oil offer monounsaturates and their attendant health benefits.

Extra-virgin olive oil is the most expensive, because it is made from the first pressing of the best olives, often hand-picked. It has the lowest acid content—no more than one percent oleic acid. Some extra-virgin oils are "cold-pressed," meaning no hot water was used to extract the oil. Many connoisseurs prefer this. Some extra-virgin oils may be unfiltered, giving them a richer color and flavor. This type excels as an oil for salads and other uncooked uses where you taste the full flavor of the oil.

Virgin olive oil is made from pressed olives, but not necessarily from the first pressing, and the olives are not as pampered. The acid content must be between one and three percent oleic acid. It can be used as an all-purpose oil, suitable for salads and cooking.

Olive oil—which used to be called "pure" olive oil—is a blend of simple refined olive oil and virgin olive oil. It may be extracted by chemicals from the third pressing. Its acid content can be anything over three percent. Many chefs prefer to reserve it for heavy cooking only.

Olive oil does not need to be refrigerated; it will turn cloudy if it is. But it is imperative to keep it in an airtight container, out of the light and away from heat, to prevent the oxidation that can turn an oil rancid. Stored this way, olive oil should keep for a year or two. It may be better, however, to get in the habit of buying only as much as you'll use in a few months. If you do buy large cans or bottles, transfer the remaining oil into progressively smaller containers as you use it up, to limit the amount of oxygen in the container that can react with the oil.

Preparation and Serving Tips

Extra-virgin olive oil is best in salads and other uncooked dishes, so its flavor can be appreciated. You may find it too expensive to use as an everyday cooking oil. A rich, fruity oil can take the place of butter. Drizzle it on or dip crusty bread in the oil, as Italians do. Even cooked vegetables will benefit from a light drizzle of olive oil in place of butter or margarine.

Delicately flavored foods can be overwhelmed by an intense olive oil. If you find this to be a problem, try one of the new "light" olive oils many Americans have embraced. They are no less caloric—the fat and calories are the same as regular olive oil—but they are lighter in taste, especially suited to the novice palate.

Italians have used olive oil for sautéing for centuries, and it holds up well to the task. Contrary to popular belief, olive oil can even be used for frying, although the oil's flavor may preclude you from doing so. Try a "light" olive oil that's not so aromatic, for the few occasions when you might fry with it.

OKRA

This unusual Southern vegetable has African roots, as does gumbo, the thick Creole soup for which it's famous. Okra exudes a unique mucilaginous juice that makes it the perfect gumbo thickener.

Health Benefits

Okra is a festival of nutrients, not the least of which is its fiber, nearly half of which is soluble. This gumbo-thickening characteristic is what makes okra a player in reducing the risk of heart disease, diabetes, and obesity. And, the insoluble fiber helps keep your intestinal tract on track.

A number of nutrients are present at or near the ten-percent-of-recommended-levels mark, including two vitamins women especially need—B_6 and folic acid. The calcium, magnesium, and manganese in okra work in concert to keep your bones strong, also particularly important for women, who are more susceptible to osteoporosis than are men. And its potassium, calcium, and magnesium work together to keep high blood pressure at bay.

NUTRIENT INFORMATION			
Okra, fresh, cooked		Vitamin A	460 IU
Serving Size: ½ cup sliced		Vitamin C	13.1 mg
Calories	25	Vitamin B$_6$	0.2 mg
Protein	1.5 g	Folic Acid	36.5 µg
Carbohydrate	5.8 g		
Fat	0.1 g	Calcium	50 mg
Saturated	0	Magnesium	46 mg
Cholesterol	0	Manganese	0.7 mg
Dietary Fiber	3.7 g	Potassium	257 mg
Sodium	4 mg		

Selection and Storage

Fresh okra is available about half the year, from late May into autumn. Pick young pods, two to four inches long; they're more tender than longer ones. If okra pods are too mature, they taste tough and stringy. They should be bright green and firm but not stiff. Pass up any that are limp, shriveled, pale, dull, or brownish.

Refrigerate okra without washing it or it will get slimy. It'll keep in your crisper drawer for a few days.

Preparation and Serving Tips

When ready to cook, wash and scrub okra well under cold running water. To serve as a vegetable, you're best off quick-steaming whole pods—for about five minutes   in a nonaluminum pan to deter discoloration. Quick-cooking keeps the vegetable crisp and prevents the infamous okra juices from gumming things up. It helps if you don't trim the stems first, so the juices won't escape.

Of course, when you're adding okra to soup, stew, or gumbo, those juices are desirable, because that's what thickens the soup. So feel free to trim the stems and cut the pods into thick slices. Still, beware of overcooked okra; it can get extremely slimy. If you want less thickening power, throw in whole okra or add it during the last ten minutes of cooking time.

Fried okra is a Southern delicacy, but unfortunately, like all fried food, it's high in fat. So if you enjoy this food, eat it sparingly.

Okra is a natural to be paired with tomatoes, peppers, and onions, all of which seem to add enough bite to counteract the gumminess of okra.

STEWED OKRA & SHRIMP

- ½ pound okra
- 1 teaspoon canola *or* vegetable oil
- ½ cup finely chopped onion
- 1 can (14½ ounces) no-salt-added stewed tomatoes, chopped, undrained

1 teaspoon thyme leaves, crushed
¼ teaspoon salt
¾ cup fresh corn kernels *or* thawed frozen cut corn
½ teaspoon hot pepper sauce
2 ounces cooked baby shrimp

Remove tip and stem ends from okra; cut into ½-inch-thick slices. Heat oil in large nonstick skillet over medium heat. Add onion; cook and stir 3 minutes. Add okra; cook and stir 3 minutes. Add tomatoes, thyme and salt; bring to a boil over high heat. Reduce heat to low. Simmer, covered, over low heat 10 minutes, stirring once. Add corn and hot pepper sauce; simmer, covered, 10 minutes. Stir in shrimp; cook and stir until heated through. *Makes 4 servings*

NUTRIENTS PER SERVING:			
Calories	107.1	Potassium	609.0 mg
Protein	6.55 g	Pyridoxine (B₆)	0.3 mg
Carbohydrate	19.16 g	Sodium	184.7 mg
Dietary Fiber	3.38 g	Vitamin C	37.33 mg
Fat	1.91 g	DIETARY EXCHANGES:	
Saturated Fat	0.23 g	Veg: 2	Bread: 0.5
Poly Fat	0.63 g	Meat: 0.5	
Mono Fat	0.79 g		
Cholesterol	27.68 mg	% OF CALORIES FROM:	
Sugar	2.16 g	PRO: 22%	CARB: 64%
Beta-Carotene	550.6 RE	FAT: 14%	
Calcium	66.67 mg		
Folate	55.83 µg		
Magnesium	66.35 mg		
Manganese	0.87 mg		

ONIONS

The onion is a member of the allium, or lily, family, which is easily identifiable in aroma as a relative of garlic, shallots, leeks, and chives. Egyptians worshipped the onion's many layers as a symbol of eternity. Today we worship the onion as one of the most useful ingredients a cook can have on hand.

Health Benefits

Like garlic, onions are just now being appreciated for their contributions to health. Research has lagged behind that of garlic, but there are promising signs that onions have similar anticancer, cholesterol-lowering properties. Onions may also play a role in preventing blood clots and alleviating the symptoms of allergies and asthma.

While dry onions are a surprising source of fiber, they are not particularly rich in any other nutrient. Green onions, on the other hand, have those green tops, which provide a wealth of vitamin A.

NUTRIENT INFORMATION Dry Onion, fresh Serving Size: ½ cup chopped		Green Onion (Scallion), fresh Serving Size: ½ cup, chopped, (stalks and bulbs)	
Calories	29	Calories	13
Protein	1 g	Protein	0.9 g
Carbohydrate	6.6 g	Carbohydrate	2.8 g
Fat	0.2 g	Fat	0.1 g
Saturated	0	Saturated	0
Cholesterol	0	Cholesterol	0
Dietary Fiber	2 g	Dietary Fiber	1.2 g
Sodium	8 mg	Sodium	2 mg
Vitamin C	6 mg	Vitamin A	2,500 IU
Vitamin B6	0.2 mg	Vitamin C	22.5 mg
		Iron	0.9 mg

Selection and Storage

"Dry" onions are not the same as "dried" onions. The term simply refers to any common onion—be it yellow, white, or red—that does not require refrigeration. They are also called "storage" onions. This distinguishes them from green onions, which are perishable.

Dry onions come in various shapes and colors, neither of which is a reliable indicator of taste or strength. The white or yellow globe onion is a pungent cooking onion that keeps its flavor when cooked. All-purpose onions, white or yellow, are milder. Sweet onions, the mildest, can be red, yellow, or white. They include the Bermuda onion, flat on one end; the Spanish onion, completely round; and the Italian onion, ovoid in shape.

For dry onions, choose firm ones with shiny, tissue-thin skins. The "necks" should be tight and dry. Avoid those that look too dry, are discolored, or have soft, wet spots.

Dry onions will keep three to four weeks if stored in a dry, dark, cool location. A hanging bag is ideal because it allows air to circulate. Don't store next to potatoes, which give off a gas that'll cause the onions to decay. Light turns an onion bitter. Onions sprout and go bad if they get too warm, but refrigeration hastens deterioration, too. Once you cut an onion, however, you should wrap it in plastic and refrigerate. Use within a day or two.

Green onions have small white bulbs topped by long, thin, green stalks. They are simply immature onions, also called "spring" onions, because that's when they are harvested. Although they are often sold as scallions, true scallions have no bulb, just long, slender, straight, green stalks. The terms green onions and scallions, however, are often used interchangeably.

Look for green onions with bright green tops that look crisp, not wilted. The bulbs should be well-formed, with no soft spots. For more pungent aroma, choose those with fatter bulbs; for a sweeter taste, pick the smaller ones.

Green onions must be refrigerated. They'll keep best in a plastic bag in the crisper drawer. Use within two or three days. Even after the tops have wilted and dried out, however, you may still be able to use the bulbs for a few days more.

Preparation and Serving Tips

To dice an onion easily: Peel the onion, then cut in half and trim the neck end, leaving the root end together. Place it flat-side down on a cutting board and cut slices down to the root end without cutting through it. Then cut horizontally through the onion. Finally, cut the onion in slices parallel to the root end. You'll end up with a perfectly diced onion.

To keep those eyes dry when chopping onions, try slicing them under running water. If you are not so adept with your knife, try running cold water over your knife after every cut. Or chill the onion for an hour before cutting it up. To get the onion smell off your fingers, rub them with lemon juice or vinegar.

Onions are the perfect seasoning for almost any cooked dish. They are milder when cooked than when raw because the smelly sulfur compounds are converted to sugar when heated. Onions sauté wonderfully, even without butter. Just use a nonstick pan and perhaps a teaspoon of olive oil. Keep the heat low and brief or the onions will scorch and turn bitter. Despite what a recipe might say, sauté onions gently for only a few minutes before adding other ingredients.

Sweet onions are ideal to serve as raw rings in salads or as slices to top hamburgers. They add bite to a three-bean salad or a plate of homegrown tomatoes.

To prepare green onions, wash well, then trim off the roots and any dry stalk leaves. Chop up what's left—bulb, stalk, and all. They work well in stir-fry dishes. They add a bite that's a bit more understated than a dry onion.

Green onions can also be served raw with dip as part of a crudité platter or as a garnish. Shred the stalks and curl them for a festive look. They'll stay curled if you refrigerate them in ice water for an hour. For a change of pace, chop up scallions, instead of dry onions, in your next tunafish salad.

ONION FOCACCIA

- 2 **tablespoons olive oil, divided**
- 1 **medium red onion, thinly sliced**
- 3 **green onions, cut into 1½-inch pieces, each piece cut lengthwise into halves**

1 **teaspoon dried rosemary leaves, crushed**
2¼ **to 2¾ cups all-purpose flour, divided**
3 **tablespoons wheat germ**
2 **tablespoons sugar**
1 **package (¼ ounce) quick-rising dry yeast**
¾ **teaspoon salt**
¾ **cup water**
⅓ **cup 1% low-fat milk**

Heat 1 tablespoon olive oil in large nonstick skillet over low heat. Add red onion; cook and stir 10 minutes until transparent. Remove pan from heat; stir in green onions and rosemary. Set aside to cool.

Combine 1¼ cups flour, wheat germ, sugar, yeast and salt in large bowl. Heat water and milk in small saucepan until very warm (127° to 130°F). Add liquid to flour mixture with remaining 1 tablespoon olive oil; beat with electric mixer on low speed until combined. Increase speed to medium; continue beating 3 minutes, scraping bowl occasionally. Stir in 1 cup flour with wooden spoon. Add as much remaining flour as necessary to make soft dough.

Turn out dough onto lightly floured surface. Knead about 8 minutes or until dough is smooth and elastic. Shape into a ball; cover with towel and let rest 10 minutes. Coat 15×10-inch pan with nonstick cooking spray.

Roll out dough to fit pan; place in prepared pan. Cover with towel; let rise in warm place 30 minutes or until slightly risen. Place oven rack in lowest position; preheat oven to 400°F.

Make indentations in dough 2 inches apart with end of wooden spoon. Spread onion mixture over top of dough; smooth out evenly with spatula, pressing in gently.

Bake 18 to 20 minutes or until golden brown. Cut into 9 pieces with serrated knife or kitchen shears. Serve warm.

Makes 9 servings

NUTRIENTS PER SERVING:		Potassium	130.5 mg
Calories	175.7	Sodium	183.8 mg
Protein	4.87 g	Vitamin A	15.35 RE
Carbohydrate	30.8 g	Vitamin C	2.67 mg
Dietary Fiber	1.84 g	Zinc	0.71 mg
Fat	3.72 g		
Saturated Fat	0.59 g	DIETARY EXCHANGES:	
Poly Fat	0.56 g	Veg: 0.5	Bread: 2
Mono Fat	2.31 g	Fat: 0.5	
Cholesterol	0.37 mg		
Sugar	4.52 g	% OF CALORIES FROM:	
Beta-Carotene	52.53 RE	PRO: 11%	CARB: 70%
Calcium	25.87 mg	FAT: 19%	
Folate	53.78 µg		
Manganese	0.72 mg		

ORANGES AND TANGERINES

Once a hard-to-get fruit, oranges are now a basic staple of the typical American diet.

Health Benefits

One orange provides about 134 percent of the recommended daily allowance for vitamin C. That's a particularly important fact for smokers, who require twice as much vitamin C as nonsmokers.

Oranges are also rich in potassium (good for warding off blood-pressure problems) and in folic acid (important for women in their childbearing years). Fiber is found in oranges—half of it soluble, half insoluble. There's even a bit of calcium.

Tangerines, on the other hand, only have a third as much vitamin C and folic acid as oranges, but they provide three times as much cancer-fighting vitamin A.

When you peel an orange, be glad if some of the white pithy part remains; it contains a lot of vitamin C and the soluble fiber pectin.

NUTRIENT INFORMATION			
Navel Orange, fresh		Tangerine, fresh	
Serving Size: 1 small		Serving Size: 1 medium	
Calories	65	Calories	37
Protein	1.4 g	Protein	0.5 g
Carbohydrate	16.3 g	Carbohydrate	9.4 g
Fat	0.1 g	Fat	0.2 g
Saturated	0	Saturated	0
Cholesterol	0	Cholesterol	0
Dietary Fiber	2 g	Dietary Fiber	2 g
Sodium	1 mg	Sodium	1 mg
Vitamin C	80.3 mg	Vitamin A	773 IU
Folic Acid	47.2 µg	Vitamin C	25.9 mg
Calcium	56 mg		
Potassium	250 mg		

Selection and Storage

This is one of the few fruits in abundance in winter. But you may get confused between the different varieties—over 100 in all—even if your supermarket carries but a few.

The California navel, with its telltale "belly-button," is a favorite eating orange, characterized by its large size, a thick skin that's easy to peel, and a flesh that segments easily with no annoying seeds.

The valencia, pride of Florida, is the premier juice orange. Though it can be eaten, it has seeds and a thin skin that's hard to peel. The blood orange is named for its distinctive red flesh. The Seville is too bitter to eat but makes the best marmalade.

Mandarin oranges are small, with thin but easily peeled skin and easily sectioned segments. They are sweeter than other oranges. Tangerines are a popular type of mandarin, with a thicker skin. Other mandarins include clementine, a cross between a tangerine and an orange; tangelo, a cross between a tangerine and a pomelo—a grapefruit relative; and the flattened-looking temple, a cross between a mandarin and an orange.

For all varieties, select firm fruit that's heavy for its size, indicating juiciness. As any Floridian will tell you, a green color and occasional blemishes are fine. Oranges are picked ripe, so you can eat them right away. If refrigerated loose, they'll keep for two weeks. Mandarins won't keep as long.

Preparation and Serving Tips

For oranges in fruit salads, pick a seedless type, such as navel. Orange sections go particularly well in spinach salads; add walnuts for crunch. Orange slices make pretty garnishes. Use orange juice to make marinades or no-fat sauces, or blend it with a banana and milk for a fruit shake.

ORANGE GLAZED CHICKEN WITH YAM & FRUIT

 4 teaspoons cornstarch, divided
 ¼ teaspoon salt
 ¼ teaspoon ground paprika
 ¼ teaspoon pepper
 4 boneless skinless chicken breast halves (4 ounces each)
 1 teaspoon canola *or* vegetable oil
 1 cup orange *or* tangerine juice
 1 medium yam, peeled
 ¼ teaspoon ground cinnamon
 4 whole cloves
 1 can (8 ounces) pineapple chunks in juice, undrained
 ½ cup chopped green onions
 1 can (11 ounces) mandarin orange segments, drained

Combine 3 teaspoons cornstarch, salt, paprika and pepper in small bowl; dust chicken with mixture.

Heat oil in large nonstick skillet over medium heat. Add chicken; brown 4 minutes on each side. Remove skillet from heat. Transfer chicken to plate; keep warm. Stir orange juice into skillet, scraping up brown bits on bottom of skillet.

Cut yam into ½-inch slices; cut each slice into quarters. Add yam, cinnamon and cloves to skillet; bring mixture to a boil over high heat. Reduce heat to low. Simmer, covered, 5 minutes, stirring once. Return chicken to skillet; simmer, covered, 7 to 8 minutes or until yam is tender and chicken is no longer pink in center.

Meanwhile, drain pineapple, reserving juice. Combine remaining 1 teaspoon cornstarch and reserved juice until smooth. Stir cornstarch mixture, pineapple and green onions into skillet. Cook and stir over medium heat until mixture boils and thickens. Add orange segments; cook and stir until heated through. Remove cloves before serving.

Makes 4 servings

NUTRIENTS PER SERVING:			
Calories	310	Potassium	976 mg
Protein	23.76 g	Sodium	195.9 mg
Carbohydrate	45.58 g	Vitamin A	143.4 RE
Dietary Fiber	1.49 g	Vitamin C	76.57 mg
Fat	3.98 g		
Saturated Fat	0.83 g	DIETARY EXCHANGES:	
Poly Fat	0.96 g	Fruit: 1.5	Bread: 1.5
Mono Fat	1.56 g	Meat: 2.5	
Cholesterol	58.31 mg		
Sugar	14.7 g	% OF CALORIES FROM:	
Beta-Carotene	823.8 RE	PRO: 30%	CARB: 58%
Calcium	54.47 mg	FAT: 11%	
Folate	55.34 µg		
Magnesium	59.23 mg		

PAPAYA

What fruit has more vitamin C than an orange, more vitamin A than apricots, and more potassium than a banana? That tropical sensation—papaya. And it's popping up at more and more supermarkets.

Health Benefits

When you talk about a nutrient-dense fruit, this is it. For the same or fewer calories than in many fruits, you get two very important antioxidant nutrients— vitamins A and C. They've both shown promise in reducing the risk of cancer, heart disease, and cataracts. And papaya's extremely generous potassium content affords protection against high blood pressure.

NUTRIENT INFORMATION			
Papaya, fresh		Vitamin A	3,061 IU
Serving Size: ½ papaya		Vitamin C	93.9 mg
Calories	59		
Protein	0.9 g		
Carbohydrate	14.9 g	Potassium	390 mg
Fat	0.2 g		
Saturated	0.1 g		
Cholesterol	0		
Dietary Fiber	1.4 g		
Sodium	4 mg		

Selection and Storage

Most of our papayas are the pear-shaped Solo variety from Hawaii. The much larger oval Mexican papaya is not as common. Sometimes a papaya is mistakenly referred to as a papaw or pawpaw, but that's an entirely different fruit. On the outside, papayas look a bit like large pears, but not on the inside, where there's a mass of black seeds.

Papayas are available year-round, although they have two true seasons—late spring and fall, when they are more abundant and the best for the price. Look for a rich golden color, with greenish-yellow undertones. Papayas ripen from the bottom up, turning more yellow as they ripen. So green should only predominate up near the stem. The skin should be smooth and firm, just yielding to pressure from your palm. Avoid any fruit that is too soft at the stem end, has a fermented odor, or is blemished or bruised.

Keep papayas at room temperature until they are mostly yellow. To speed ripening, place in a perforated paper bag. Once ripe, refrigerate. Handle gently, as they bruise easily.

Preparation and Serving Tips

Wash papaya well under cool, running water. Then slice in half lengthwise. Scoop out the seeds and discard, or rinse them and save them to eat; they have a peppery taste that works well in salad dressings. Peel the papaya and cut into slices or wedges, or scoop out the flesh like you would melon balls for a fresh fruit salad.

For best flavor, serve papaya cool but not right from the refrigerator. It makes a nice addition to green salads or can be served in slices on a plate, sprinkled with lime juice. For a refreshing light lunch, serve a scooped-out papaya half, filled with low-fat cottage cheese or seafood salad.

Papayas can be cooked into pies. They also make delicious chutney and preserves.

The meat tenderizer ingredient papain comes from papayas. But you can only get its effect from an unripe papaya. Try it Caribbean-style: Grill meat wrapped in papaya leaves, or cut up a green papaya into your usual meat marinade.

PAPAYA SNOWCAPS

  2 **ripe papayas**
 ¼ **cup shredded sweetened coconut, toasted**
  2 **green-tipped bananas**
  1 **tablespoon lime juice**
  2 **egg whites, at room temperature**
 ¼ **teaspoon cream of tartar**
  1 **tablespoon sugar**
  1 **tablespoon honey**

Preheat oven to 325°F. Cut each papaya lengthwise into halves; discard seeds. Cut off thin slice from round side of each half so halves sit upright without rolling. Place on baking sheet; sprinkle coconut over papayas. Peel and slice bananas; toss with lime juice. Arrange bananas on top of coconut.

To make meringue, beat egg whites in medium bowl with electric mixer until foamy. Add cream of tartar, beating on high speed until mixture forms soft peaks. Continue beating, gradually adding sugar and honey in thin stream until mixture is stiff and glossy. Spoon meringue on each papaya half, spreading to edge of papaya to seal.

Bake 20 minutes or until meringue is golden brown. Serve immediately. ***Makes 4 servings***

NUTRIENTS PER SERVING:

Calories	237	Potassium	673 mg
Protein	3.49 g	Sodium	53.49 mg
Carbohydrate	51.6 g	Vitamin A	69.16 RE
Dietary Fiber	4.93 g	Vitamin C	155.1 mg
Fat	2.83 g		
Saturated Fat	0.11 g	DIETARY EXCHANGES:	
Poly Fat	0.05 g	Fruit: 3.5	Fat: 0.5
Mono Fat	0.02 g		
Cholesterol	0 mg	% OF CALORIES FROM:	
Sugar	17.81 g	PRO: 6%	CARB: 84%
Beta-Carotene	415 RE	FAT: 10%	
Calcium	63.2 mg		
Folate	12.11 µg		
Magnesium	70.35 mg		

PASTA

It's the Mediterranean wonder food, existing in that region long before Marco Polo traveled to China. In fact, pasta is the cornerstone of a healthy diet for many different cultures.

Health Benefits

Pasta has finally shed its fattening image, which was so undeserved. Just by glancing at the nutrients listed here, you can tell pasta is a health food. Indeed, it is the ideal carbo-loading food for athletes, packing in complex carbohydrates with just the right amount of protein and essentially no fat. To help process that carbohydrate into energy, pasta even brings along its own B vitamins. Whole-wheat pasta is particularly rich in minerals and fiber.

All this is true for anyone, not just athletes. Diabetics, especially, benefit from pasta because it is digested slowly, allowing them to avoid unwanted peaks in blood sugar.

NUTRIENT INFORMATION

Whole Wheat Spaghetti, cooked Serving Size: 1 cup (2 oz uncooked)		Elbow Macaroni, enriched, cooked Serving Size: 1 cup (2 oz uncooked)	
Calories	174	Calories	197
Protein	7.5 g	Protein	6.7 g
Carbohydrate	37.2 g	Carbohydrate	39.7 g
Fat	0.8 g	Fat	0.9 g
Saturated	0.1 g	Saturated	0.1 g
Cholesterol	0	Cholesterol	0
Dietary Fiber	5.4 g	Dietary Fiber	1.4 g
Sodium	4 mg	Sodium	1 mg
Thiamin	0.2 mg	Thiamin	0.3 mg
Riboflavin	0.1 mg	Riboflavin	0.1 mg
Niacin	1 mg	Niacin	2.3 mg
Copper	0.2 mg	Copper	0.1 mg
Iron	1.5 mg	Iron	2 mg
Magnesium	42 mg	Magnesium	25 mg
Manganese	1.9 mg	Manganese	0.4 mg
Phosphorus	124 mg	Zinc	0.7 mg
Zinc	1.1 mg		

Selection and Storage

Golden semolina pasta, made from durum wheat, is naturally higher in nutrients, and its protein is of better quality than other wheats. But durum flour, or semolina, is refined like white flour, so it's missing the nutritious bran and germ. So although it's not the type of pasta used in traditional cultures, the whole-wheat pasta has the nutrition edge. It packs a fabulous fiber punch—mostly the insoluble kind—triple that of regular pasta.

Enriched pasta adds back nutrients lost during milling, but it only adds back three B vitamins and iron, not fiber. Granted, these four nutrients are present in greater amounts than in whole-wheat pasta, but other B vitamins and minerals are not, including hard-to-get copper, magnesium, and zinc.

High-protein pasta is 50 percent higher in protein than regular pasta. Noodles, by government definition, must be made with eggs. Those that include the yolk contain about 50 milligrams of cholesterol in a one cup serving. Total protein is comparable to pasta's. Fresh pasta usually contains fat and cholesterol in amounts similar to noodles.

Spinach pasta and pastas colored red from beets or tomatoes are pretty and make dishes more interesting, but don't expect much of a nutritional bonus. The exception: Spinach pasta rivals whole wheat in fiber content.

What shape to buy? That's entirely up to you. The Italians have created over 600 shapes, while Americans must make do with 150 or so. Some sauces work well with tubular types like ziti or mostaccioli, while others are better with thin cappellini. Spiral-shaped rotelle holds sauce particularly well. Farfalle, or bow-ties, are fun for kids. Experiment ad infinitum and you'll never be bored. You can even opt for specialty flavored pastas, like wild mushroom, chili, squid ink, lobster, and spicy sesame—but be prepared to pay up to six times more.

The dried pasta you get at the supermarket is fine stored in your cupboards for months, especially if you have transferred it to airtight containers. Clear glass jars make a pretty display, but you'll lose B vitamins. Keep it cool and dry and away from light and air.

Fresh pasta is light-years ahead in taste and texture, but it isn't as practical. It must be eaten fresh, preferably right away. If not, refrigerate it.

Preparation and Serving Tips

Cooking pasta may seem simple, but note these finer points:

• Start with a large pot of water. Pasta needs room to move around or it gets sticky. Use four to six quarts of water per pound of pasta.

• Add a pinch of salt. It's not just for flavor; it makes the water boil at a slightly higher temperature, so the pasta cooks faster and is less likely to stick.

• Add pasta gradually after the water reaches a rolling boil. This ensures the water won't cool down as you add it, which would slow the cooking.

• Don't overcook pasta. If you do, the starch granules absorb too much water and rupture, releasing starch and making it sticky. A dash of olive oil in the water keeps it from sticking, but purists object to this because the sauce then slides off. Pasta is best cooked al dente—tender but chewy. Five to ten minutes does it, depending on the pasta shape. Test for doneness by biting it—you should be able to see a small inner core that's still starchy. The time-honored Italian way to test spaghetti is to throw a strand against the wall; it should stick only to the count of 2 or 3, then fall. It's a little messy, but it works!

• Drain pasta immediately, or it continues to cook. Do not rinse; you'll lose valuable nutrients. To prevent sticking, here's another Italian trick: Mix a little of the sauce in with the pasta and toss.

You can't go wrong basing your diet on pasta. You *can* go wrong with what you put on top of it, however. Forget heavy, fat-laden Alfredo cream sauce or pesto sauce swimming in oil. Often, the simpler, the better. There's nothing more delicious than piping hot spaghetti topped with uncooked chopped homegrown tomatoes, fresh basil or arugula, and freshly grated Parmesan cheese.

If you are not fond of the taste or chewiness of whole-wheat pasta, try mixing it with regular pasta, for at least half the benefit. As you get used to it, increase the proportion.

Add your favorite vegetables to a no-oil marinara sauce for pasta primavera—carrots, broccoli, and cauliflower make a knockout cruciferous/antioxidant combination that's surprisingly filling for not many calories. Try zucchini and mushrooms for lighter summer fare.

Don't limit yourself to tomato sauce. Try a light drizzle of extra-virgin olive oil, lots of crushed garlic, and a dusting of Romano cheese.

BROCCOLI–FILLED MANICOTTI WITH JALAPEÑO PEPPER CHEESE SAUCE

     8 manicotti shells
        Nonstick cooking spray
     1 cup chopped onion
     1 cup chopped red or green bell pepper
     3 cloves garlic, minced
     2 tablespoons chopped jalapeño peppers✽
  1¾ cups skim milk, divided
     4 teaspoons cornstarch
   ¾ cup (3 ounces) shredded reduced fat Monterey Jack
        cheese
     1 package (16 ounces) frozen chopped broccoli, thawed
        and well drained
     1 carton (15 ounces) low fat ricotta cheese, drained
     2 egg whites
   ⅛ teaspoon ground red pepper
   ⅛ teaspoon black pepper

463

Cook manicotti according to package directions in salted water; drain. Rinse under cold water; drain.

Meanwhile, preheat oven to 350°F. Coat 13×9-inch baking dish with nonstick cooking spray; set aside. Coat medium saucepan with nonstick cooking spray. Add onion, bell pepper, garlic and jalapeño peppers; cook and stir over medium heat about 3 minutes or until vegetables are tender. Add 1½ cups milk; bring to a boil over high heat.

Combine remaining ¼ cup milk and cornstarch in small bowl until smooth. Stir into mixture in saucepan. Cook and stir over medium heat until mixture boils and thickens. Cook and stir 2 minutes more. Add Monterey Jack cheese; stir until cheese melts.

Press out any excess liquid from broccoli. Combine broccoli, ricotta cheese, egg whites, ground red pepper and black pepper in medium bowl. Spoon scant ⅓ cup broccoli mixture into each manicotti shell; place in prepared baking dish. Pour sauce over filled shells. Cover with foil; bake 25 to 30 minutes or until heated through.   ***Makes 4 servings***

✽ Chili peppers can sting and irritate the skin; wear rubber gloves when handling peppers and do not touch eyes. Wash hands after handling chili peppers.

NUTRIENTS PER SERVING:

Calories	358.1	Niacin (B$_3$)	1.76 mg
Protein	35.96 g	Potassium	616.4 mg
Carbohydrate	47.97 g	Riboflavin (B$_2$)	0.67 mg
Dietary Fiber	7.37 g	Sodium	403.5 mg
Fat	5.18 g	Thiamin (B$_1$)	0.32 mg
Saturated Fat	2.61 g	Vitamin C	101.0 mg
Poly Fat	0.50 g	Zinc	1.37 mg
Mono Fat	0.18 g		
Cholesterol	28.33 mg	DIETARY EXCHANGES:	
Sugar	8.6 g	Milk: 0.5	Veg: 4
Beta-Carotene	77.83 µg	Bread: 1.5	Meat: 2
Calcium	632.1 mg		
Copper	0.24 mg	% OF CALORIES FROM:	
Folate	95.86 µg	PRO: 38%	CARB: 50%
Magnesium	61.64 mg	FAT: 12%	

PEACHES

Its origins may be Chinese, but the peach is America's favorite summer fruit. It's a sweet delight.

Health Benefits

Peaches don't break any records for nutrient content, but fresh peaches do provide respectable amounts of the antioxidant vitamins A and C; potassium, which is helpful in controlling high blood pressure; and both soluble and insoluble fiber. Processing robs canned peaches of vitamin C.

NUTRIENT INFORMATION			
Peach, fresh		Sodium	0
Serving Size: 1 small			
Calories	37	Vitamin A	465 IU
Protein	0.6 g	Vitamin C	5.7 mg
Carbohydrate	9.7 g		
Fat	0.1 g	Potassium	171 mg
Saturated	0		
Cholesterol	0		
Dietary Fiber	1.8 g		

Selection and Storage

Peach varieties fall into two categories, freestone and clingstone, self-descriptive names for how easily the flesh separates from the pit. Most peaches sold fresh are freestone. Not only are they easier to eat, but they're juicier. Most canned peaches are clingstone because they're firmer.

Not all peaches have yellow flesh inside. White peaches are common in Italy. Not all peaches have fuzz, either. Today's peach growers are breeding the fuzz away or removing it with mechanical brushes, due to its unpopularity.

Peaches have a fairly long season, mid-spring to mid-fall. It peaks in the summertime, when local fruit reigns. In winter, imported peaches are available.

You should always pick peaches individually, carefully looking them over for blemishes and bruises. Choose plump, well-shaped fruit with a creamy golden color and a well-defined crease. A green undertone is a sure sign of being underripe. A reddish blush indicates variety, not ripeness. Avoid peaches that are rock hard; they were picked too soon to ripen on their own. Select those that feel soft along the seam. But don't squeeze them; they bruise and decay too easily.

Ripen peaches at room temperature in a ventilated paper bag. They're ripe when just soft and when you can smell that sweet aroma. Don't let them get overripe, though, or they'll be mealy. Refrigerate once ripe.

Preparation and Serving Tips

Peaches don't last long. They ripen quickly or don't ripen at all. Eat them as soon as they're ripe, or cut them up for fruit salad, sprinkling with lemon juice to prevent browning. If you must refrigerate them for a few days, let them reach room temperature before eating.

Wash peaches well under running water, gently scrubbing the skin to remove pesticides. Freestone peaches are destoned easily by cutting in half and twisting free. Ripe peaches can be skinned easily, too.

Peaches are a natural sliced over cereal and waffles. They make great cobblers and pies, as well. A classy dessert is traditional Peach Melba—vanilla ice milk topped with poached peach slices and raspberry sauce. Or, try grilled peaches at your next cookout.

PEACH AND BLUEBERRY CRISP

3 **cups fresh *or* thawed frozen sliced peeled peaches, undrained**
1 **cup fresh *or* thawed frozen blueberries, undrained**
2 **tablespoons granulated sugar**
¼ **teaspoon ground nutmeg**

2 tablespoons uncooked rolled oats
2 tablespoons crisp rice cereal
2 tablespoons all-purpose flour
1 tablespoon packed brown sugar
1 tablespoon reduced calorie margarine, melted
⅛ teaspoon ground cinnamon

Preheat oven to 375°F. Combine peaches and blueberries in ungreased 8-inch round baking pan. Combine granulated sugar and nutmeg in small bowl. Sprinkle over fruit; toss gently to combine.

Combine oats, rice cereal, flour, brown sugar, margarine and cinnamon in small bowl. Sprinkle over fruit. Bake, uncovered, 35 to 40 minutes or until peaches are tender and topping is golden brown.   ***Makes 4 servings***

NUTRIENTS PER SERVING:			
Calories	152.9	Potassium	310.9 mg
Protein	2.02 g	Sodium	45.53 mg
Carbohydrate	34.45 g	Thiamin (B₁)	0.11 mg
Dietary Fiber	3.14 g	Vitamin D	0.38 µg
Fat	1.93 g	Vitamin E	0.35 mg
Saturated Fat	0.35 g	Vitamin K	0.02 µg
Poly Fat	0.86 g	Zinc	0.35 mg
Mono Fat	0.67 g		
Cholesterol	0 mg	DIETARY EXCHANGES:	
Sugar	20.04 g	Fruit: 1.5	Bread: 1
Calcium	14.66 mg		
Copper	0.14 mg	% OF CALORIES FROM:	
Folate	9.05 µg	PRO: 5%	CARB: 84%
Magnesium	16.99 mg	FAT: 11%	

PEARS

Pears first appear in late summer, continuing through fall and winter. Lucky for us, their season is long.

Health Benefits

The fiber in other fruit pales in comparison to that in a pear eaten with the skin. Much of its fiber is insoluble, making the pear a natural laxative whose gritty fiber may help lessen the number of cancerous polyps in the colon.

Pears provide a decent amount of copper, potassium, and, if you eat the skin, vitamin C. They're also an excellent source of boron, needed for proper functioning of calcium and magnesium.

```
NUTRIENT INFORMATION
Pear, fresh                          Sodium          1 mg
Serving Size: 1 medium
Calories          98                 Vitamin C       6.6 mg
Protein           0.7 g
Carbohydrate      25.1 g             Copper          0.2 mg
Fat               0.7 g              Potassium       208 mg
  Saturated       0
Cholesterol       0
Dietary Fiber     5.8 g
```

Selection and Storage

First to appear is the juicy Bartlett, the most common variety, fresh or canned. The traditional Bartlett is golden yellow with a red blush. The red Bartlett is deep maroon.

The d'Anjou pear reigns in fall and winter. It is rounder, greener, and firmer, though not quite as sweet, as the Bartlett. It's an all-purpose pear, as is Bosc, which has an elongated neck and unusual dull-russet coloring. It is crunchier than other pears and holds its shape when cooked. Seckel, the runt of pears, is also russeted but very sweet.

Comice is the premier dessert pear—sweet and juicy. It is yellow-green and squatty, with a bulbous body and no neck. It is bred to have less fiber than other common varieties, as grittiness is considered undesirable in a gift-box pear.

Asian pears are increasingly popular. They look and crunch like apples, but their flavor is all pear.

Pears are picked before they're ripe. Left on the tree, they get mealy. Off the tree, the starch converts to sugar. You can't always tell a ripe pear from its color; fragrance and touch are better indicators. Because a pear ripens from the inside out, once the outside seems perfect, the inside is on its way to rotting. So don't buy pears ripe; buy them firm, but not rock hard. Ripen in a ventilated paper bag, taking care not to pile them up or let them sit on one side too long, because they bruise easily. Eat them when they just barely yield to gentle pressure. Don't wait—their ripeness is fleeting.

Preparation and Serving Tips

To get a pear's full nutritional value, be sure to eat the skin. Of course, wash it well first.

Pears and cheese are a classic combo for dessert, European-style. If still a little firm, pear slices work well in salads with blue cheese crumbled on top.

Of all the fruits, pears are arguably the best for cooking, becoming even more sweet and creamy. Cook them when still firm. The traditional method is poaching; try it in wine or juice.

POACHED PEARS IN CINNAMON-APRICOT SAUCE

- 1 can (5½ ounces) apricot nectar
- 1 tablespoon sugar
- 1 teaspoon lemon juice
- ½ teaspoon ground cinnamon
- ¼ teaspoon grated lemon peel
- ⅛ teaspoon ground cloves
- 2 large pears

Combine apricot nectar, sugar, lemon juice, cinnamon, lemon peel and cloves in large skillet. Bring to a boil over medium-high heat.

Meanwhile, cut pears lengthwise into halves, leaving stem attached to one half. Remove cores. Cut pears lengthwise into thin slices, taking care not to cut through stem end. Add pears to skillet with nectar mixture; bring to a boil over medium-high heat. Reduce heat to medium-low. Simmer, covered, 6 to 8 minutes or until pears are just tender. Carefully remove pears from skillet, reserving liquid.

Simmer liquid in skillet, uncovered, over medium heat 2 to 3 minutes or until mixture slightly thickens, stirring occasionally. Fan out pears; spoon sauce over pears. Serve pears warmed or chilled. *Makes 4 servings*

NUTRIENTS PER SERVING:			
Calories	84.29	Potassium	152.4 mg
Protein	0.49 g	Sodium	1.46 mg
Carbohydrate	21.68 g	Vitamin C	17.21 mg
Dietary Fiber	2.56 g		
Fat	0.39 g	DIETARY EXCHANGES:	
Saturated Fat	0.03 g	Fruit: 1.5	
Poly Fat	0.09 g		
Mono Fat	0.09 g	% OF CALORIES FROM:	
Cholesterol	0	PRO: 2%	CARB: 94%
Sugar	11.77 g	FAT: 4%	
Beta-Carotene	51.41 µg		
Calcium	16.11 mg		
Copper	0.13 mg		

PEAS, GREEN

Green peas, or garden peas, are legumes just like dried peas, except they're eaten still immature. As with all legumes, they're chock full of nutrients.

Health Benefits

Green peas have more than twice the protein of most vegetables and lots of fiber, mostly the insoluble kind. In addition, they provide a myriad of other nutrients in amounts at or near ten percent of recommended levels. That's particularly important for iron, since it's hard to find iron-rich foods.

Snow peas and other edible-podded peas don't contain the same amount of protein nor all the nutrients green peas do. But they are an excellent source of iron and vitamin C, needed to keep your immune system functioning fine.

NUTRIENT INFORMATION

Green Peas, fresh, cooked Serving Size: ½ cup		Snow Peas, fresh, cooked Serving Size: ½ cup	
Calories	67	Calories	34
Protein	4.3 g	Protein	2.6 g
Carbohydrate	12.5 g	Carbohydrate	5.6 g
Fat	0.2 g	Fat	0.2 g
Saturated	0	Saturated	0
Cholesterol	0	Cholesterol	0
Dietary Fiber	2.4 g	Dietary Fiber	1.4 g
Sodium	2 mg	Sodium	3 mg
Vitamin A	478 IU	Vitamin C	38.3 mg
Vitamin C	11.4 mg	Thiamin	0.1 mg
Niacin	1.6 mg		
Folic Acid	50.7 µg	Iron	1.6 mg
		Magnesium	21 mg
Iron	1.2 mg	Potassium	192 mg
Magnesium	31 mg		
Potassium	217 mg		

Selection and Storage

Fresh green peas are only available in April and May. Choose firm, bright-green pods that are plump, but not large. Avoid yellow or blemished pods. Keep in mind that a pound of pea pods yields about a cup of shelled peas.

Snow peas, also called Chinese pea pods, are increasingly available fresh in supermarkets year-round. Look for shiny, flat pods. Pick the smallest ones for sweetness and tenderness. Avoid cracked, overly large, limp, or dull pods.

Sugar snap peas, available at farmer's markets in late spring and early summer, are edible pods like snow peas but are sweet like green peas, being a cross between the two. Select plump, bright-green pods.

Fresh peas only keep for two or three days in the refrigerator. The sooner you eat them, the better, as the sugar in them quickly turns to starch.

Preparation and Serving Tips

Wash peas just before shelling and cooking. To shell, pinch off the ends, pull down the string on the inside, and pop out the peas. Steam for a very short time—six to eight minutes, tops. They'll retain their flavor and vitamin C if still bright green and a bit crisp.

Snow peas just need to be washed and to have their ends trimmed. Remove the string from both sides of the sugar snap pea pod. Both are delicious raw, in salads or as crudité with dip. Snow peas are perfect in stir-frys; they need only be cooked lightly—a minute or two. Try peas with mushrooms or onions. Add peas to unexpected dishes, like spaghetti sauce, macaroni and cheese, or tuna casserole.

If you can't get fresh—and often you can't—frozen peas are a decent substitute. To use in salads, thaw but don't cook them.

ROSEMARY PEAS AND CARROTS

    2   **cups frozen peas**∗
 1⅓   **cups julienned carrots**
    1   **tablespoon reduced calorie margarine**
   ¼   **cup chopped red onion**
    1   **teaspoon lemon juice**
   ½   **teaspoon dried rosemary leaves, crushed**
   ⅛   **teaspoon pepper**

Bring 1 cup water to a boil in small saucepan over high heat. Add peas and carrots; return to a boil. Reduce heat to medium-low. Simmer, covered, 5 to 7 minutes or until vegetables are crisp-tender. Drain.

Meanwhile, melt margarine in medium saucepan over medium heat. Add onion; cook and stir about 3 minutes or until tender. Stir in lemon juice, rosemary and pepper. Add peas and carrots; toss to combine. *Makes 4 servings*

✻ Substitute shelled fresh peas for frozen. Add to boiling water 5 minutes before adding carrots.

NUTRIENTS PER SERVING:			
Calories	100	Potassium	355.1 mg
Protein	4.8 g	Sodium	47.75 mg
Carbohydrate	17.34 g	Vitamin A	1,112 RE
Dietary Fiber	4.08 g	Vitamin C	16.2 mg
Fat	1.71 g		
Saturated Fat	0.3 g	DIETARY EXCHANGES:	
Poly Fat	0.77 g	Veg: 3	Fat: 0.5
Mono Fat	0.55 g		
Cholesterol	0	% OF CALORIES FROM:	
Sugar	7.41 g	PRO: 18%	CARB: 67%
Beta-Carotene	1,082 RE	FAT: 15%	
Calcium	36.14 mg		
Folate	57.71 µg		
Iron	1.5 mg		

PEPPERS

If there is confusion regarding the pepper, it started back in Columbus' time, when explorers misnamed it because they thought it tasted like black peppercorns. It is, in fact, a completely different plant.

Health Benefits

All peppers are good sources of vitamins A and C, but those that are red are simply bursting with these antioxidant nutrients. A single pepper, sweet or hot, nearly meets a day's needs for vitamin A and far exceeds it for vitamin C, if eaten raw. That's reason to munch away.

Hot peppers may have powers beyond their nutritional content. Their fire comes from capsaicin, which acts on pain receptors, not taste buds, in our mouths. Capsaicin predominates in the white membranes of peppers, often imparting its "heat" to the seeds as well.

Whether hot peppers are good or bad for you is not clear. At least one study has found capsaicin to benefit people suffering migraines. And it's been shown to act as an anticoagulant, perhaps helping prevent heart attacks and strokes.

But capsaicin has confounded researchers by exhibiting both anticancer and procancer effects. And too much cayenne pepper may irritate your bladder. On the other hand, though you may have heard that hot foods like peppers can cause ulcers, you've heard wrong. There's no proof they even irritate existing ulcers.

"Easy does it" may be the best advice. If hot peppers bother you, cut back. It takes time to develop an affinity and immunity to capsaicin's fire. Some people never do.

Selection and Storage

Sweet peppers differ from hot peppers by having no capsaicin, hence no heat. They do have a pleasant bite, though.

The bell pepper is most common. You may be surprised to learn that a green bell pepper is simply a red, yellow, or purple pepper before it's completely ripe. As it matures, it turns various shades of yellow and orange, until it is completely red. Because nongreen peppers are more ripe, they are more perishable and more difficult to keep fresh. Therefore, they carry a premium price. But many people favor their milder taste and vivid colors.

The cubanelle, or Italian frying pepper, is long, narrow, and pale green, yellow, or red. A bit more intense in flavor, it is preferred for roasting or sautéing.

Hot peppers (or chili peppers, or chiles—the Mexican word for peppers) come in over 200 varieties. They are popular the world over, though many Americans are neophytes when it comes to tolerating the heat.

NUTRIENT INFORMATION			
Sweet Bell Pepper, fresh		**Hot Chili Pepper, fresh**	
Serving Size: 1 pepper		**Serving Size: 1 pepper**	
Calories	18	Calories	18
Protein	0.6 g	Protein	0.9 g
Carbohydrate	3.9 g	Carbohydrate	4.3 g
Fat	0.3 g	Fat	0.1 g
Saturated	0.1 g	Saturated	0
Cholesterol	0	Cholesterol	0
Dietary Fiber	1.3 g	Dietary Fiber	na
Sodium	2 mg	Sodium	3 mg
Vitamin A		Vitamin A	
green pepper	392 IU	green pepper	346 IU
red pepper	4,218 IU	red pepper	4,838 IU
Vitamin C		Vitamin C	109.1 mg
green pepper	94.7 mg		
red pepper	141 mg		
Iron	0.9 mg		

Red peppers, being more ripe, are usually hotter than green peppers. Still, shape is a better indicator than color when trying to tell which peppers are hot and which are not. Rule of thumb: the smaller, the hotter.

The poblano, or ancho chile, is frequently used in Tex-Mex cuisine. It is only mildly hot and is fatter in shape than most hot peppers, so it works best for the popular stuffed-pepper dish chiles rellenos. Anaheim chiles are also fairly mild. You'll find them canned as "green chiles." Jalapeno is a popular moderately hot pepper. Among the hottest are cayenne and serrano chiles.

With all peppers, look for a full shape with a glossy sheen and no shriveling, cracks, or soft spots. Bell peppers should feel heavy for their size, indicating fully developed, thick walls.

Store sweet peppers in the refrigerator crisper drawer in a plastic bag to hold in moisture. Green peppers can stay firm for a week, but the other colors will go soft after three or four days. Hot peppers do better when they are refrigerated in a perforated paper bag.

Preparation and Serving Tips

Wash bell peppers well just before using; mild, diluted dish detergent will help get rid of some of the pesticides and wax on supermarket peppers. To core, cut into quarters, then trim away the stem and white membrane and wash away the seeds.

To cool the fire of hot peppers, cut away the white membrane lining the inside, discarding the seeds. Wear gloves when you do this, or you'll get oils on your fingers that will be difficult to remove. If you then rub your eyes, it will sting and burn. As a precaution, wash your hands and all utensils and cutting boards with soap and water after cutting hot chiles.

Bell peppers are delicious raw with dip. Cut into rings for a festive look in salads. Diced, they add delightful crunch and color to sandwich spreads such as tunafish or egg salad. When cooked, bell peppers develop a stronger flavor. Don't overcook, or they'll be bitter. They work well in stir-frys.

Hot peppers are great on pizza or in scrambled eggs, cornbread, tomato sauce, almost anything. A great way to add seasoning, as hot as you like it, is salsa, which recently passed ketchup as the most popular condiment in the United States, evidence of the evolving ethnicity of American taste buds.

What to do if you accidentally swallow more than your palate can handle? Here's unusual advice: Don't drink water, drink milk. Water cannot put out the fire in your mouth. It just spreads it around, making it worse. But research from the Taste and Smell Clinic in Washington D.C. shows that a dairy protein, casein, acts like detergent, literally washing away capsaicin and quenching the inferno. Eating a slice of bread, to absorb the capsaicin instead of spreading it around, also helps.

Chicken Rolls Stuffed with Peppers

- 4 boneless skinless chicken breast halves (about 1¼ pounds)
- ½ teaspoon onion powder
- ¼ teaspoon garlic powder
- 2 cups thin red, yellow *and/or* green bell pepper strips
- 1½ teaspoons olive oil, divided
- ¼ teaspoon dried oregano leaves, crushed
- ¼ teaspoon dried thyme leaves, crushed
- ⅛ teaspoon black pepper
- 1 tablespoon grated Romano cheese
- 1 tablespoon fine dry bread crumbs

Preheat oven to 350°F. Pound chicken breasts between two sheets of waxed paper with flat side of meat mallet to about ¼-inch thickness. Store chicken in refrigerator until needed.

Combine 1 cup water, onion powder, and garlic powder in small saucepan; bring to a boil over high heat. Add bell peppers; return to a boil. Reduce heat to medium-low. Simmer, covered, 2 to 3 minutes or until bell peppers are crisp-tender. Drain.

NUTRIENTS PER SERVING:			
Calories	208.9	Potassium	432.6 mg
Protein	29.01 g	Sodium	119.2 mg
Carbohydrate	9.07 g	Vitamin A	83.94 RE
Dietary Fiber	1.99 g	Vitamin C	101.1 mg
Fat	6.01 g		
Saturated Fat	1.75 g	DIETARY EXCHANGES:	
Poly Fat	0.96 g	Veg: 1.5	Meat: 3
Mono Fat	2.62 g		
Cholesterol	76.34 mg	% OF CALORIES FROM:	
Sugar	2.79 g	PRO: 56%	CARB: 18%
Beta-Carotene	60.04 µg	FAT: 26%	
Calcium	67.27 mg		
Cobalamin (B₁₂)	0.33 µg		
Folate	28.15 µg		

Combine ½ teaspoon oil, oregano, thyme and black pepper in small bowl. Spread mixture over one side of flattened chicken breasts; arrange bell peppers on top. Roll up chicken; secure with wooden toothpicks or metal skewers. Place chicken, seam side down, in ungreased 8-inch square baking dish. Brush chicken with remaining 1 teaspoon oil.

Combine Romano cheese and bread crumbs in small cup; sprinkle over chicken. Bake, uncovered, 20 to 25 minutes or until chicken is golden brown and no longer pink in center. Remove toothpicks before serving. ***Makes 4 servings***

PINEAPPLE

The pineapple, so named by explorers because it looked like a giant pinecone, is loved the world over. The best—and most expensive—come from Hawaii. Although pineapples from Puerto Rico, Mexico, and elsewhere are cheaper, they aren't as juicy and flavorful as those from Hawaii.

Health Benefits

Pineapple is a sweet way to get your manganese, that bone-strengthening mineral. Just one cup exceeds a day's recommended amount by 30 percent. At the same time, you get a decent amount of copper, thiamin, and fiber, not to mention more than a third of the requirement for vitamin C.

Selection and Storage

When shopping for pineapple, let your nose be your guide. A ripe pineapple emits a sweet aroma from its base, except when cold. It shouldn't smell sour or fermented.

Color is not a reliable guide. Ripe pineapples vary in color by variety. The Smooth Cayenne from Hawaii is golden yellow when ripe. The Red Spanish from Puerto Rico is reddish-brown, while the Sugar Loaf is green even when ripe.

NUTRIENT INFORMATION			
Pineapple, fresh		Dietary Fiber	1.9 g
Serving Size: 1 cup, diced		Sodium	1 mg
Calories	77		
Protein	0.6 g	Vitamin C	23.9 mg
Carbohydrate	19.2 g	Thiamin	0.1 mg
Fat	0.7 g		
Saturated	0	Copper	0.2 mg
Cholesterol	0	Manganese	2.6 mg

Don't rely on plucking a leaf from the middle. You can do this with all but the most unripe pineapples. And it can just as easily mean it's rotten—hardly a foolproof method.

Choose a large pineapple that feels heavy for its size, indicating juiciness and a lot of pulp. The leaves should be smallish and vivid green, not brown or wilted. The eyes should stand out, not be sunken. Avoid rock-hard pineapples and those with surface damage. A ripe one yields slightly when pressed.

Once a pineapple is picked, it's as sweet as it will get. It does no good to let it "ripen" at home. It will only rot. Buy pineapple ripe and eat it as soon as you can. Until then, refrigerate it.

Preparation and Serving Tips

Core a pineapple and peel the outside first, then cut into slices. Or cut into quarters first, then scoop out the inside without peeling at all. Use whatever method works without waste. Refrigerate pieces. Pineapple tastes best slightly cool.

Here's a unique dessert treat: fruit kebabs that alternate pineapple, strawberries, and other fruit on skewers. Or grill pineapple skewered with chicken chunks and vegetables. Try pineapple to give brown rice some zing.

Pineapple contains an enzyme that breaks down protein. It's only found in fresh pineapple. That's why you can add canned pineapple to gelatin, but if you try to add fresh, the gelatin won't set.

To tenderize meat, add chunks to your marinade. Let it sit only ten minutes—any longer will leave your meat mushy.

MARINATED PINEAPPLE DESSERT

    1   can (20 ounces) pineapple chunks in juice, undrained
    2   tablespoons honey
    1   stick cinnamon, broken in pieces
    1   tablespoon lemon juice
    1   teaspoon vanilla
  ½   teaspoon grated lemon peel
1½   cups strawberries, cut into halves, *or* blueberries
  ¼   cup toasted flaked coconut*

Combine pineapple with juice, honey, cinnamon, lemon juice, vanilla and lemon peel in small saucepan. Bring to a boil over medium-high heat. Pour mixture into medium bowl; refrigerate, covered, at least 4 hours or up to 24 hours.

Drain pineapple mixture; reserve liquid. Remove cinnamon pieces. Arrange pineapple and strawberries in four dessert dishes. Pour reserved liquid over fruit. Sprinkle with coconut before serving.   *Makes 4 servings*

* To toast coconut, spread on baking sheet. Bake in preheated 300°F oven 4 to 6 minutes or until light golden brown, stirring frequently. Remove from pan to cool.

NUTRIENTS PER SERVING:			
Calories	167.4	Manganese	1.75 mg
Protein	1.22 g	Potassium	293 mg
Carbohydrate	37.67 g	Sodium	14.52 mg
Dietary Fiber	2.04 g	Thiamin (B₁)	0.15 mg
Fat	2.61 g	Vitamin C	47.25 mg
Saturated Fat	0.02 g		
Poly Fat	0.15 g	DIETARY EXCHANGES:	
Mono Fat	0.04 g	Fruit: 2.5	Fat: 0.5
Cholesterol	0		
Sugar	33.76 g	% OF CALORIES FROM:	
Calcium	29.02 mg	PRO: 3%	CARB: 84%
Folate	17.51 µg	FAT: 13%	

PLUMS

If you can't find a plum you like, you haven't tried hard enough. There are over 200 varieties in the United States alone, some quite different from others. It pays to be adventurous and explore unfamiliar plums.

Health Benefits

If you eat a couple of plums at a time—and who can't, since most are so small—you'll get more than a fair dose of vitamins A and C, the B vitamin riboflavin, potassium, and fiber. None is in amounts to bowl you over, but they're important all the same.

NUTRIENT INFORMATION			
Plum, fresh		Vitamin A	426 IU
Serving Size: 2 medium		Vitamin C	12.6 mg
Calories	72	Riboflavin	0.1 mg
Protein	1 g		
Carbohydrate	17.2 g	Potassium	226 mg
Fat	0.8 g		
Saturated	0.1 g		
Cholesterol	0		
Dietary Fiber	2.5 g		
Sodium	0		

Selection and Storage

Plums are a summer pitted fruit, called a drupe, with a long season—May through October. Like their relatives the peaches, some plums cling to their pits and some have "free" stones.

Plums are generally either Japanese or European in origin. The Japanese type are usually superior for eating. Many European types are used for stewing, canning, or preserves or for turning into prunes.

Plum skins come in a rainbow of colors: red, purple, black, green, blue, and even yellow. Plum flesh is surprisingly colorful, too. It can be yellow, orange, green, or red.

There's no room here to chronicle the characteristics of every type of plum, but here are a few eating plums you're likely to encounter in your local market: Santa Rosa, Friar, Red Beauty, El Dorado, Greengage, and Kelsey.

When choosing plums, look for plump fruit with a bright or deep color, covered with a powdery "bloom"—its natural protection. If it yields to gentle palm pressure, it's ripe. If not, as long as it isn't rock hard, it will ripen at home. But it won't get sweeter, just softer. So, if you don't mind your plums a bit crunchy, eat them whenever you like.

To ripen plums, place them in a loosely closed paper bag at room temperature. Check on them frequently so they won't get shriveled or moldy. When slightly soft, refrigerate or eat them.

Preparation and Serving Tips

Don't wash plums until you're ready to eat them, or you'll wash away the protective bloom. Like most fruits, they taste best at room temperature or slightly cooler.

Although Japanese plums are best eaten out of hand, most European varieties are excellent for cooking. They're easy to pit—being freestone—and their firmer flesh holds together better. Try famous Damson plums or Beach plums for preserves.

A compote of plums and other fruits, such as apricots, is a traditional way to warm up your winter. Poach plum halves, skin on. Purée plums without the skins to serve with poultry or game. Plum sauce is a treat on ice milk or mixed into low-fat yogurt.

FRESH PLUM COFFEE CAKE

2¼ **cups all-purpose flour, divided**
 ¼ **cup packed brown sugar**
 ½ **teaspoon ground cinnamon**
  1 **tablespoon margarine, softened to room temperature**
1½ **teaspoons baking powder**

½ teaspoon baking soda
¼ teaspoon salt
1 cup lemon low fat yogurt
⅔ cup granulated sugar
2 egg whites
1 egg
1 teaspoon grated lemon peel
4 medium plums, seeded, cut into ¼-inch-thick slices

Preheat oven to 350°F. Coat 9-inch square pan with non-stick cooking spray; set aside. For streusel topping, mix ¼ cup flour, brown sugar, cinnamon and margarine in small bowl with fork until crumbs form; set aside.

Mix remaining 2 cups flour, baking powder, baking soda and salt in large bowl. Beat yogurt, granulated sugar, egg whites, egg and lemon peel in medium bowl with electric mixer until well blended. Stir yogurt mixture into flour mixture until ingredients are combined.

Pour batter into prepared pan. Arrange plums on top of batter; sprinkle streusel topping evenly over plums. Bake 30 to 35 minutes or until wooden toothpick inserted in center of cake comes out clean. Cool in pan on wire rack 10 minutes. Serve warm.   *Makes 16 servings*

NUTRIENTS PER SERVING:			
Calories	147.8	Potassium	99.7 mg
Protein	3.46 g	Riboflavin (B$_2$)	0.17 mg
Carbohydrate	30.17 g	Sodium	133.5 mg
Dietary Fiber	0.82 g	Vitamin A	19.99 RE
Fat	1.55 g	Vitamin C	1.75 mg
Saturated Fat	0.27 g		
Poly Fat	0.36 g	DIETARY EXCHANGES:	
Mono Fat	0.52 g	Bread: 2	
Cholesterol	14.15 mg		
Sugar	11.8 g	% OF CALORIES FROM:	
Calcium	35.81 mg	PRO: 9%	CARB: 81%
Folate	6.59 µg	FAT: 9%	

PORK, LEAN

Pork has a bad reputation that it used to deserve. But no more. Recent analysis provides proof that, through breeding, today's hogs are leaner than in the past. The average pork cut is 34 percent leaner than in 1963.

Health Benefits

Lean pork is nutrient-dense—it provides a lot of nutrients for the calories. Of course, it provides high-quality protein. But it really shines as the best source for the entire gamut of B vitamins, falling short only in folic acid. B vitamins are important for processing carbohydrates, proteins, and fats into energy to fuel your body. Pork is also an important source of zinc, a mineral often in short supply that is essential for proper wound healing and immune functioning.

Surprisingly, today's "new" pork contains only a third of the iron it had before. It still makes a significant contribution, however, because most of it is well-absorbed heme iron.

NUTRIENT INFORMATION
**Boneless Top Loin Pork Chop,
  broiled (trimmed)**
**Serving Size: 3 oz (5 oz before
  cooking)**

Calories	173	Riboflavin	0.3 mg
Protein	26.5 g	Niacin	4.4 mg
Carbohydrate	0	Vitamin B$_6$	0.3 mg
Fat	6.6 g	Vitamin B$_{12}$	0.6 µg
Saturated	2.3 g		
Cholesterol	68 mg	Iron	0.7 mg
Dietary Fiber	0	Phosphorus	209 mg
Sodium	55 mg	Potassium	357 mg
Thiamin	0.8 mg	Zinc	2 mg

Selection and Storage

While pork is leaner, on average, some cuts are definitely leaner than others. Choose wisely. The best cuts are from the loin, such as: top loin chop or roast, center loin chop, and sirloin chop or roast. The leanest by far is tenderloin, at only 133 calories and 4 grams of fat in a 3-ounce serving.

Boneless rib roast and rib chop are moderately lean. Even bacon and ham can fit into a healthy diet, if you choose Canadian-style bacon and 95 percent lean ham.

When buying pork, look for meat that's pink to slightly gray, with as little exterior fat as possible, or else you're paying for waste. Cook it within the next two days, or else wrap it in heavy freezer paper and freeze it.

Preparation and Serving Tips

Since most of pork's fat is on the outside, not marbled as in beef, you can trim it. Do it before cooking.

Use cooking methods that do not add fat; try broiling, roasting, or grilling. Braising is OK if the meat is well-trimmed and the liquid used is broth or wine.

Don't make the mistake of overcooking pork, despite what Mom taught you. The *Trichinella* organism that causes trichinosis has been virtually eliminated from hogs in the United States today and poses little threat. It's killed at temperatures as low as 137 degrees Fahrenheit. The U.S. Department of Agriculture currently recommends cooking pork to 160 degrees Fahrenheit to be safe. That's low enough to allow a bit of pink and juiciness to be retained.

When cooking pork chops, rub with garlic first for flavor. Medallions of pork tenderloin is an extremely tasty and lean dish; try stuffing them with peeled garlic cloves and seasoning with tarragon.

TWICE COOKED PORK STIR-FRY

- 6 ounces boneless pork tenderloin
- 1 tablespoon vegetable oil
- ½ cup sliced onion
- 1 clove garlic, minced
- 2 cups shredded cabbage
- 1 cup julienned carrots
- ¾ cup thinly sliced red bell pepper
- 1 cup sliced mushrooms
- 1 teaspoon dried basil leaves, crushed
- ¼ teaspoon salt
- ⅛ to ¼ teaspoon black pepper
- ½ cup defatted low sodium chicken broth✳
- 2 teaspoons cornstarch
- 4 cups cooked brown rice

Place pork on microwave-safe plate; cover and microwave at MEDIUM-HIGH (70% power) 5 to 7 minutes or until pork is just slightly pink in center. Let cool; cut into thin strips.

NUTRIENTS PER SERVING:			
Calories	348.5	Niacin (B_3)	5.91 mg
Protein	16.27 g	Pyridoxine (B_6)	0.6 mg
Carbohydrate	55.56 g	Riboflavin (B_2)	0.3 mg
Dietary Fiber	5.99 g	Sodium	187.9 mg
Fat	7.08 g	Thiamin (B_1)	0.58 mg
Saturated Fat	1.37 g	Zinc	2.56 mg
Poly Fat	2.94 g		
Mono Fat	2.18 g	DIETARY EXCHANGES:	
Cholesterol	30.25 mg	Veg: 2	Bread: 3
Sugar	5.11 g	Meat: 1	Fat: 0.5
Beta-Carotene	4,675 RE		
Calcium	68.78 mg	% OF CALORIES FROM:	
Folate	50.88 µg	PRO: 19%	CARB: 63%
Iron	2.28 mg	FAT: 18%	

Heat oil in large skillet or wok over medium-high heat. Stir-fry onion and garlic 2 to 3 minutes or until onion is translucent. Add cabbage, carrots, bell pepper, mushrooms, pork, basil, salt and black pepper; stir-fry about 5 minutes or until vegetables are crisp-tender.

Combine chicken broth and cornstarch in small cup until smooth. Add to skillet; cook and stir about 1 minute or until mixture is slightly thickened. Serve over rice.

Makes 4 servings

* To defat chicken broth, skim fat from surface of broth with spoon. Or, place can of broth in refrigerator at least 2 hours ahead of time. Before using, remove fat that has hardened on surface of broth.

POTATOES

Whoever coined the phrase "the lowly potato" wasn't talking about its nutrient values.

Health Benefits

With the glaring exception of vitamin A, a potato has just about every nutrient, including a fistful of fiber. Did you know potatoes are rich in vitamin C? Don't forget iron and copper. They're also a standout in potassium, putting other high-potassium foods to shame. A potato a day is good news for your blood pressure and heart health. Better put a spud or two in your future.

NUTRIENT INFORMATION

White Potato, fresh, baked (with skin)			
Serving Size: 1 large baking potato			
Calories	220	Vitamin C	26.1 mg
		Thiamin	0.2 mg
		Niacin	3.3 mg
		Vitamin B₆	0.7 mg
Protein	4.7 g	Copper	0.6 mg
Carbohydrate	51 g	Iron	2.8 mg
Fat	0.2 g	Magnesium	55 mg
Saturated	0.1 g	Manganese	0.5 mg
Cholesterol	0	Phosphorus	115 mg
Dietary Fiber	4 g	Potassium	844 mg
Sodium	16 mg		

Selection and Storage

Boiling potatoes are red or white. They're small and round, with thin skins that look waxy, signaling more moisture and less starch. Baking potatoes, also known as russets or Idahos, are large and long, with skin that's brown and dry. Their lack of moisture makes them bake up fluffy. Long, white, all-purpose potatoes are also known as Maine, Eastern, or, curiously, California potatoes. New potatoes are not a variety of potato, just small, young potatoes of any variety that have yet to mature to full starchiness. They look waxy, with thin, undeveloped skin, often partially rubbed away.

Choose firm potatoes, with no soft or dark spots. Pass over green-tinged potatoes; they contain toxic alkaloids, such as solanine. Avoid any that are sprouting; they're old. If you buy potatoes in bags, open the bags right away and discard any rotting potatoes. A single bad potato can spoil a bagful.

Store potatoes in a dry, cool, dark, ventilated location. Light causes production of toxic solanine. Too much moisture causes rotting. Don't refrigerate, or the starch converts to sugar. Don't store with onions; both go bad faster. Mature potatoes keep for weeks; new potatoes only a week or so.

Preparation and Serving Tips

Don't wash potatoes until ready to cook, then scrub well with a vegetable brush under running water. Cut out sprouts and bad spots. If the potato is green or too soft, throw it out.

Baking a potato takes an hour in a conventional oven, but only five minutes in a microwave (12 minutes for four potatoes). Prick the skin for a fluffier potato. If you're baking them in a conventional oven, don't wrap them in foil unless you like steamed, mushy potatoes. Boil potatoes whole to reduce nutrient loss. Try a mint sprig in the water.

Remember, it's not the potato that can cause problems, it's what you put on it. Limit potatoes slathered in cheese. Instead, eat them plain or top them with low-fat yogurt or fat-free "sour cream" plus chopped dill, parsley, or scallions. Pile broccoli or other veggies on top.

New potatoes are delicious boiled and drizzled lightly with olive oil, then dusted liberally with dill weed.

POTATO PANCAKES

1½ pounds russet potatoes, grated
½ cup onion, grated
2 tablespoons chopped chives
¼ teaspoon salt
¼ teaspoon pepper
Nonstick cooking spray
½ cup applesauce

Combine potatoes, onion, chives, salt and pepper in medium bowl; mix well. Coat large nonstick skillet with cooking spray. Heat over medium heat until water droplets sprinkled on skillet bounce off surface.

Drop potato mixture by ⅓ cupfuls into skillet; flatten with spatula. Cook over medium-high heat 4 to 5 minutes on each side or until pancakes are cooked through. Serve with applesauce. *Makes 6 servings*

NUTRIENTS PER SERVING:			
Calories	126.4	Copper	0.28 mg
Protein	2.58 g	Iron	0.56 mg
Carbohydrate	29.77 g	Potassium	500.8 mg
Dietary Fiber	0.57 g	Sodium	97.58 mg
Fat	0.15 g	Vitamin C	18.93 mg
Saturated Fat	0.04 g		
Poly Fat	0.06 g	DIETARY EXCHANGES:	
Mono Fat	0.01 g	Fruit: 0.5	Bread: 1.5
Cholesterol	0		
Sugar	0.36 g	% OF CALORIES FROM:	
Beta-Carotene	41.88 RE	PRO: 8%	CARB: 91%
Calcium	10.67 mg	FAT: 1%	

PRUNES

Prunes are a sweet way to add fiber to your diet. Because they are dried, you tend to eat more of them than whole fruit, so they become a concentrated source of calories and nutrients.

Health Benefits

First and foremost, you think of the prune to relieve constipation. And that it does. Not only does each prune you eat sneak in more than half a gram of fiber, but it contains more than a gram of sorbitol as well. Sorbitol is a sugar alcohol that our bodies do not absorb well. Large amounts of it can cause diarrhea, accounting for the effect large numbers of prunes are known to have. But that's not all. Prunes also contain the laxative chemical diphenylisatin. No wonder they prevent constipation. So snack away, but don't go overboard.

Prunes also have a reputation for being rich in iron. In reality, they're a decent, but not spectacular, source. Not being a green or yellow vegetable, prunes get overlooked as a vitamin A source. But a serving provides more than ten percent of recommended levels. Potassium is another pleasant surprise you get from eating prunes.

NUTRIENT INFORMATION			
Prunes, dried		Vitamin A	668 IU
Serving Size: 4 medium			
Calories	80	Iron	0.8 g
Protein	0.9 g	Potassium	250 mg
Carbohydrate	21.1 g		
Fat	0.2 g		
Saturated	0		
Cholesterol	0		
Dietary Fiber	2.3 g		
Sodium	1 mg		

Selection and Storage

In case you've forgotten, prunes are simply dried plums. But don't try drying the plums you have at home. Only certain plums are good for making prunes, and they must be left on the tree longer for maximum sweetness.

When buying, look for well-sealed packages that keep moisture in, such as those that are vacuum-sealed. Choose pitted or unpitted, as you prefer. After opening, be sure to seal the package up well or transfer to an airtight container or plastic bag. You can store them in a cool, dry location or in the refrigerator. They'll keep for several months.

Preparation and Serving Tips

You can eat them out of the box, of course. They make a particularly portable snack. Combine them with dried apricots for a delightful mix of sweet and tang. Or mix them up with nuts and seeds for a healthy "trail mix." But watch out—the calories add up fast.

If you're not crazy about eating prunes whole, try prune bits in your baking. They'll add sweetness, flavor, and fiber to brownies, cookies, cakes, breads, even pancakes.

Purée pitted prunes in your food processor to make a great fat substitute to use in baked goods. Try substituting prune purée, in equal measure, for some of the fat in your recipes for baked goods.

To revive prunes that have dried out, microwave briefly, or simmer on the stove in water with a slice or two of apple.

PRUNE ZUCCHINI BREAD

- ⅔ **cup pitted prunes**
- 3 **tablespoons water**
- 1 **cup sugar**
- ½ **cup orange juice**
- 1 **teaspoon grated orange peel**
- 2 **cups grated zucchini**

1½ cups all-purpose flour
1½ cups whole wheat flour
 2 teaspoons pumpkin pie spice
 1 teaspoon baking powder
 1 teaspoon baking soda
 ¼ teaspoon salt
 ¼ cup plain low fat yogurt

Preheat oven to 350°F. Coat 9×5-inch loaf pan with non-stick cooking spray; set aside. For prune purée, combine prunes and water in food processor or blender; process until smooth. Combine prune purée, sugar, orange juice and orange peel in large bowl; mix well. Stir in zucchini; set aside.

Combine all-purpose flour, whole wheat flour, pumpkin pie spice, baking powder, baking soda and salt in medium bowl. Stir half of flour mixture into zucchini mixture, then stir in half of yogurt. Repeat with remaining flour mixture and yogurt; stir until blended. Pour batter into prepared pan.

Bake 1 hour and 15 minutes or until wooden toothpick inserted in center of loaf comes out clean. Cool in pan 10 minutes. Remove from pan; cool completely on wire rack. For best flavor, store bread, wrapped in plastic, overnight before serving it.   *Makes 1 loaf (12 servings)*

NUTRIENTS PER SERVING:			
Calories	187.2	Iron	1.52 mg
Protein	4.34 g		
Carbohydrate	43.06 g	Potassium	179.9 mg
Dietary Fiber	3.01 g	Sodium	146.9 mg
Fat	0.62 g	Vitamin A	13.8 RE
Saturated Fat	0.13 g		
Poly Fat	0.2 g	DIETARY EXCHANGES:	
Mono Fat	0.08 g	Fruit: 1.5	Bread: 1.5
Cholesterol	0.29 mg		
Sugar	17.61 g	% OF CALORIES FROM:	
Beta-Carotene	56.98 RE	PRO: 9%	CARB: 88%
Calcium	28.97 mg	FAT: 3%	
Folate	21.62 µg		

PUMPKIN

The pumpkin is an American original. This national symbol of Halloween seems to have been relegated to being used as a holiday ornament or being served up as pumpkin pie at Thanksgiving. That's too bad, because the pumpkin, a member of the varied squash family, has an understated taste that lends itself well to a variety of dishes.

Health Benefits

The distinctive bright orange color of a pumpkin is a dead giveaway that it's a good source of that all-important antioxidant beta-carotene. We've said it before, but we'll say it again: Research shows that people who eat a diet rich in beta-carotene are less likely to develop certain cancers than are people who fail to include such foods in their diets.

NUTRIENT INFORMATION			
Pumpkin, cooked		Vitamin A	1,320 IU
Serving Size: ½ cup mashed		Niacin	0.5 mg
Calories	102	Vitamin C	5.7 mg
Protein	0.9 g		
Carbohydrate	6.0 g	Calcium	18 mg
Fat	0.1 g	Potassium	181 mg
Saturated	0		
Fiber	0.6 g		
Cholesterol	0 mg		
Sodium	2 mg		

Selection and Storage

Look for a pumpkin that is free of cracks or soft spots and has a deep orange color. Though large pumpkins make the best jack-o'-lanterns, they don't always make the best edible squash. Very large pumpkins tend to be tough and stringy.

A whole pumpkin can keep well for up to a month, if you store it in a cool, dry spot. If you cut it, wrap it and place it in the refrigerator; it should keep for about one week.

To prepare pumpkin, first wash off any dirt from the surface. Cut away the skin, remove the seeds, then slice, dice, or cut the pulp into chunks. You might want to save the seeds; they make a great snack if you roast them.

If you prefer the quick and simple method of preparing pumpkin, you can always opt for canned. It's just as nutritious as the fresh variety. And for pies and purées, some say it tastes just as good.

Preparation and Serving Tips

Pumpkin pie is, without a doubt, Americans' favorite way of preparing pumpkin. But if it's prepared in the traditional way with heavy cream and whole eggs, you will have transformed a virtually fat-free food into one that provides almost half its calories from fat. Instead, substitute evaporated skim milk for the cream and use only one egg yolk for every two eggs that the recipe calls for. You'll cut the fat to about 30 percent of calories, and we bet no one will know the difference.

CRUSTLESS PUMPKIN PIE

- ¼ cup coarsely crushed corn flakes (½ cup uncrushed)
- ¼ cup *plus* 1 tablespoon packed brown sugar, divided
- 1 teaspoon ground cinnamon, divided
- ¼ teaspoon plus ⅛ teaspoon ground ginger, divided
- ¾ cup evaporated skim milk
- 1 teaspoon cornstarch
- ¼ teaspoon nutmeg
- ¾ cup canned pumpkin
- 2 tablespoons corn syrup
- ⅓ cup egg substitute

Preheat oven to 350°F. For topping, combine corn flakes, 1 tablespoon brown sugar, ½ teaspoon cinnamon and ⅛ teaspoon ginger. Mix well; set aside.

For custard mixture, heat milk in small saucepan over medium heat. *Do not boil.* Combine remaining ¼ cup brown sugar, ½ teaspoon cinnamon, ¼ teaspoon ginger, cornstarch and nutmeg in small bowl; mix well.

Place pumpkin in large bowl; stir in sugar mixture and corn syrup until well mixed. Stir in hot milk; mix well. Add egg substitute; stir until smooth. Pour custard into four 6-ounce ovenproof custard cups or ramekins. Place cups in baking pan; carefully add boiling water to ¾-inch depth. Sprinkle topping evenly over custard. Bake 35 to 40 minutes or until knife blade inserted in center of custard comes out clean.

Makes 4 servings

NUTRIENTS PER SERVING:		Folate	30.97 µg
Calories	172	Iron	2.56 mg
Protein	6.12 g		
Carbohydrate	37.23 g	Potassium	367 mg
Dietary Fiber	0.99 g	Sodium	132.7 mg
Fat	0.31 g	Vitamin A	1,210 RE
Saturated Fat	0.17 g		
Poly Fat	0.02 g	DIETARY EXCHANGES:	
Mono Fat	0.06 g	Milk: 0.5	Bread: 2
Cholesterol	1.91 mg		
Sugar	20.39 g	% OF CALORIES FROM:	
Beta-Carotene	95.96 RE	PRO: 14%	CARB: 85%
Calcium	184.2 mg	FAT: 2%	

RAISINS

Raisins have been prepared for thousands of years, and they remain a favorite. In the simplest of terms, raisins are dried grapes. Most of the raisins in the United States, both dark and golden, come from dried Thompson seedless grapes that are either sun dried or dried in ovens. Both are dried in the same way, but golden are dried for a shorter period of time, thus their plumper texture, and they are treated with sulphur dioxide to help maintain their naturally light color.

The sweeter, more intensely flavored Zante grape is used to make currants, which are used mainly in baked goods. This is not to be confused with the tiny blackberry, related to the gooseberry, that is also called a currant.

Health Benefits

Raisins, like other dried fruit, are a good source of iron—an important thing to know if your leaning toward a more vegetarian-style diet. They are also an excellent source of potassium, a nutrient that just might help you keep hypertension at bay, if you get enough of it.

NUTRIENT INFORMATION			
Raisins, seedless		Niacin	0.6 mg
Serving Size: ½ cup			
Calories	217	Calcium	35.5 mg
Protein	2.3 g	Copper	2.2 mg
Carbohydrate	57 g	Iron	1.5 mg
Fat	0.3 g	Potassium	544 mg
Saturated	0.1 g		
Cholesterol	0		
Dietary Fiber	1.7 g		
Sodium	8 mg		

Selection and Storage

Raisins packaged in boxes and bags are available year-round. Choose raisins sold in tightly sealed bags or boxes rather than in open bins. Once you open them, reseal them tightly to keep out air. When exposed to air, raisins will dry out, and sugar will crystalize on the surface. If you store them in the refrigerator, raisins will keep for up to one year; they'll last even longer in the freezer.

Preparation and Serving Tips

Raisins are the perfect portable no-fuss, no-muss snack food. They don't require refrigeration to stay fresh for a short period of time, and they make no mess.

Raisins are also delicious added to low-fat yogurt or added to your own low-fat trail mix of dried fruit, puffed rice, popcorn, and a sprinkling of nuts and sunflower seeds.

While they're great simply eaten straight from the box, raisins are also delicious added to muffins, biscuits, scones, and breads or sprinkled as a topping over hot cereals. If, by the time you reach in the refrigerator for raisins, they've dried out, you can plump them up by steaming them over boiling water for about five minutes. If you simply want to plump them for baking, you can let them stand in hot water, fruit juice, wine, brandy, or liqueur for about five minutes.

Though not commonly added to meat dishes in American cookery, raisins are popular ingredients in many Indian and Middle-Eastern dishes, including curry and couscous.

STREUSEL TOPPED APPLE–RAISIN CAKE

   Streusel (recipe follows)
   All-purpose flour
2 cups all-purpose flour
1 teaspoon baking powder
1 teaspoon baking soda
1 teaspoon ground cinnamon
½ teaspoon ground nutmeg
4 tablespoons margarine, softened
1 cup granulated sugar
2 eggs
2 egg whites
2 cups shredded cored peeled apples
¾ cup dark raisins

Preheat oven to 350°F. Prepare Streusel; set aside. Coat 9-inch springform pan with nonstick cooking spray. Sprinkle lightly with flour; tap side of pan to evenly coat bottom and side.

Combine 2 cups flour, baking powder, baking soda, cinnamon and nutmeg in medium bowl; set aside. Beat margarine and sugar in large bowl until well blended. Blend in eggs and egg whites; mix well. Stir in apples. Add flour mixture; mix well. Stir in raisins.

Pour batter into prepared pan; sprinkle with Streusel. Bake about 50 minutes or until wooden toothpick inserted in center of cake comes out clean. Cool in pan on wire rack 15 minutes. Remove side of pan. Serve warm. ***Makes 12 servings***

STREUSEL

- 3 tablespoons packed light brown sugar
- 3 tablespoons all-purpose flour
- 1 tablespoon cold margarine

Combine brown sugar and flour in small bowl. Cut in margarine with pastry blender or 2 knives until mixture resembles coarse crumbs.

NUTRIENTS PER SERVING:

Calories	252.5	Magnesium	11.34 mg
Protein	4.37 g		
Carbohydrate	47.18 g	Potassium	147.4 mg
Dietary Fiber	1.5 g	Sodium	173.2 mg
Fat	5.91 g	Vitamin A	74.89 RE
Saturated Fat	1.26 g	Vitamin C	1.41 mg
Poly Fat	1.72 g		
Mono Fat	2.43 g	DIETARY EXCHANGES:	
Cholesterol	35.5 mg	Fruit: 1	Bread: 2.5
Sugar	27.01 g	Fat: 1	
Beta-Carotene	11.87 RE		
Calcium	25.56 mg	% OF CALORIES FROM:	
Folate	10.9 µg	PRO: 7%	CARB: 73%
Iron	1.6 mg	FAT: 21%	

RASPBERRIES

This delicately fragile and exquisitely expensive berry is actually a member of the rose family. Though we usually think of raspberries as being red, they also come in golden and black. Their flavors are similar. Raspberries are generally available May through November. They are grown mainly in California and are at their peak in June and July. Imported raspberries may be available at other times of the year.

Health Benefits

Besides being a great source of the antioxidant vitamin C, raspberries are also a good source of fiber. And much of that fiber is in the form of pectin, a substance known to help lower blood cholesterol. Moreover, raspberries fall into the same category as strawberries and cherries as a fruit that contains the phytochemical ellagic acid, believed to have anticancer properties.

NUTRIENT INFORMATION

Raspberries		Sodium	0 mg
Serving Size: ½ cup			
Calories	30	Niacin	0.6 mg
Protein	0.6 g	Vitamin C	39 mg
Carbohydrate	7.1 g		
Fat	0.3 g	Manganese	0.6 mg
Saturated	0		
Cholesterol	0		
Dietary Fiber	1.7 g		

Selection and Storage

Because they are so fragile, choose and use raspberries with care. When you're looking through the selection at the market, look for berries that are brightly colored and have no hulls attached. If the green hull is still on the berry, it will be tart. Steer clear of berries that look shriveled or have visible mold. They should be plump, firm, well shaped, and evenly colored, with no green. They should be packed in a single layer container and should have a clean, slightly sweet fragrance. When you get them home, don't expect them to keep in the refrigerator more than a day or two. It's best if you eat them as soon as possible.

Don't try to cut or slice raspberries. They have a hollow core and will fall apart in your hands.

Preparation and Serving Tips

Just before you serve them, take chilled raspberries and rinse them under cool water. Whole, chilled raspberries make an elegant topping for frozen desserts or slices of angel-food cake. Make a raspberry purée to pour generously (it's terrifically low in calories) over a fruit salad, cake, pancakes, or waffles. If you're in a celebratory mood, pour champagne over chilled, ripe raspberries in a tall champagne glass. Raspberries, combined with blueberries and a sprig of fresh mint, make a colorfully contrasting (and edible) garnish for any dish.

Frozen raspberries packed in light syrup can be used to make a frozen dessert. Combine frozen raspberries with one-percent milk and fresh lemon juice. Purée the berries first. Then give all the ingredients a whirl on low speed in the food processor. Freeze the mixture, then run it through the food processor. Freeze again overnight.

RASPBERRY SWIRL CHEESECAKE

    2 tablespoons vanilla wafer cookie crumbs
    2 containers (12 ounces each) nonfat cream cheese,
        softened
 ⅔ cup sugar
    2 eggs
    2 tablespoons cornstarch
    2 teaspoons vanilla
    1 cup low fat sour cream
    1 pint raspberries, divided
      Mint sprigs for garnish

Preheat oven to 400°F. Coat bottom and 1 inch up side of 9-inch springform pan with nonstick cooking spray; coat with cookie crumbs. Beat cream cheese in large bowl with electric mixer until fluffy. Beat in sugar. Add eggs, cornstarch and vanilla; beat until smooth. Mix in sour cream until well combined. Pour batter into prepared pan.

Place 1 cup raspberries in food processor or blender; process until smooth. Strain purée; discard seeds. Spoon purée onto cheesecake; swirl into batter with knife.

Bake 45 to 50 minutes or until cheesecake is set around edge but slightly soft in center. Turn off oven; let cheesecake cool in oven about 3 hours with oven door slightly opened.

Refrigerate cheesecake overnight. Remove side of pan; place cheesecake on serving plate. Garnish with remaining 1 cup raspberries and mint sprigs.   *Makes 14 servings*

NUTRIENTS PER SERVING:			
Calories	135.7	Folate	7.86 µg
Protein	8.83 g	Magnesium	4.05 mg
Carbohydrate	16.53 g	Potassium	35.97 mg
Dietary Fiber	0.8 g	Sodium	325.7 mg
Fat	2.57 g	Vitamin C	4.4 mg
Saturated Fat	0.25 g		
Poly Fat	0.18 g	DIETARY EXCHANGES:	
Mono Fat	0.33 g	Bread: 1	Meat: 1
Cholesterol	46.11 mg		
Sugar	10.34 g	% OF CALORIES FROM:	
Beta-Carotene	13.71 RE	PRO: 28%	CARB: 53%
Calcium	7.82 mg	FAT: 19%	

RHUBARB

Rhubarb has been grown for thousands of years and used for medicinal purposes in India, China, Mongolia, and Siberia. Rhubarb looks like pink celery, but it tastes quite different. It has a tart, acidic flavor that is usually toned down by cooking it with a fairly large dose of sugar. In fact, rhubarb is best known as an ingredient in rhubarb pie. Although it is actually a vegetable, rhubarb is used like a fruit. Whatever you do, don't eat the leaves. They contain a high level of oxalic acid; enough to be toxic. Rhubarb season peaks in May, but rhubarb is best in late winter through late spring.

Health Benefits

The calcium in rhubarb cannot be absorbed because of the oxalic acid the plant contains. Rhubarb is, however, a good source of potassium and the B vitamin niacin.

Selection and Storage

Whether you buy it loose or prepackaged in cellophane bags, choose crisp, brightly colored stalks. If leaves are attached, be sure they are fresh and green. The stalks should be medium size. Younger, smaller stalks are usually more tender than mature ones. Color is a prime clue to taste. There are actually two crops of rhubarb each season. One is light pink, the other a darker red. Light pink stalks are less acidic and more tender than the darker red stalks.

Fresh rhubarb is highly perishable, but you can store rhubarb in a bag in the refrigerator for a day or two. You can also freeze it, if you blanch it first.

NUTRIENT INFORMATION		Dietary Fiber	0.4 g
Rhubarb		Sodium	2 mg
Serving Size: ½ cup, diced,			
cooked		Niacin	0.2 mg
Calories	13		
Protein	0.6 g	Potassium	175 mg
Carbohydrate	2.8 g		
Fat	0.1 g		
Saturated	na		
Cholesterol	0		

Preparation and Serving Tips

Light-pink stalks of rhubarb don't need to be peeled. But the darker-red variety tends to be stringy; you will need to peel it and remove the strings as you would do for celery.

In addition to being a pie ingredient, rhubarb also makes delicious sauces, jams, and pudding. When you add a lot of sugar to rhubarb to make it palatable, you of course add calories. There's no getting around the fact that rhubarb must be sweetened, but you can lessen the need for sugar by stewing it in orange juice or pineapple juice first. Other flavoring ideas for rhubarb: orange zest, rose water, ginger, or cinnamon. Generally, rhubarb will cook in about 20 to 35 minutes depending on the thickness of the stalks.

RHUBARB AND STRAWBERRY SAUCE

1 cup rhubarb, cut into ½-inch slices
2 tablespoons water
½ teaspoon ground cinnamon
½ cup sliced strawberries
3 to 4 tablespoons sugar

Bring rhubarb, water and cinnamon to a boil in small saucepan over high heat. Reduce heat to low. Simmer, uncovered, about 10 minutes or until rhubarb is soft. Stir in strawberries and sugar; cook 1 to 2 minutes or until sugar is dissolved.

Serve sauce warm or chilled over vanilla low fat yogurt, fruit or angel food cake. *Makes 8 servings (about 2 tablespoons per serving)*

NUTRIENTS PER SERVING:		Folate	2.74 µg
Calories	23.29	Niacin (B₃)	0.07 mg
Protein	0.2 g	Potassium	60 mg
Carbohydrate	5.96 g	Sodium	0.8 mg
Dietary Fiber	0.52 g		
Fat	0.07 g	DIETARY EXCHANGES:	
Saturated Fat	0.01 g	Fruit: 0.5	
Poly Fat	0.03 g		
Mono Fat	0.01 g	% OF CALORIES FROM:	
Cholesterol	0 mg	PRO: 3%	CARB: 94%
Sugar	4.78 g	FAT: 2%	
Calcium	16.18 mg		

RICE

Rice is the backbone of the diets of over one-half of the world's population. It's a common enough sight at American tables as well. Still, rice has hardly reached the status it has in Asian countries such as Japan and China, where each person consumes, on average, 200 to 400 pounds of rice a year. In some parts of Asia, the word "to eat" is literally translated to mean "to eat rice." By comparison, in the United States, we consume up to about 21 pounds per person, per year.

Do the Asian countries know something we don't? For one, rice is part of the formula that keeps native Asian diets so low in fat. While we tend to view rice as a side dish to a meat-centered meal, they view rice itself as the focus of the meal, with other dishes merely complementing its presence.

Health Benefits

Rice is an excellent source of complex carbohydrates and, if it's enriched, a good source of several B vitamins. Brown rice provides three times the fiber of white rice. Recent research has shown that rice bran, a small amount of which remains on brown rice, lowers cholesterol. And rice-bran oil, which is usually available in health-food stores, also has cholesterol-lowering abilities. The carbohydrate of processed white rice, on the other hand, is readily digested and raises blood glucose as rapidly and as high as white bread and almost as efficiently as glucose in a glucose tolerance test.

Selection and Storage

Though there are over 7,000 varieties of rice grown around the world, only a few are readily found in the United States. The most broad categorization is to break rice down according to grain size—long, medium, or short. Long grain is the most popular in this country. When cooked, the grains tend to

NUTRIENT INFORMATION

Rice, white, long-grain Serving Size: ½ cup, cooked		Rice, brown, long-grain Serving Size: ½ cup, cooked	
Calories	131	Calories	109
Protein	2.7 g	Protein	2.5 g
Carbohydrate	28.5 g	Carbohydrate	22.5 g
Fat	0.3 g	Fat	0.9 g
Saturated	0.1 g	Saturated	
Cholesterol	0		0.2 g
Dietary Fiber	0.5 g	Cholesterol	0
Sodium	2 mg	Dietary Fiber	1.7 g
		Sodium	5 mg
Iron	1.1 mg		
Manganese	0.5 mg	Magnesium	42 mg
		Manganese	0.9 mg
Niacin	1.5 mg		
Pantothenic Acid	0.4 mg	Niacin	1.5 mg
Thiamin	0.2 mg		

be fluffy and dry and to separate readily. Medium grain is popular in some Asian and Latin-American cultures. Though it is fairly fluffy right after cooking, it tends to clump together once it begins to cool. Short-grain rice, also known as glutinous rice, has fat, almost round grains that have a higher starch content than the other-size grains. When cooked, it becomes moist and sticky, with the grains clumping together—perfect for eating with chopsticks.

The more common varieties of rice can be further categorized into brown rice and white rice. Brown rice is the whole grain with only the outer husk removed. It is tan in color, has a chewy texture, and has what some people describe as a nut-like flavor.

White rice should be stored in an airtight container in a cool, dark, dry place where it will keep almost indefinitely. Brown rice, on the other hand, is much more perishable. It keeps only about six months—slightly longer if you refrigerate it in an airtight container.

It's becoming increasingly easy to find more-exotic aromatic varieties of rice such as basmati, jasmine, and arborio.

Wild rice, one of the most expensive varieties, is not a rice at all but a member of the grass family. It has a rich flavor and is higher in protein than other types of rice.

You're better off buying a box of rice and seasoning it yourself than buying ready-made rice mixes. Mixes tend to be very high in sodium and many have unnecessarily added fat.

Preparation and Serving Tips

If the rice is bought from bins, as it is in Asia, it must be washed to remove dust and dirt. Rice packaged in the United States usually does not need to be washed before cooking. Indeed, if the packaged rice was fortified, rinsing could wash away some of the B vitamins. It's not a bad idea to rinse imported rices. They are not enriched, so you don't have to worry about losing nutrients, and they may be dirty or dusty.

Cooking times for rice vary depending upon the variety and the size of the grain. Long-grain white rice takes about 20 minutes to cook. Place ½ cup uncooked rice in one cup of boiling water, cover, and let simmer.

Long-grain brown rice takes a bit longer—25 to 30 minutes—to become tender. As with white rice, place ½ cup uncooked rice in one cup of boiling water, cover, and let simmer. Short-grain brown rice takes about 40 minutes to prepare.

Wild rice has the longest preparation time. It takes up to 50 minutes to cook ½ cup of wild rice in two cups of water. The aromatic varieties such as arborio take only 15 minutes to cook. Some require a smaller ratio of water to rice. Check the package instructions.

Water isn't the only cooking medium you can use to prepare rice. You can use seasoned broth or stock, fruit juice, or tomato juice. Just remember that when you add acid to the cooking water, the rice will take longer to cook. And always dilute it to half strength with water.

Though rice is often served as a stand-alone side dish, it's even better stir-fried and mixed with vegetables. Or try it as a cold salad with peas, red peppers, and a warm vinaigrette dressing.

The sky's the limit when it comes to seasoning cooked rice. Just remember that heartier-flavored rice demands little in the way of dressing up. Save that extra dose of herbs for plain white rice. Here are just a few of the herbs and spices to try: curry, soy sauce (try a lower-sodium variety if you are sodium sensitive), sesame oil, hot peppers, turmeric, cumin, fresh cilantro, basil, parsley, or oregano.

BROWN RICE AND VEGETABLES

    Nonstick cooking spray
½ cup chopped onion
3 cloves garlic, minced
1 teaspoon dried thyme leaves, crushed
1 cup sliced mushrooms
1 medium zucchini, sliced
1 cup chopped carrots
¼ cup thinly sliced celery
2 cups uncooked brown rice

NUTRIENTS PER SERVING:			
Calories	504.4	Niacin (B₃)	6.73 mg
Protein	22.46 g	Potassium	688 mg
Carbohydrate	82.85 g	Pyridoxine (B₆)	0.69 mg
Dietary Fiber	8.4 g	Riboflavin (B₂)	0.31 mg
Fat	10.57 g	Sodium	109.4 mg
Saturated Fat	2.13 g	Thiamin (B₁)	0.58 mg
Poly Fat	4.75 g	Vitamin C	9.08 mg
Mono Fat	2.7 g	Zinc	3.49 mg
Cholesterol	2.47 mg		
Sugar	3.12 g	DIETARY EXCHANGES:	
Beta-Carotene	4,796 RE	Veg: 1.5	Bread: 5.0
Calcium	252.4 mg	Meat: 1	Fat: 1
Copper	0.69 mg		
Folate	60.78 µg	% OF CALORIES FROM:	
Iron	10.43 mg	PRO: 17%	CARB: 64%
Magnesium	221.7 mg	FAT: 18%	
Manganese	4.56 mg		

1   **package (10 ½ ounces) firm tofu, cut into ½-inch cubes**
½   **teaspoon pepper**
1   **can (about 14 ounces) defatted low sodium chicken broth✲**
2   **tablespoons grated Parmesan cheese**

Coat large saucepan with cooking spray; heat over medium heat. Add onion, garlic and thyme; cook and stir about 3 minutes or until onion is tender. Add mushrooms, zucchini, carrots and celery; cook and stir 10 to 12 minutes or until vegetables are almost tender.

Stir in rice, tofu and pepper. Add chicken broth; bring to a boil over high heat. Reduce heat to low. Simmer, covered, 50 to 60 minutes or until rice is tender and liquid is absorbed. Stir in Parmesan just before serving.   *Makes 4 servings*

✲ To defat chicken broth, skim fat from surface of broth with spoon. Or, place can of broth in refrigerator at least 2 hours ahead of time. Before using, remove fat that has hardened on surface of broth.

RUTABAGAS

The rutabaga, a close relative of the turnip, is probably one of the least attractive vegetables. It might not be your first choice, with its large form; bumpy, irregular shape; and thick wax coating (to retain moisture). But inside that unattractive package is a surprisingly sweet, mild-flavored vegetable that acts as a complement to other, somewhat heartier flavors.

Rutabagas, also known as Swedish or Russian turnips, are generally available all year but have a long peak season through the fall and winter months.

Health Benefits

As cruciferous vegetables, rutabagas are one of the foods thought to help reduce the risk of cancer. They are also a good source of vitamin C, especially if you eat them raw, and a good source of potassium, a mineral believed to help ward off high blood pressure and strokes.

NUTRIENT INFORMATION			
Rutabagas		Vitamin C	18.6 mg
Serving Size: ½ cup, cooked			
Calories	29	Calcium	36 mg
Protein	0.9 g	Potassium	244 mg
Carbohydrate	6.6 g		
Fat	0.1 g		
Saturated	0		
Cholesterol	0		
Dietary Fiber	1.6 g		
Sodium	15 mg		

Selection and Storage

Look for smooth-skinned, firm, uncracked rutabagas that are small but heavy for their size. Smaller rutabagas tend to be sweeter. Large rutabagas tend to be pulpy and stringy. These root vegetables are almost always trimmed of their tops and are usually coated with a thick film of wax to hold moisture in.

Though they are sometimes confused with turnips, they are considerably larger than turnips and have a tan skin with a dark-purple cap. Rutabagas store well. They should keep in the refrigerator for at least two weeks.

Preparation and Serving Tips

Always wash and peel rutabagas before cooking. Peel them with a paring knife rather than a vegetable peeler; the skin is tough and you want to be sure to remove the wax coating. Rutabagas tend to develop a stronger flavor the longer they're cooked. The amount of time required to prepare rutabagas varies with the vegetable's age. Older, larger rutabagas take longer to cook than smaller, more tender roots. But generally, if you cook them in boiling water, they should take about 15 to 20 minutes to become tender.

Because they have a mildly sweet flavor, rutabagas work well with spices such as nutmeg, ginger, and cloves. They can be prepared much the same as sweet potatoes. Rutabaga strips can be used in vegetable stir-fries, and mashed or puréed rutabagas can be served as a substitute for mashed potatoes.

Generally speaking, because they have a heartier flavor than say, potatoes, they work best when served with full-flavored foods such as beef. They tend to overwhelm the more delicate flavors of fish or poultry.

MASHED RUTABAGAS AND POTATOES

  1 **pound rutabagas, peeled, cut into ½-inch pieces**
  ½ **pound potatoes, peeled, cut into ½-inch pieces**
  ¼ **cup 1% low fat milk**
  ¼ **teaspoon ground nutmeg**
  1 **tablespoon chopped parsley**

Place rutabagas and potatoes in large saucepan; add enough water to cover vegetables. Bring to a boil over high heat. Cook, uncovered, 15 minutes or until vegetables are fork-tender. Drain well; transfer to medium bowl.

Mash vegetables with potato masher or electric mixer. Blend in milk and nutmeg until smooth. Stir in chopped parsley before serving.   *Makes 4 servings*

NUTRIENTS PER SERVING:			
Calories	92.58	Magnesium	36.13 mg
Protein	2.66 g	Potassium	515.7 mg
Carbohydrate	20.25 g	Sodium	29.95 mg
Dietary Fiber	3.46 g	Vitamin A	14.26 RE
Fat	0.61 g	Vitamin C	28.62 mg
Saturated Fat	0.26 g	Zinc	0.54 mg
Poly Fat	0.13 g	DIETARY EXCHANGES:	
Mono Fat	0.12 g	Veg: 2	Bread: 0.5
Cholesterol	1.13 mg		
Sugar	0.7 g	% OF CALORIES FROM:	
Calcium	68.79 mg	PRO: 11%	CARB: 83%
Folate	23.52 µg	FAT: 6%	

SALAD GREENS

When you make a salad, don't overlook salad greens other than lettuce. Wonderfully flavorful greens like raddichio, arugula, endive, chicory, and escarole add new tastes and textures to really make a salad stand out. Most of these "other" salad greens are more expensive than lettuce and have stronger flavors, so you may want to use them to complement lettuce, rather than as a salad base.

Health Benefits

As with lettuce, the darker the color of the salad green, the more nutritious it is. Beta-carotene is the chief disease-fighting nutrient found in abundance in some of the darker-colored greens like endive and chicory. Chicory is also a very good source of vitamin C, another one of the antioxidant nutrients. Some of the greens, including arugula and watercress, are members of the cruciferous family, giving them even more ammunition to help you reduce your risk of disease.

NUTRIENT INFORMATION			
Endive		Dietary Fiber	1.0 g
Serving Size: 1 cup, chopped		Sodium	12 mg
Calories	8		
Protein	0.6 g	Vitamin A	1,026 IU
Carbohydrate	1.6 g	Folic Acid	71 µg
Fat	0.2 g		
Saturated	0		
Cholesterol	0		

Selection and Storage

These less-recognizable greens come in an even wider variety of sizes, shapes, and colors than their salad-making cohorts of the lettuce family. Most varieties are available year-round, though prices may vary during different times of the year.

As you would when shopping for lettuce, avoid salad greens that have begun to wilt or that have brown-edged or slimy leaves. Once they have reached this point, there's no bringing them back to life. You want salad greens that are displayed on ice or at least in a refrigerated area. They should have vivid colors, and the leaves should be firm, and when appropriate, crisp. If you don't use them right away, store them in the refrigerator crisper drawer, roots intact, in plastic bags.

Here are some of the more common varieties of these less-than-common salad greens:

Arugula: Also known as rocket or roquette, these small, flat leaves have what has been described as a hot, peppery flavor. Though arugula is quite popular in Italy, most American palates are not used to its bold flavor. The older and larger the leaves, the more mustard-like the flavor becomes. You're more likely to find it in ethnic markets than in the supermarket. One of the more delicate greens, it will keep in the refrigerator for only a day or two.

Chicory: This curly-leaved green is sometimes mistakenly called curly endive. The dark-green leaves have a bitter taste, but they work well in salads that have well-seasoned dressings. Chicory is available all year and is best when eaten fresh. Roasted chicory comes from the roasted ground roots and is used as a coffee extender. This coffee-chicory blend is most popular in Louisiana.

Endive: Belgian endive and white chicory are also names for this characteristically pale salad green. Endive is grown specifically to be lacking in color. The small, cigar-shaped head has tightly packed leaves that have a somewhat bitter flavor. Endive should stay fresh in the refrigerator for three to four days. It is generally available September through May.

Escarole: A close cousin to chicory, escarole is actually a type of endive. It has broad, slightly curved green leaves and has a milder flavor than Belgian endive. It is available year-round, but the peak season is June through October.

Radicchio: Though it looks something like a miniature head of red cabbage, this salad green is actually a member of the varied chicory family. It is treated much the same as chicory but has a less bitter flavor. Radicchio heads will keep for up to a week in the refrigerator. Radicchio is available all year, with a peak season from mid-winter to early spring.

Watercress: This delicate green, which is a member of the mustard family, is sold in "bouquets" or trimmed and sealed in vacuum packs. Choose a bunch that has dark-green, glossy leaves. Unopened packs should last for up to three days in the refrigerator. Place bunches in a plastic bag and use within a day or two.

Preparation and Serving Tips

Because most salad greens are either loose leaf or individual bunches of leaves grouped together, dirt and grit tend to settle in between the leaves. Wash them well before use. Cut off the roots and swish the leaves in a large bowl of water. You may want to repeat the process a few times to be sure no trace of grime is left behind. Most will keep for a few days if you put them in a plastic bag and store them in the crisper drawer.

Besides being used in salads, several of these salad greens can also be grilled, sautéed, or baked as cooking greens.

As a general rule, the stronger and more bitter the salad green, the stronger the flavor of the dressing should be. Warm mustard or garlic-based dressings work well with strong-flavored salad greens.

For a different look, watercress or arugula can be used to make a nice garnish. Watercress can also be used to make a light sauce to be served with fish and is a delicious base for soup. The other larger-leaf greens make attractive beds for fruit or chicken salad.

ORANGE AND GREEN SALAD

3 slices whole wheat bread, cut into ½-inch cubes
   Olive oil cooking spray
1 clove garlic, minced
3 tablespoons frozen orange juice concentrate, thawed
3 tablespoons balsamic vinegar
2 teaspoons honey
1 clove garlic, crushed
½ teaspoon grated orange peel
½ teaspoon olive oil
6 cups torn washed mixed salad greens, such as escarole, chicory, arugula, radicchio, romaine, spinach and watercress
2 navel oranges, peeled, seeded, cut into thin slices
½ cup thinly sliced red onion

Preheat oven to 250°F. For croutons, spread bread cubes in shallow baking pan. Coat lightly with cooking spray; sprinkle

NUTRIENTS PER SERVING:			
Calories	113.1	Potassium	574. mg
Protein	4.6 g	Sodium	115.2 mg
Carbohydrate	23.11 g	Vitamin C	100.3 mg
Dietary Fiber	4.27 g	Vitamin K	67.55 µg
Fat	1.28 g		
Saturated Fat	0.15 g	DIETARY EXCHANGES:	
Poly Fat	0.27 g	Veg: 1.5	Fruit: 0.5
Mono Fat	0.39 g	Bread: 0.5	
Cholesterol	0		
Sugar	3.18 g	% OF CALORIES FROM:	
Beta-Carotene	2,061 RE	PRO: 15%	CARB:
Calcium	245.4 mg	76%	
Folate	87.99 µg	FAT: 9%	
Iron	5.33 mg		

with minced garlic. Bake 10 minutes. Stir bread cubes; coat lightly with cooking spray. Bake 5 minutes more or until croutons are browned and crisp. Let cool to room temperature.

For dressing, combine orange juice concentrate, vinegar, honey, crushed garlic, orange peel and oil in medium bowl until smooth. Let stand, covered, 1 hour to allow flavors to blend.

Combine salad greens, oranges and onion in large bowl. Just before serving, remove crushed garlic clove from dressing. Pour dressing over salad; toss gently to coat. Sprinkle with croutons.   *Makes 6 servings*

Note: Dressing may be stored, covered, in refrigerator up to 4 days.

SEEDS

Seeds are the "eggs" that contain the nutrients needed to nourish the growth of another plant. So their high nutritional content is no surprise. Though seeds from pumpkin, squash, and sunflower are usually consumed as snacks, the nutrition punch they pack make them better suited to be the main attraction. Their only drawback is that they provide about 80 percent of their calories as fat. Though the fat is mostly of the unsaturated variety, it's still a heavy dose for a single food.

Health Benefits

With their gold mine of healthy minerals and their niacin and folic-acid contents, seeds are an excellent nutrition package. They are among the better plant sources of iron and zinc. In fact, one ounce of pumpkin seeds contains almost twice as much iron as three ounces of skinless chicken breast. And they provide more fiber per ounce than nuts. They are also good sources of protein. Sesame seeds are a surprising source of the bone-building mineral calcium. And they are a rich source of vitamin E.

NUTRIENT INFORMATION			
Sunflower Seed Kernels, oil roasted		Folic Acid	67 µg
		Niacin	1.2 mg
Serving Size: 1 oz, oil roasted		Vitamin E	14 mg
Calories	176		
Protein	6.1 g	Copper	0.5 mg
Carbohydrate	4.2 g	Iron	1.9 mg
Fat	16.3 g	Magnesium	36 mg
Saturated	1.7 g	Manganese	0.6 mg
Cholesterol	0	Phosphorus	323 mg
Dietary Fiber	1.7 g	Zinc	1.5 mg
Sodium	1 mg		

Selection and Storage

Seeds are often sold in bulk, both with the hull in place and the kernel separated out. Make sure they are fresh. Because of their high fat content, seeds are vulnerable to rancidity. If they're exposed to heat, light, or humidity, they're likely to become rancid much quicker. A quick sniff of the seed bin should tell you if the contents are fresh or not. Seeds with the hulls intact should keep several months if stored in a cool, dry place. Seed kernels will keep for a slightly shorter period.

Hulled pumpkin seeds are a popular ingredient in Mexican cooking. Pumpkin and squash seeds are similar in appearance—white to yellowish in color—and they have a relatively thin hull. Sunflower seeds have a distinctive hard black-and-white-striped hull.

Preparation and Serving Tips

As a snack, go easy, because of the high fat content. But, in moderation, seeds can be mixed in with cereals or trail mix or eaten by themselves.

A sprinkling of seed kernels over fruits, vegetables, pastas, or salads adds a touch of crunchy texture and flavor. Sesame seeds are especially attractive as toppers for breads, rolls, salads, and stir-fries.

SHELLFISH

Shellfish is a broad category of seafood delicacies made up of the crustaceans, including crabs, crayfish, lobster, and shrimp, and the mollusks, such as clams and oysters. They have full-bodied flavors that are distinctive from their milder-tasting finfish neighbors of the sea. Though shellfish are generally more expensive than finfish, they are delicious, and in our opinion, well worth the price. But you'll need to take special care in handling your precious cargo to ensure that it does not spoil.

Health Benefits

Shellfish may carry the reputation of being high in cholesterol, but the fact is, most provide no more cholesterol than lean beef or chicken. And they are terrifically low in fat. Like finfish, shellfish are low in saturated fat and provide a dose of the healthy omega-3 fatty acids, which are believed to help reduce the risk of heart disease and help alleviate the symptoms of some devastating conditions, such as psoriasis and migraines.

NUTRIENT INFORMATION			
Shrimp, cooked		Niacin	2.2 mg
Serving Size: 3 oz		Vitamin B$_{12}$	1.3 µg
Calories	84		
Protein	17.8 g	Copper	0.2 mg
Carbohydrate	0	Iron	2.6 mg
Fat	0.9 g	Zinc	1.3 mg
Saturated	0.1 g		
Cholesterol	166 mg		
Dietary Fiber	0		
Sodium	190 mg		

Selection and Storage

Clams: Like most other crustaceans, it's important that the clams you cook are live. How to tell: They are tightly closed, or, if open, they close automatically when you lightly tap the shell. Any clam with an open shell that won't shut is dead and should be thrown out. For soft-shell clams, merely touch the protruding neck; if it moves, it's still alive. You can store live clams in the refrigerator for a couple of days. Fresh clams are available on the East Coast and in the Pacific Northwest all year. In California, clam season runs from November through April.

Crabs: They are the second-most-eaten shellfish in the United States after shrimp. Though there are several varieties of crab, including Dungeness, King, Snow, Blue, and Stone, all have a distinctive, almost sweet flavor. Crabs are sold either live or as cooked meat. All live crabs should be used the day you buy them. Cooked meat can be stored for a couple of days in the refrigerator. Hard-shelled crabs are available year-round; soft shell from April to mid-September.

Crayfish: These crustaceans look like tiny lobsters, but they are a different species. Also known as crawfish or crawdads, these creatures are quite popular in France, New Zealand, Scandinavia, and Louisiana. As with crabs, crayfish should be purchased live and should be cooked the same day. Like lobsters, they turn bright red when they are boiled. They can be prepared in just about any dish suitable for lobster, but the meat is not as dense or as intensely flavored. Crayfish are an exception to the low-cholesterol rule. They contain about 175 milligrams per 3½ ounces.

Lobster: Prior to the 20th century, lobster was so common that it was used as fish bait. Now, it is the most premium-priced, prized member of the crustacean family. Buy your lobster live. Lobsters begin to deteriorate rapidly once they die and become perfect breeding grounds for bacteria. You'll need to either cook them live or immediately after killing. Fresh lobster is available all year, but it is a better buy during the spring and summer. Lobsters are usually categorized according to size: Jumbo lobsters weigh more than two pounds, large lobsters weigh 1½ to 2 pounds, and quarters weigh from 1¼ to 1½ pounds.

Oysters: You either love them or you hate them. And if you eat them raw, you run a significant risk of getting seriously ill, because they could have been harvested from contaminated waters. Be sure to follow the same "live preparation" guidelines as for clams. In other words, purchase them only if their shells are tightly shut or if they close when you lightly tap on their shells. Fresh oysters are available year-round. The smaller the oyster, the more tender it is likely to be.

Shrimp: This most popular of crustaceans comes in hundreds of species, which can be broken down into two groups: warm-water or cold-water shrimp. Generally speaking, the colder the water, the smaller and more tasty the shrimp. Look for shrimp that smells fresh and doesn't smell of ammonia. Shrimp come in a variety of sizes that range from miniature to colossal. Usually, the larger the shrimp, the higher the price.

Preparation and Serving Tips

The key to good shellfish is freshness. It's also the key to avoiding illness when eating them. Most shellfish deteriorates rapidly once they die. So you need to buy from reputable markets that you know and trust.

Shrimp, lobster, and crab can simply be boiled with seasonings and served. Their flavors stand alone. However, oysters and clams will require shucking, or opening of the shell. If you've never done it before, get someone to demonstrate or get the retailer to do it for you. Many a finger has been sliced by a slip of the knife while shucking shells.

Shellfish are also common ingredients in a tremendous variety of dishes from many ethnic cuisines, including Italian, Greek, French, and Spanish. Some of the herbs and spices that work well with shellfish are dill, fennel, mace, marjoram, parsley, cayenne pepper, and saffron.

Cooked shrimp and crabmeat are excellent as part of a cold salad or as appetizers with a spicy dip. And all shellfish make wonderful ingredients in seafood soups.

SCALLOP AND ARTICHOKE HEART CASSEROLE

- 1 **package (9 ounces) frozen artichoke hearts, cooked and drained**
- 1 **pound scallops**
- 1 **teaspoon canola *or* vegetable oil**
- ¼ **cup chopped red bell pepper**
- ¼ **cup sliced green onion tops**
- ¼ **cup all-purpose flour**
- 2 **cups 1% low-fat milk**
- 1 **teaspoon dried tarragon leaves, crushed**
- ¼ **teaspoon salt**
- ¼ **teaspoon white pepper**
- 1 **tablespoon chopped parsley**
  Dash paprika

Cut large artichoke hearts lengthwise into halves. Arrange artichoke hearts in even layer in 8-inch square baking dish.

Rinse scallops; pat dry with paper towel. If scallops are large, cut into halves. Arrange scallops evenly over artichokes.

Preheat oven to 350°F. Heat oil in medium saucepan over medium-low heat. Add bell pepper and green onions; cook and stir 5 minutes or until tender. Stir in flour. Gradually stir in milk until smooth. Add tarragon, salt and white pepper; cook and stir over medium heat 10 minutes or until sauce boils and thickens.

Pour hot sauce over scallops. Bake, uncovered, 25 minutes or until bubbling and scallops are opaque. Sprinkle with chopped parsley and paprika before serving.

Makes 4 servings

NUTRIENTS PER SERVING:

Calories	226.7	Potassium	846.2 mg
Protein	26.4 g	Riboflavin (B$_2$)	0.38 mg
Carbohydrate	23.19 g	Sodium	438.3 mg
Dietary Fiber	3.73 g	Vitamin C	23.69 mg
Fat	3.66 g	Zinc	2 mg
Saturated Fat	1.02 g		
Poly Fat	0.77 g	DIETARY EXCHANGES:	
Mono Fat	1.1 g	Milk: 0.5	Veg: 2
Cholesterol	42.80 mg	Meat: 2.5	
Sugar	6.92 g		
Beta-Carotene	43.28 µg	% OF CALORIES FROM:	
Calcium	217.7 mg	PRO: 46%	CARB: 40%
Cobalamin (B$_{12}$)	2.18 µg	FAT: 14%	
Folate	44.43 µg		
Iron	1.96 mg		

SPINACH

It seems Popeye had the right idea. Spinach is one of the nutrition superstars of the vegetable family. It's loaded with vitamins and minerals, some of which are hard to find in many other foods, and it's surprisingly high in fiber—offering at least twice as much as most other cooking or salad greens. But it seems to carry an undeserved reputation as an unappetizing dish. That may be because people tend to overcook it to a drab-colored mush. And when served raw, it can be gritty if it's not washed thoroughly beforehand. But prepare it right and it's a delicious nutrition-packed salad or cooking green.

Health Benefits

Like other greens, spinach is an excellent source of vitamin A in the form of beta-carotene, a powerful disease-fighting nutrient that has been shown, among other things, to reduce the risk of developing cataracts. Its deep-green color is the tip-off to the beta-carotene content. Served raw, spinach is a good source of vitamin C. Overcook it, and you lose most of the vitamin. Though spinach is rich in calcium, most of the calcium cannot be absorbed because the oxalic acid in spinach tends to bind it up.

NUTRIENT INFORMATION			
Spinach, raw		Vitamin A	3,760 IU
Serving Size: 1 cup		Folic Acid	108 µg
Calories	12	Vitamin C	16 mg
Protein	1.6 g		
Carbohydrate	2.0 g	Iron	1.6 mg
Fat	0.2 g	Manganese	0.6 mg
Saturated	0	Potassium	312 mg
Cholesterol	0		
Dietary Fiber	4 g		
Sodium	44 mg		

Selection and Storage

Spinach comes in two basic varieties, curly leaved or smooth. They taste the same, but it's harder to get dirt and grit out of the curly-leaved variety. So-called New Zealand spinach is not really spinach at all, but a different variety of plant. It is, however, nutritionally similar to true spinach.

Choose spinach with leaves that are crisp and dark green. Avoid them if they are limp and yellowing. Refrigerate them in a plastic bag as is, and they should keep for three to four days. Wait until you're ready to prepare them before you wash. If you wash and store them, the leaves will deteriorate rapidly.

Preparation and Serving Tips

Wash all fresh spinach leaves carefully and thoroughly, repeating the rinsing process two or three times. Even the smallest speck of grit left on spinach leaves can ruin an otherwise perfect dish.

Fresh spinach salads are a classic served with a warm dressing that slightly wilts the leaves. Omit the common bacon and egg yolks and use mushrooms and garbanzo beans instead.

Spinach should be simmered with very little water for a short period of time, about five to ten minutes. Top it off with lemon juice, seasoned vinegar, sautéed garlic, or nutmeg.

SWEET–SOUR SPINACH

    2 pounds fresh spinach
    1 tablespoon all-purpose flour
 1½ teaspoons granulated sugar
   ⅛ teaspoon pepper
   ½ cup cider vinegar

Wash spinach well to remove sand and grit; remove stems and bruised leaves. Place spinach and ½ cup water in Dutch oven or large saucepan. Cook, covered, over low heat 15 minutes or until tender. Drain spinach; return to pan. Cover; set aside.

Combine flour, sugar and pepper in small saucepan. Blend in vinegar and ¼ cup water until smooth. Cook and stir over medium heat 3 minutes or until sauce boils and thickens. Pour over spinach; toss gently to coat. Serve hot.

Makes 4 servings

NUTRIENTS PER SERVING:

Calories	53.01	Iron	6.55 mg
Protein	5.4 g	Manganese	1.65 mg
Carbohydrate	11.58 g	Potassium	846.2 mg
Dietary Fiber	5.96 g	Sodium	122.2 mg
Fat	0.48 g	Vitamin A	1,429 RE
Saturated Fat	0.08 g	Vitamin C	17.17 mg
Poly Fat	0.2 g		
Mono Fat	0.01 g	DIETARY EXCHANGES:	
Cholesterol	0	Veg: 2	
Sugar	1.48 g		
Beta-Carotene	1,524 RE	% OF CALORIES FROM:	
Copper	0.32 mg	PRO: 30%	CARB: 64%
Folate	254.8 µg	FAT: 6%	

SQUASH

Squash are actually the fruits of the various members of the gourd family. It's believed that this delectable edible was eaten as far back as 5500 B.C. in Mexico. There is a wide variety of squash in a wide array of colors and sizes. But basically, squash can be divided into two broad categories: winter squash and summer squash. Summer varieties include chayote, yellow crookneck, and zucchini. Winter varieties include banana, buttercup, butternut, calabaza, delicata, golden nugget, hubbard, sweet dumpling, spaghetti, and turban. Summer squash tend to have thin, edible skins and soft seeds. Winter squash, on the other hand, have hard, thick skins that are not eaten.

Health Benefits

Though all varieties of squash are good nutrition choices for your dinner table, the winter varieties, with their darker flesh, tend to be more nutrient dense. They generally contain more beta-carotene and more of several B vitamins than the tasty, but lighter summer squash. Butternut squash even rivals mangoes and cantaloupe in terms of beta-carotene content.

Selection and Storage

Despite the seasonal-sounding names, most squash is available all year. Still, winter squash is best from early fall to late winter. Look for smaller squash that are brightly colored and free of spots, bruises, and mold.

The hard skin of winter squash acts as a protector, allowing it to be stored longer than summer squash—a month or more in a dark, cool place. An added bonus: The beta-carotene content actually increases during storage. Summer squash will only keep for a few days in the crisper of the refrigerator.

NUTRIENT INFORMATION

Squash, Crookneck, cooked Serving Size: ½ cup		Squash, Butternut, cooked Serving Size: ½ cup	
Calories	18	Calories	41
Protein	0.8 g	Protein	0.9 g
Carbohydrate	3.9 g	Carbohydrate	10.7 g
Fat	0.3 g	Fat	0.1 g
Saturated	0.1 g	Saturated	0
Cholesterol	0	Dietary Fiber	2.8 g
Dietary Fiber	1.3 g	Cholesterol	0
Sodium	1 mg	Sodium	4 mg
Niacin	0.5 mg	Vitamin A	7,141 IU
Calcium	24 mg	Niacin	1.0 mg
Potassium	173 mg	Pantothenic Acid	0.4 mg
Manganese	0.2 mg	Vitamin C	15.4 mg
		Calcium	42 mg
		Potassium	290 mg

Preparation and Serving Tips

After the seeds have been removed (whether or not you peel winter squash is up to you), winter squash can be baked, steamed, sautéed, or simmered. You'll need a good knife, preferably a chef's knife, to cut through the tough outer skin.

Summer squash, on the other hand, is easily sliced and can be cooked with skin, seeds, and all.

One of the more interesting squashes is the winter variety spaghetti squash. When it is cooked, the flesh separates into spaghetti-like strands that can actually be served instead of spaghetti or noodles for about 75 percent fewer calories. It takes a little practice to prepare; be sure you get instructions. The flavor it adds to dishes is worth the extra effort.

Here are a few savory squash-seasoning suggestions: allspice, basil, cardamom, chervil, cinnamon, cloves, curry, fennel, marjoram, nutmeg, poppy seed, sage, sesame seeds, and tarragon.

BAKED ACORN SQUASH

2 medium acorn squash (about 2¼ pounds)
⅓ cup reduced calorie pancake syrup
1 Granny Smith apple, peeled, cored, coarsely chopped
¼ cup seedless raisins
⅛ teaspoon ground nutmeg
1½ teaspoons cornstarch
2 tablespoons water

Preheat oven to 400°F. Cut squash into halves with large knife. Scoop out and discard seeds. Place squash, cut side down, in 13×9-inch baking dish. Add 1 cup water to baking dish; bake 35 to 45 minutes or until fork-tender. Turn squash cut side up.

Meanwhile, heat pancake syrup in medium saucepan over medium heat. Add apple, raisins and nutmeg; cook and stir about 8 minutes or until apples are almost crisp-tender. Combine cornstarch and 2 tablespoons water in small cup until smooth; stir into saucepan. Cook and stir over medium-high heat until mixture boils and thickens. Cook and stir 2 minutes more. Divide mixture evenly among squash halves. Return squash to oven; bake 10 minutes more or until heated through. *Makes 4 servings*

NUTRIENTS PER SERVING:			
Calories	196.3	Niacin (B₃)	2.18 mg
Protein	2.27 g	Potassium	713.8 mg
Carbohydrate	52 g	Sodium	152.2 mg
Dietary Fiber	5.54 g	Vitamin C	33.9 mg
Fat	0.36 g		
Saturated Fat	0.09 g	DIETARY EXCHANGES:	
Poly Fat	0.12 g	Fruit: 1	Bread: 2
Mono Fat	0.02 g		
Cholesterol	0 mg	% OF CALORIES FROM:	
Sugar	24.39 g	PRO: 4%	CARB: 94%
Beta-Carotene	1,037 µg	FAT: 1%	
Calcium	93.95 mg		

STRAWBERRIES

These luscious berries are the most popular of the berries. Actually a member of the rose family, strawberries have grown wild for centuries in North America and in Europe. They were cultivated six centuries ago and have been a prized fruit ever since. Strawberries are unique in that they are the only fruit that has seeds on the outside rather than on the inside.

These delicate, heart-shaped berries range in size from tiny wild varieties to the larger, juicier cultivated ones. Generally, the smaller varieties are more flavorful. But today's berries have been bred with durability in mind, not flavor. Still, in peak spring and summer months, April to June, you can find superbly sweet strawberries from farmers' markets and green grocers if you know what to look for.

Health Benefits

Strawberries are a super source of vitamin C, even better than oranges or grapefruit. Only guava offers significantly more of this free-radical fighter. Strawberries are also a good source of fiber and potassium, one of the important nutrients that may keep you from becoming a stroke statistic. Also, strawberries are one of the few fruits that contain the phyto-chemical ellagic acid, which may help to reduce your risk of cancer.

NUTRIENT INFORMATION
Strawberries
Serving Size: 1 cup

Calories	45	Vitamin C	84.5 mg
Protein	0.9 g	Calcium	21 mg
Carbohydrate	11 g	Manganese	0.4 mg
Fat	0.6 g	Pantothenic Acid	0.5 mg
Saturated	0	Potassium	247 mg
Cholesterol	0		
Dietary Fiber	2.2 g		
Sodium	2 mg		

Selection and Storage

Look for strawberries that are ruby red, evenly colored, and plump. The leafy tops should look fresh and green. Smaller fruit tend to be the sweetest. Avoid berries that are packed in containers with juice stains or are packed tightly with plastic wrap. And walk on by if they appear soft or mushy or if mold is beginning to grow on them.

Strawberries begin to spoil quickly. So, it's best to buy them on the same day you plan to serve them. However, they can keep in the refrigerator for a day or two if you store them loosely covered in the bottom of the refrigerator.

Strawberries are harder to find and of poorer quality in the winter months. Don't try to freeze strawberries; they tend to become mushy. You can, however, freeze strawberry purée.

Preparation and Serving Tips

Strawberries are superb served *au naturel*. But they also make classy toppers to cakes, puddings, pies, and frozen desserts. If strawberries get overripe, try puréeing them (you can strain the seeds, if you wish) for use in fruit drinks or to drizzle over fruit salad or desserts.

STRAWBERRY BUTTERMILK SHORTCAKE

- 1   cup all-purpose flour
- 3   tablespoons sugar
- 1   teaspoon baking powder
- ¼   teaspoon baking soda
- ¼   teaspoon ground ginger
- 1½ tablespoons canola *or* vegetable oil
- ⅓   cup plus 1 tablespoon low-fat buttermilk
- 1   pint strawberries, hulled, sliced
- 1   cup vanilla *or* strawberry low-fat yogurt

Preheat oven to 425°F. Coat baking sheet with nonstick cooking spray; set aside. Sift flour, sugar, baking powder, baking soda and ginger together into large bowl. Stir in oil until mixture resembles coarse crumbs. Add buttermilk, stirring just until ingredients are moistened and mixture holds together.

Turn out dough onto floured work surface; flour hands lightly. (Dough will be slightly sticky.) Quickly shape dough into 1-inch-thick disc. Cut out four rounds with floured 2½-inch biscuit cutter or rim of drinking glass, piecing together dough scraps to form last biscuit. Place biscuits on prepared baking sheet. Bake 15 minutes or until wooden toothpick inserted near center comes out clean.

To serve, split warm biscuits horizontally into halves. Place bottom halves on individual serving plates. Arrange strawberries on top of biscuits; spoon yogurt over strawberries. Cover with biscuit tops.   *Makes 4 servings*

NUTRIENTS PER SERVING:

Calories	289.4	Niacin (B$_3$)	2.06 mg
Protein	7.56 g	Potassium	343.9 mg
Carbohydrate	49.99 g	Sodium	200.5 mg
Dietary Fiber	3.05 g	Vitamin C	48.47 mg
Fat	6.95 g	Vitamin K	55.46 µg
Saturated Fat	1.02 g	Zinc	0.91 mg
Poly Fat	1.83 g		
Mono Fat	3.33 g	DIETARY EXCHANGES:	
Cholesterol	4.23 mg	Milk: 1	Fruit: 1
Sugar	14.34 g	Bread: 1.5	
Calcium	142.6 mg		
Folate	30.51 µg	% OF CALORIES FROM:	
Magnesium	27.42 mg	PRO: 10%	CARB: 68%
		FAT: 21%	

SWEET POTATOES

In some households in the United States, sweet potatoes are only served once a year—at Thanksgiving. What a waste! Sweet potatoes are one of the unsung heroes of healthy eating. For only a few calories, you get a laundry list of nutrients in more than respectable amounts. Though it's often called a yam, a sweet potato is a different vegetable. It's an edible root that is a member of the morning-glory family. The only place you're likely to find true yams is at ethnic markets. Despite the fact that sweet potatoes are featured only at Thanksgiving, they are available all year. You should take advantage.

Health Benefits

If we held a beta-carotene contest, sweet potatoes would just about tie carrots for first place. That makes them top-notch foods for fighting disease. Sweet potatoes are also an excellent source of potassium and a surprisingly good source of vitamin C; a small four-ounce potato provides almost half of the daily recommended allowance of this powerful free-radical fighter.

NUTRIENT INFORMATION			
Sweet Potatoes, baked		Pantothenic Acid	0.7 mg
Serving Size: 1 potato (4 oz)		Vitamin B$_6$	0.3 mg
Calories	118	Vitamin C	28.1 mg
Protein	2.0 g	Vitamin E	4.5 mg
Carbohydrate	27.7 g		
Fat	0.1 g	Calcium	32 mg
Saturated	0	Magnesium	23 mg
Cholesterol	0	Potassium	397 mg
Dietary Fiber	2.3 g	Copper	0.2 mg
Sodium	10 mg	Manganese	0.6 mg
Vitamin A	24,877 mg		
Folic Acid	25.7 µg		

Selection and Storage

There are many varieties of sweet potato, but the kinds you find in the market can basically be broken down into two groups: moist, orange-fleshed sweet potatoes and dry, yellow-fleshed sweet potatoes. The yellow variety has a thin, light colored skin and pale yellow flesh. When cooked, it is dry and resembles a baking potato in texture. The orange variety has a thicker, darker skin, with bright orange flesh. It is much sweeter and moister.

Whichever variety you choose, look for potatoes that are small to medium in size with smooth, unbruised skin. Avoid those that have a white stringy "beard" attached. It's a sure sign that the potato is overmature and is probably tough and stringy.

Though they are available year-round, peak season for freshly harvested sweet potatoes is mid-fall to late winter.

Though sweet potatoes look hardy, they actually are quite fragile and spoil easily. Any cut or bruise on the surface quickly spreads and ruins the whole potato. Do not refrigerate them. It speeds up the deterioration.

Preparation and Serving Tips

The dry variety can be used in just about any recipe that normally calls for white potatoes. The darker, sweeter varieties are what you candy at Thanksgiving. The sweet variety also works well mashed, souffléd, or as the basis for the traditional Southern sweet-potato pie.

When you cook sweet potatoes, drop them in boiling water unpeeled. Leaving the peel intact helps prevent precious nutrients from being lost and keeps the natural sugar in.

SWEET POTATO BISQUE

  1 **pound sweet potatoes, peeled**
  2 **teaspoons margarine**
 ½ **cup minced onion**
  1 **teaspoon curry powder**
 ½ **teaspoon ground coriander**
 ¼ **teaspoon salt**
 ⅔ **cup unsweetened apple juice**
  1 **cup low-fat buttermilk**
 ¼ **cup water**
    Plain low-fat yogurt for garnish (optional)

Bring 2 quarts water and potatoes to a boil in large saucepan over high heat. Cook, uncovered, 40 minutes or until potatoes are fork-tender. Drain; run under cold water until cool enough to handle.

Meanwhile, melt margarine in small saucepan over medium heat. Add onion; cook and stir 2 minutes. Stir in curry, coriander and salt; cook and stir about 45 seconds. Remove saucepan from heat; stir in apple juice. Set aside until potatoes have cooled.

Cut potatoes into pieces. Combine potatoes, buttermilk and onion mixture in food processor or blender; process until smooth. Pour soup back into large saucepan; stir in ¼ cup water to thin to desired consistency. (If soup is too thick, add 1 to 2 more tablespoons water). Cook and stir over medium heat until heated through. *Do not boil.* Garnish each serving with dollop of yogurt.   ***Makes 4 servings***

NUTRIENTS PER SERVING:			
Calories	159.6	Potassium	490.4 mg
Protein	3.88 g	Sodium	230.5 mg
Carbohydrate	30.9 g	Vitamin A	1,958 RE
Dietary Fiber	3.79 g	Vitamin C	24.09 mg
Fat	2.63 g		
Saturated Fat	0.73 g	DIETARY EXCHANGES:	
Poly Fat	0.67 g	Fruit: 0.5	Bread: 1.5
Mono Fat	1 g	Fat: 0.5	
Cholesterol	2.25 mg		
Sugar	7.54 g	% OF CALORIES FROM:	
Beta-Carotene	2,374 µg	PRO: 10%	CARB: 76%
Calcium	105 mg	FAT: 15%	
Folate	26.92 µg		

SWISS CHARD

Swiss Chard, also known simply as chard or as the sea-kale beet, is a member of the beet family. It is similar to spinach. Indeed, the leaves are a perfect substitute for spinach in recipes. The stalks are typically prepared separately and cooked like asparagus or celery. You'll find it in two varieties red stemmed and white stemmed. The red stemmed variety has darker green leaves and a stronger flavor than the white stemmed does, though the white stemmed is the more common variety of the two.

Health Benefits

Like other members of the greens group, chard is a good source of vitamin A in the form of its precursor, beta-carotene. It's also a very good source of a second antioxidant, vitamin C. Like spinach, it's not as good a source of calcium and iron as the nutrition numbers suggest. Because it is rich in oxalic acid, it's thought that only a small percentage of these two minerals are actually available to the body. But it is still an excellent source of magnesium and potassium. Chard's only nutrition drawback is that it is one of the vegetables highest in sodium. Keep that in mind if you're watching your sodium intake.

NUTRIENT INFORMATION			
Swiss Chard, cooked		Niacin	0.3 mg
Serving Size: 1/2 cup		Vitamin C	15.8 mg
Calories	18		
Protein	1.7 g	Calcium	51 mg
Carbohydrate	3.6 g	Iron	2 mg
Fat	0.1 g	Magnesium	76 mg
Saturated	0	Potassium	483 mg
Cholesterol	0		
Dietary Fiber	0.8 g		
Sodium	158 mg		
Vitamin A	2,762 mg		

Selection and Storage

Chard is available only in the summer. Look for small, tender green leaves and fresh, crisp stalks. Avoid leaves that are yellow. They are old and may have an off flavor. Store fresh leaves, unwashed, in a plastic bag in the refrigerator and they should keep for up to three days.

Preparation and Serving Tips

As with spinach and most other greens, chard should be rinsed well before preparation. If not, you may bite into an unappetizing bit of grit or dirt when you put fork to mouth. But be sure you rinse it just before you're ready to cook. If you put chard in the refrigerator damp, it will deteriorate rapidly.

In the United States, the leaves are the most commonly eaten part of chard. In Europe, however, the stalk is considered the better tasting part of the plant, and varieties have been developed especially for their tender stalks.

Chard makes a tasty ingredient in soups, salads, and mixed dishes like casserole or quiches. Steamed chard tastes wonderful with a little sautéed onion and garlic.

The stems take a little longer to cook than the leaves, and they should be prepared separately. Chard leaves cook quickly—in about four to five minutes in a very small amount of water. Don't cook chard in an iron pot, or it will become discolored.

CHARD STIR–FRY

- ¾ **pound Swiss chard, red or white**
- 2 **cloves garlic, minced**
- 4 **green onions**
- 1 **tablespoon cornstarch**
- 2 **teaspoons onion powder**
- 1 **teaspoon paprika**
- ¼ **teaspoon pepper**
- ½ **cup low sodium vegetable juice**
- 2 **teaspoons canola *or* vegetable oil**
- ½ **pound mushrooms, sliced**
- 2 **medium tomatoes, cored, cut into ½-inch-thick wedges**
- 2 **slices Canadian bacon, cut into julienne strips**

Rinse chard, shaking off excess water. Cut out rib sections; coarsely chop ribs and stems. Place in medium bowl; toss with garlic. Stack chard leaves; cut crosswise into ½-inch strips. Set aside.

Slice green onions, separating white parts from green tops. Add white parts to chard stem mixture. Combine cornstarch, onion powder, paprika and pepper in 1-cup measure; stir in vegetable juice until smooth.

Heat oil in wok or large nonstick skillet over medium-high heat. Add chard stem mixture; stir-fry 1 minute. Add mushrooms; stir-fry 1 minute. Add chard leaves; stir-fry 2 minutes or until wilted. Stir cornstarch mixture; add to wok with tomatoes, green onion tops and Canadian bacon. Cook and stir about 3 minutes or until sauce thickens and mixture is heated through. *Makes 4 servings*

NUTRIENTS PER SERVING:			
Calories	108.5	Niacin (B₃)	4.17 mg
Protein	6.51 g	Potassium	973.4 mg
Carbohydrate	14.21 g	Riboflavin (B₂)	0.41 mg
Dietary Fiber	3.43 g	Sodium	348.7 mg
Fat	3.86 g	Thiamin (B₁)	0.24 mg
Saturated Fat	0.57 g	Vitamin C	41.58 mg
Poly Fat	0.99 g	Vitamin D	0.10 µg
Mono Fat	1.85 g	Vitamin E	0.48 mg
Cholesterol	6.75 mg	Vitamin K	18.71 µg
Sugar	5.09 mg	Zinc	1.04 mg
Beta-Carotene	375.7 µg		
Calcium	72.71 mg	DIETARY EXCHANGES:	
Folate	29.82 µg	Veg: 3	Fat: 0.5
Iron	3.5 mg		
Magnesium	92.33 mg	% OF CALORIES FROM:	
		PRO: 22%	CARB: 48%
		FAT: 30%	

TOFU

Nationally, tofu consumption has doubled over the past ten years. But there are still a lot of hard-line resisters. Even tofu believers concede that the white blocks sometimes sold floating in pans of water are rather unappetizing. But the right preparation can turn tofu around.

Tofu is made from soybeans that have been soaked, mashed, cooked, and filtered to produce soy milk. The milk is then curdled using a coagulant or jelling compounds such as magnesium chloride or calcium sulfate. The curds that form are pressed into blocks as the whey drains off.

Health Benefits

Because tofu comes from soybeans, it offers similar nutritional and health benefits. It is an excellent source of protein, is low in sodium, contains no cholesterol, and is very low in saturated fat and also contains the same antiestrogen compounds researchers have suggested may play a role in the low incidence of breast cancer in women in Asian countries. Only tofu made with calcium sulfate is a good source of calcium.

NUTRIENT INFORMATION			
Tofu		Calcium	130 mg
Serving Size: 4½ oz		Copper	0.2 mg
Calories	94	Magnesium	127 mg
Protein	10 g	Manganese	0.8 mg
Carbohydrate	2.3 g		
Fat	5.9 g		
Saturated	0.9 g		
Cholesterol	0		
Dietary Fiber	1.5 g		
Sodium	9 mg		

Selection and Storage

Tofu can be purchased one of three ways: in bulk, water-packed, and aseptically packaged. If you buy tofu that is sold unwrapped, floating in water, there are a few safety precautions you should take. Because of its ability to harbor bacteria, tofu should always be refrigerated. Don't buy it if you find it in the unrefrigerated-produce section. Though food poisoning from tofu is thought to be rare, there's no need to tempt fate. When you get it home, refrigerate it in water and change the water daily. Water-packed tofu will have a "sell-by" date stamped on the package. To store it at home, open the package and replace the water with fresh water. Change the water daily. Aseptically packaged tofu will keep without refrigeration for up to ten months. But you'll need to refrigerate it once it's opened and then use it within a day or two.

Preparation and Serving Tips

While nutritionists and vegetarians rave over tofu's versatility and nutritional attributes, many cooks are at a loss as to what to do with the white chunks of bean curd. But the versatility of this culinary chameleon lies in its ability to take on flavors and spices of the dishes in which it's used.

You can choose from soft, firm, or extra-firm tofu. Soft is best used as a substitute for cream or mayonnaise or in pureeing and blending. Firm tofu holds it shape better and works well as a substitute for ricotta cheese. Extra-firm tofu is a good meat substitute for tossing and shaping in a vegetable stir-fry.

TOFU STUFFED SHELLS

    1   can (15 ounces) no-salt-added tomato purée
    ½   pound mushrooms, thinly sliced
    ½   cup shredded carrot
    2   cloves garlic, minced
    1   tablespoon Italian seasoning
    1   tablespoon sugar
    ¼   cup water
   12   jumbo macaroni shells
    1   package (14 ounces) firm tofu, drained
    ½   cup chopped green onions
    2   tablespoons grated Parmesan cheese
    2   tablespoons minced parsley
    1   tablespoon dried basil leaves, crushed

½ **teaspoon salt**
¼ **teaspoon pepper**
½ **cup (2 ounces) shredded part-skim mozzarella cheese**

For sauce, combine tomato purée, mushrooms, carrot, garlic, Italian seasoning, sugar and water in medium saucepan. Bring to a boil over medium heat. Reduce heat to low. Simmer, covered, 20 minutes, stirring occasionally.

Meanwhile, cook shells according to package directions, omitting salt. Drain shells; rinse under cold water. Drain upside down on paper towels. Rinse tofu under cold water. Cut into 4 pieces; drain on several layers of paper towels, gently pressing out excess liquid. Preheat oven to 350°F.

Mash tofu in medium bowl to resemble small curds. Stir in green onions, Parmesan, parsley, basil, salt and pepper. Stuff shells with tofu mixture (about 1 heaping tablespoon per shell). Spread thin layer of sauce in bottom of 11½×8-inch baking pan. Place shells, seam side up, in single layer in pan. Pour remaining sauce evenly over shells. Cover pan tightly with foil; bake 30 minutes. Remove foil; sprinkle with mozzarella. Bake, uncovered, 5 to 10 minutes more or until cheese melts and sauce is hot and bubbly. *Makes 4 servings*

NUTRIENTS PER SERVING:			
Calories	421.8	Niacin (B₃)	5.96 mg
Protein	30.43 g	Potassium	1,072 mg
Carbohydrate	53.01 g	Sodium	450.9 mg
Dietary Fiber	6.75 g	Vitamin C	49.61 mg
Fat	12.83 g	Zinc	3.16 mg
Saturated Fat	2.09 g		
Poly Fat	5.58 g	DIETARY EXCHANGES:	
Mono Fat	2.35 g	Veg: 2.5	Bread: 2.5
Cholesterol	7.46 mg	Meat: 2.5	
Sugar	5.9 g		
Beta-Carotene	439 µg	% OF CALORIES FROM:	
Calcium	332.1 mg	PRO: 27%	CARB: 47%
Copper	0.99 mg	FAT: 26%	
Folate	67.02 µg		
Iron	14.74 mg		
Magnesium	160 mg		

TOMATOES

Related to the potato, bell pepper, and eggplant, tomatoes are members of the nightshade family. Though it's thought of as a vegetable, the tomato is botanically classified as a fruit. We consume tomatoes raw, steamed, fried, stewed, crushed, puréed, and reduced to a sauce. In fact, tomatoes are one of the most frequently consumed "vegetables" in the United States, and one of our most significant dietary sources of vitamin C. Dozens of varieties of tomatoes are available that come in a wide range of sizes, colors, and shapes.

Health Benefits

While it's not bursting at the seams with a variety of vitamins and minerals, the tomato is an excellent source of vitamin C and, as such, contributes to your intake of that all-important antioxidant nutrient. It also contains beta-carotene and several other members of the carotenoid family that may have their own disease-preventing properties. Tomatoes also offer a good dose of potassium.

NUTRIENT INFORMATION			
Tomatoes		Sodium	10 mg
Serving Size: 1 tomato			
Calories	24	Vitamin A	1,133 IU
Protein	1.1 g	Vitamin C	22 mg
Carbohydrate	5.3 g		
Fat	0.3 g	Potassium	254 mg
Saturated	0		
Cholesterol	0		
Dietary Fiber	1 g		

Selection and Storage

Tomatoes generally fall into three groups: cherry tomatoes, plum tomatoes, and round slicing tomatoes. Cherry tomatoes are small, bite-sized, perfectly round, and red or yellow in color. Plum tomatoes, also known as Italian plum, are egg-shaped and may also be red or yellow in color. Slicing tomatoes are large, round varieties that are perfect for slicing.

Though fresh tomatoes are available year-round, their peak season is from June to September. The best-tasting tomatoes are "vine-ripened," that is, they have been allowed to become ripe on the vine rather than being picked green and treated. However, to find them, you'll probably have to shop at farmers' markets or green grocers or grow your own. Moreover, there is no standard definition for the term "vine-ripened." So, know your vendor to be sure you can trust the claim.

Generally, look for tomatoes that are firm and well-shaped and that have a noticeable fragrance. They should be heavy for their size and yield to slight pressure when gently squeezed.

A common mistake is to store tomatoes in the refrigerator. Cold temperatures will ruin the taste and texture of a good tomato. Wait until you're just ready to serve before you slice them; once cut, the flavor tends to gradually fade.

Preparation and Serving Tips

Most salads seem incomplete without a ripe, red tomato sliced or quartered into it. But sliced tomatoes make a delicious salad by themselves—laying on a bed of radicchio, drizzled with a flavored vinaigrette, and garnished with a sprig of watercress.

Chopped tomatoes also add flavor and color to soups, stews, vegetables, and casseroles.

ITALIAN BREAD SALAD

- 3 slices (½-inch-thick) day-old whole wheat bread
- ½ cup low-fat buttermilk
- 1 small clove garlic, minced
- 1 tablespoon minced fresh dill *or* 1 teaspoon dried dill weed
- 1½ teaspoons onion powder
- ¼ teaspoon pepper

2 **large tomatoes, cored, cut into 1-inch cubes**
1 **small cucumber, peeled, cut into halves, seeded, thinly sliced**
1 **small rib celery, thinly sliced**
2 **tablespoons minced parsley**
⅛ **teaspoon salt**

Preheat oven to 400°F. Cut bread into 1-inch pieces. Place on baking sheet; bake 5 to 7 minutes or until lightly toasted and dry, stirring occasionally. Remove from pan; let cool.

For dressing, combine buttermilk, garlic, dill, onion powder, and pepper in small jar with tight-fitting lid; shake well. Let stand 15 minutes to allow flavors to blend.

Combine tomatoes, cucumber, celery, and parsley in large bowl. Sprinkle with salt; toss well. Just before serving, toss toasted bread with vegetables. Shake dressing; pour over salad and toss to coat. Serve immediately. *Makes 4 servings*

NUTRIENTS PER SERVING:

Calories	92.21	Potassium	370.5 mg
Protein	4.29 g	Sodium	220 mg
Carbohydrate	17.35 g	Thiamin (B₁)	0.15 mg
Dietary Fiber	0.86 g	Vitamin C	19.15 mg
Fat	1.5 g	Vitamin K	15.38 µg
Saturated Fat	0.42 g		
Poly Fat	0.35 g	DIETARY EXCHANGES:	
Mono Fat	0.48 g	Veg: 0.5	Bread: 1
Cholesterol	1.13 mg		
Sugar	3.19 g	% OF CALORIES FROM:	
Beta-Carotene	69.68 µg	PRO: 17%	CARB: 69%
Calcium	72.98 mg	FAT: 14%	
Folate	33.94 µg		

TURKEY

Turkey is another one of those nutritious foods that, in many households, appears on the dinner table only at holiday times, such as Thanksgiving. In fact, about 90 percent of all turkeys are sold during the months of November and December. But turkey is as versatile as chicken and just as nutritious. It's even slightly lower in fat. So don't limit its appearance to only one or two holidays each year. It's a healthy food any time.

Health Benefits

The white meat of a turkey is just about the lowest-fat meat you can find. Most of the fat in turkey is found below the skin. But if you remove the skin, fat provides only about 20 percent of turkey's calories. Turkey is also a good source of several vitamins and minerals, including iron, zinc, potassium, phosphorus, vitamin B_{12}, and niacin.

NUTRIENT INFORMATION			
Turkey, light meat (hen), cooked		Pantothenic Acid	0.8 mg
Serving Size: 4¼ oz		Vitamin B_6	0.6 mg
Calories	192	Vitamin B_{12}	0.4 µg
Protein	35.6 g		
Carbohydrate	0	Iron	1.6 mg
Fat	4.5 g	Magnesium	33 mg
Saturated	1.4 g	Phosphorus	260 mg
Cholesterol	81 mg	Potassium	361 mg
Dietary Fiber	0	Zinc	2.3 mg
Sodium	71 mg		
Niacin	1.4 mg		

Selection and Storage

There are generally three types of turkeys you'll find in the market. Toms are large male turkeys that usually weigh up to 20 pounds. Hens, female turkeys, weigh about 8 to 16 pounds. Fryer-roasters are turkeys of either sex that weigh between 5 and 8 pounds. Some turkeys are self-basting and have been injected with butter or vegetable oil.

Ground turkey is also available, but much of it is high in fat. For a truly low-fat ground turkey, look for "ground turkey breast."

If you buy a fresh bird, it should have a "sell by" date on it. It should stay fresh for a day or two after the date, but no more. Frozen turkeys should be frozen *solid*; the wrapping should be well sealed, and the turkey should have no freezer burn. To help choose the size turkey that is best for you, figure about ½ pound per person—more if it's a small bird.

Put the bird in the coldest part of the refrigerator. It's best to let it thaw in the refrigerator. It will take anywhere from one to two days to thaw a small 8-to 12-pound turkey, four to five days for a 20-pounder.

Preparation and Serving Tips

When you handle raw turkey, be sure to wash your hands thoroughly with soap and warm water before you touch any other food or utensil. Turkey is likely to be contaminated with *salmonella* bacteria, which is destroyed in cooking.

If you buy a turkey with a pop-up button to indicate when it's done, you'll have no problem knowing when it's turkey time. Otherwise, test the bird by checking to see if the leg moves up and down easily and the hip joint is loose. Or, pierce the thickest part of the thigh with a fork. If the juices run clear, the turkey is done.

Turkey can be used in any dish that calls for chicken and works well by itself using seasonings such as turmeric, thyme, sage, or saffron.

MEXICAN TURKEY TENDERLOIN WITH CHUNKY TOMATO SAUCE

- 1   teaspoon ground cumin
- ¾   teaspoon garlic powder
- 1   pound turkey breast tenderloin, cut into 4 pieces
- 2   tablespoons vinegar
- 2   teaspoons sugar
- 2   teaspoons cornstarch

- 1 **cup coarsely chopped tomatoes**
- 1 **cup chopped zucchini**
- ⅓ **cup chopped onion**
- 1 **tablespoon chopped fresh cilantro** *or* **1 teaspoon dried cilantro leaves, crushed**
- 1 **tablespoon chopped jalapeño pepper**＊

Preheat broiler. Combine cumin and garlic powder in small bowl; rub mixture on both sides of turkey. Place turkey on broiler pan. Broil 4 inches below heat 5 minutes. Turn and broil about 5 minutes more or until juices run clear and turkey is no longer pink in center.

Meanwhile, combine vinegar, sugar and cornstarch in small saucepan until smooth. Stir in tomatoes, zucchini, onion, cilantro and jalapeño pepper. Cook and stir over medium heat until mixture boils and thickens. Cook and stir 2 minutes more. Spoon over turkey.   *Makes 4 servings*

＊ Chili peppers can sting and irritate the skin; wear rubber gloves when handling peppers and do not touch eyes. Wash hands after handling chili peppers.

NUTRIENTS PER SERVING:

Calories	150.7	Niacin (B₃)	5.43 mg
Protein	22.63 g	Potassium	472.8 mg
Carbohydrate	9.07 g	Pyridoxine (B₆)	0.48 mg
Dietary Fiber	1.23 g	Sodium	84.38 mg
Fat	2.69 g	Vitamin C	14.74 mg
Saturated Fat	0.78 g	Zinc	1.65 mg
Poly Fat	0.72 g		
Mono Fat	0.44 g	DIETARY EXCHANGES:	
Cholesterol	49.55 mg	Veg: 1	Meat: 2.5
Sugar	4.57 g		
Beta-Carotene	96.39 µg	% OF CALORIES FROM:	
Calcium	31.55 mg	PRO: 60%	CARB: 24%
Cobalamin (B₁₂)	0.27 µg	FAT: 16%	
Copper	0.11 mg		
Folate	22.36 µg		
Iron	1.87 mg		

TURNIP GREENS

These leafy greens from the turnip root are an outstanding member of the nutritious greens club. Though older leaves are among the most bitter-tasting greens, young leaves actually have a sweet taste. You won't often find turnip greens with the turnip roots attached. Generally, plants grown for the leaves don't have well-developed turnip roots. The greens are a familiar staple on Southern tables.

Health Benefits

As a member of both the greens and cruciferous-vegetable clubs, turnip greens are a must-try food for disease prevention. As we've mentioned more than once, researchers have found that people who eat a lot of vegetables from the cruciferous family have a lower risk of developing some cancers than people who seldom eat them. Turnip greens are an excellent source of beta-carotene—once again, that deep-green color is your clue. And they are a surprisingly good source of calcium. Though the calcium in some other greens that are high in oxalic acid is not completely available, the calcium in cruciferous greens, such as the turnip green, appears to be readily available. Turnip greens also offer more than two grams of fiber per serving—not too shabby. That's more than some cereals that boast of hearty grains.

NUTRIENT INFORMATION			
Turnip Greens, cooked		Vitamin A	3,959 IU
Serving Size: ½ cup		Folic Acid	85 µg
Calories	15	Vitamin C	20 mg
Protein	0.8 g		
Carbohydrate	3.1 g	Calcium	99 mg
Fat	0.2 g	Copper	0.2 mg
Saturated	0	Manganese	0.2 mg
Dietary Fiber	2.2 g		
Cholesterol	0		
Sodium	21 mg		

Selection and Storage

Look for young, crisp, tender leaves with a nice green color.
Store them as is in a plastic bag in the refrigerator. They
should keep for up to three days. They are available year-
round but are usually at their peak October through February.

Preparation and Serving Tips

Thoroughly wash turnip greens before you prepare them,
and remove any thick ribs that may be tough. As with other
greens, they are likely to have grit and dirt hidden in their leaves.

Turnip greens are best eaten cooked. They are usually too
bitter and tough to be used as a raw ingredient in salads.
Turnip greens, like other greens, cook down a great deal, so
allow about one pound of raw leaves for ½ cup cooked. Use a
small amount of water and cook for a minimum amount of
time to preserve the vitamin C.

Turnip greens add character to hearty soups and stews and
are a real standout braised with stock or sautéed with a little
olive oil and seasoned with fresh marjoram.

SWEET–SOUR TURNIP GREEN SALAD

    2 cups shredded stemmed washed turnip greens
    2 cups washed mixed salad greens
    1 cup sliced plum tomatoes *or* quartered cherry tomatoes
    ½ cup shredded carrot
    ⅓ cup sliced green onions
    8 tablespoons water, divided
    2 teaspoons all-purpose flour
    1 tablespoon packed brown sugar
    ½ teaspoon celery seeds
       Dash pepper
    1 tablespoon white wine vinegar

Combine turnip greens, salad greens, tomatoes and carrot
in salad bowl; set aside. Combine green onions and 2 table-

spoons water in small saucepan. Bring to a boil over high heat. Reduce heat to medium. Cook, covered, 2 to 3 minutes or until onions are tender.

Mix remaining 6 tablespoons water and flour in small bowl until smooth. Stir into green onions in saucepan. Add brown sugar, celery seeds and pepper; cook and stir until mixture boils and thickens. Cook and stir 1 minute more. Stir in vinegar. Pour hot dressing over salad; toss to coat. Serve immediately. *Makes 4 servings*

NUTRIENTS PER SERVING:

Calories	48.89	Manganese	0.44 mg
Protein	1.96 g	Potassium	402.2 mg
Carbohydrate	10.9 g	Sodium	40.52 mg
Dietary Fiber	2.71 g	Vitamin C	28.75 mg
Fat	0.44 g	Vitamin K	237.2 µg
Saturated Fat	0.07 g		
Poly Fat	0.16 g	DIETARY EXCHANGES:	
Mono Fat	0.08 g	Veg: 2	
Cholesterol	0		
Sugar	2.74 g	% OF CALORIES FROM:	
Beta-Carotene	668.7 µg	PRO: 14%	CARB: 79%
Calcium	76.65 mg	FAT: 7%	
Folate	92.37 µg		

TURNIPS

The lowly turnip has a history of being the food of peasants. But it deserves better. With its mildly pungent flavor, this root vegetable makes a tasty and nutritious addition to a variety of dishes. Sometimes confused with the rutabaga, the turnip is actually from a different botanical family. The turnip is small to medium sized and has a white peel and flesh with a purple-ringed top. Rutabagas are much larger and have yellow-colored flesh.

Health Benefits

Turnips are an excellent source of fiber, providing as much as many of the highest high-fiber cereals. It also provides vitamin C and niacin, with a little calcium and potassium thrown in for good measure. Turnips are also one of the respected members of the cruciferous family.

NUTRIENT INFORMATION			
Turnips, cooked		Sodium	39 mg
Serving Size: ½ cup			
Calories	14	Niacin	2.3 mg
Protein	0.6 g	Vitamin C	9 mg
Carbohydrate	3.8 g		
Fat	0.1 g	Calcium	18 mg
Saturated	0	Potassium	106 mg
Cholesterol	0		
Dietary Fiber	4.8 g		

Selection and Storage

You'll find turnips in the market both with and without the greens attached. If the greens are attached, look for those that are fresh and green, not wilted and yellowing. Choose the smallest turnips, and check for those that are heavy for their size. The smaller roots are more tender and have a sweeter, milder flavor than the larger ones, which can be pulpy and strong flavored. Turnips will keep in the refrigerator for a week or more if sealed in plastic. Though turnips are generally available year-round, the peak season is October through February.

Preparation and Serving Tips

Wash and trim turnips before you prepare them. Small, tender turnips can be cooked with the peel on. But if you do decide to peel them, use a vegetable peeler instead of a knife to keep as much flesh as possible.

Turnips can be steamed or boiled and take from 15 to 25 minutes to cook, depending on the size and maturity of the root. Like other cruciferous vegetables, the flavor of turnips tends to become stronger the longer it is cooked.

Because of their somewhat pungent flavor, turnips tend to overpower chicken or fish dishes; they are better complements to the heartier flavors of beef, ham, or pork.

Julienned strips of carrots and turnips simmered in well-seasoned stock make a deliciously different side dish. Or make mashed potatoes with a twist, blending puréed turnips and potatoes. To add a little zip to slaw, try grating raw turnip in with cabbage and carrots. Turnips cut into cubes make flavorful additions to stews, soups, and casseroles.

HERBED DUCHESS TURNIPS

   2 cups peeled turnip cubes
1½ cups peeled potato slices
   1 cup carrot slices
   2 egg whites
   2 teaspoons reduced calorie margarine
   1 teaspoon onion powder
   ½ teaspoon dried marjoram leaves, crushed
   ¼ teaspoon salt
   ⅛ teaspoon pepper

Bring 2 cups water to a boil in medium saucepan over high heat. Add turnips, potatoes and carrots; return to a boil. Reduce heat to medium-low. Simmer, covered, 30 to 35 minutes or until vegetables are very tender. Drain well; transfer vegetables to large bowl.

Preheat oven to 375°F. Coat baking sheet with nonstick cooking spray; set aside. Beat vegetables with electric mixer at medium-low speed until mashed. Add egg whites, margarine, onion powder, marjoram, salt and pepper; beat at medium speed until mixture is nearly smooth. (Mixture should have consistency of mashed potatoes.)

Spoon mixture into pastry bag with large open star tip. Pipe mixture into 12 mounds on prepared baking sheet. Bake 12 to 14 minutes or until heated through. *Makes 4 servings*

* Or, spoon mixture into mounds on prepared baking sheet; bake as directed above.

NUTRIENTS PER SERVING:

Calories	119.9	Niacin (B₃)	1.66 mg
Protein	4.16 g	Potassium	512.3 mg
Carbohydrate	24.78 g	Pyridoxine (B₆)	0.33 mg
Dietary Fiber	3.59 g	Sodium	235.8 mg
Fat	1.16 g	Vitamin C	18.25 mg
Saturated Fat	0.2 g	Vitamin D	0.25 µg
Poly Fat	0.53 g	Zinc	0.47 mg
Mono Fat	0.36 g		
Cholesterol	0	DIETARY EXCHANGES:	
Sugar	4.33 g	Veg: 2	Bread: 1
Beta-Carotene	1,200 µg		
Calcium	37.21 mg	% OF CALORIES FROM:	
Copper	0.21 mg	PRO: 13%	CARB: 79%
Folate	19.32 µg	FAT: 8%	

WHEAT GERM

Wheat germ, a health-food basic, is the embryo of the wheat kernel. And as such, it has a well-deserved reputation for being a powerhouse of nutrients. The germ is the portion of the wheat that is removed when wheat is processed into refined flour.

Health Benefits

Wheat germ is definitely a nutrition standout. It's one of the best sources of folic acid. That's good news, since the government is now recommending that all women of childbearing age get sufficient amounts of this nutrient to prevent certain birth defects. And it's a good source of a number of minerals including iron and zinc.

```
NUTRIENT INFORMATION
Wheat Germ                          Thiamin            0.5 mg
Serving Size: 1 oz, toasted         Vitamin B6         0.3 mg
Calories          108               Vitamin E          4.0 mg
Protein           8.3 gm
Carbohydrate      14.1 gm           Calcium            13 mg
Fat               3.0 gm            Copper             0.2 mg
  Saturated       0.5 gm            Iron               2.6 mg
Cholesterol       0                 Magnesium          91 mg
Dietary Fiber     3.7 gm            Manganese          5.7 mg
Sodium            1 mg              Phosphorus         325 mg
                                    Potassium          269 mg
Folic Acid        100 µg            Zinc               4.7 mg
Pantothenic Acid  0.4 mg
Riboflavin        0.2 mg
```

Selection and Storage

Because of its fat content, wheat germ easily goes rancid, especially if it's raw. Always store opened wheat germ in the refrigerator in a tightly sealed container. If you buy it in jars, store it in the refrigerator in its original container. Fresh wheat germ should smell like toasted nuts, not musty. Unopened, a sealed jar of wheat germ will keep for about one year on the shelf. Refrigerate it after you open the jar. It can keep up to nine months in the refrigerator if the jar is resealed tightly.

Preparation and Serving Tips

You can buy wheat germ already toasted, but if you want to toast raw wheat germ yourself, here's how: Sprinkle the raw wheat germ onto a cookie sheet, and toast in a preheated (300 degrees Fahrenheit) oven for about 15 minutes, stirring the kernels several times.

Wheat germ makes a nutritious, and often undetected, addition to a wide variety of dishes, including breads, pancakes, waffles, cookies, cereals, and milk shakes. It can also be used as a meat extender in meat loaf or meatballs—it ups the nutrient content and lowers the fat. And it's a lower-fat alternative to granola that can be added to yogurt and cereals.

Here are some tips for adding wheat germ to recipes: In muffins and quick breads, replace up to one-half cup flour with wheat germ. In cookies, replace up to one cup flour with wheat germ. In pie shell recipes, you can replace up to one-half cup flour with wheat germ in a two-crust recipe. Wheat germ tends to absorb extra moisture, so you may want to try adding one to two tablespoons of water for every ¼ cup of wheat germ that you add to a recipe.

WHEAT GERM PANCAKES WITH APRICOT-ORANGE SAUCE

- ½ cup orange juice
- 1 tablespoon cornstarch
- 1 tablespoon honey
- ¼ teaspoon ground nutmeg
- 1 can (5½ ounces) apricot nectar
- 2 seedless small oranges, peeled, sectioned
- 1 cup whole wheat flour
- ¼ cup all-purpose flour
- 2 tablespoons toasted wheat germ
- 2 teaspoons packed brown sugar
- 1½ teaspoons baking powder
- 1 cup plus 3 tablespoons skim milk
- 1 tablespoon canola or vegetable oil
- 2 egg whites
  Nonstick cooking spray

For apricot-orange sauce, combine orange juice, cornstarch, honey and nutmeg in small saucepan until smooth. Stir in apricot nectar. Cook and stir over medium heat until mixture boils and thickens. Cook and stir 2 minutes more. Stir in orange sections; cover to keep warm.

Combine whole wheat flour, all-purpose flour, wheat germ, sugar and baking powder in medium bowl. Combine milk and oil in small bowl. Add milk mixture to flour mixture; stir just until combined. Beat egg whites in small bowl with electric mixer until whites form stiff (but not dry) peaks. Gently fold into batter.

Coat nonstick griddle or heavy skillet with nonstick cooking spray. Heat over medium heat until water droplets sprinkled on griddle bounce off surface. Drop 2 tablespoons batter onto hot griddle for each pancake; spread to form 3-inch rounds. Cook 2 to 3 minutes or until tops of pancakes are bubbly and appear dry. Turn; cook 1 to 2 minutes more or until bottoms of pancakes are lightly browned. Serve with warm apricot sauce.

Makes 6 servings (2 pancakes per serving)

NUTRIENTS PER SERVING:			
Calories	205.7	Niacin (B₃)	2.09 mg
Protein	7.31 g	Riboflavin (B₂)	0.23 mg
Carbohydrate	39.04 g	Sodium	128.7 mg
Dietary Fiber	4.3 g	Thiamin (B₁)	0.25 mg
Fat	3.17 g	Vitamin C	42.72 mg
Saturated Fat	0.37 g	Vitamin D	0.51 µg
Poly Fat	1.02 g	Vitamin E	0.99 mg
Mono Fat	1.47 g	Vitamin K	10.37 µg
Cholesterol	0.79 mg	Zinc	1.18 mg
Sugar	11.79 g		
Beta-Carotene	34.27 µg	DIETARY EXCHANGES:	
Calcium	106.5 mg	Fruit: 0.5	Bread: 2
Chromium	0	Fat: 0.5	
Cobalamin (B₁₂)	0.21 µg		
Copper	0.18 mg	% OF CALORIES FROM:	
Folate	44.61 µg	PRO: 14%	CARB: 73%
Iron	1.43 mg	FAT: 13%	
Manganese	1.15 mg		

YOGURT, LOW-FAT

Yogurt was a long-established staple in Eastern Europe and the Middle East before it reached our shores. And there was a time when yogurt eaters in this country were considered "health nuts." Our attitudes have changed considerably. Today, yogurt is commonly consumed by men, women, and children of all ages in the United States. Walk into any supermarket today, and you'll see that the varieties and flavors of this nutritious food take up considerable space in the refrigerated dairy section.

Health Benefits

Yogurt may not be the miracle food that some have claimed, but it certainly has a lot to offer in the health department. Besides being an excellent source of bone-building calcium, it's believed that the bacterial cultures, *Lactobacillicus bulgaricus* and *Streptococcus thermophilus*, used to make yogurt, carry their own health benefits. For example, research has suggested that eating yogurt regularly helps boost immune function, warding off colds and possibly cancer. It's also thought that the friendly bacteria that yogurt offers help prevent and cure diarrhea. One study found that women who were plagued with chronic vaginal yeast infections found protection by eating a daily dose of bacteria-toting yogurt. But don't look to frozen yogurt as an option; most frozen yogurt contains little of the healthful bacteria.

NUTRIENT INFORMATION			
Yogurt, low-fat, vanilla			
Serving Size: 8 oz			
Calories	194	Pantothenic Acid	1.3 mg
Protein	11.2 gm	Riboflavin	0.5 mg
Carbohydrate	31.3 gm	Vitamin B12	1.3 µg
Fat	2.8 gm	Calcium	389 mg
Saturated	2.8 gm		
Cholesterol	11 mg	Magnesium	37 mg
Dietary Fiber	0	Phosphorus	306 mg
Sodium	149 mg	Potassium	498 mg
		Zinc	1.9 mg

Selection and Storage

There is a dizzying array of brands and flavors of yogurts in most supermarkets. But there are three basic traits to look for. Choose a yogurt that is either low fat or fat free. It should contain no more than three grams of fat per eight-ounce carton. Second, look for yogurt that contains live, active bacterial cultures. And third, choose plain, vanilla, lemon, or any one of the yogurts without a jam-like fruit mixture added. The mixture adds little nutrition and a lot of calories.

Yogurt must always be refrigerated. Each carton should have a "sell by" date stamped on it. It should keep in the refrigerator for up to ten days after that date, but when you re-open the carton, be sure to check that the yogurt has not begun to sour or curdle.

Preparation and Serving Tips

Yogurt can be enjoyed as a low-fat dessert; just add sliced berries, nuts, wheat germ, bananas, low-fat granola, or bran cereal. Yogurt also works well as a low-fat substitute in a lot of recipes that call for high-fat ingredients such as sour cream or cream. Yogurt is especially well-suited as a base for dips and salad dressings.

GARDEN POTATO SALAD WITH BASIL-YOGURT DRESSING

- 6 new potatoes, quartered
- 8 ounces asparagus, cut into 1-inch slices
- 1¼ cups red, yellow or green bell pepper strips
- ⅔ cup plain low-fat yogurt
- ¼ cup sliced green onions
- 2 tablespoons chopped pitted ripe olives
- 1½ tablespoons chopped fresh basil *or* 1½ teaspoons dried basil leaves, crushed
- 1 tablespoon chopped fresh thyme *or* 1 teaspoon dried thyme leaves, crushed
- 1 tablespoon white vinegar
- 2 teaspoons sugar
  Dash ground red pepper

Bring 3 cups water to a boil in large saucepan over high heat. Add potatoes; return to a boil. Reduce heat to medium-low. Simmer, covered, 8 minutes. Add asparagus and bell peppers; return to a boil over high heat. Reduce heat to medium-low. Simmer, covered, about 3 minutes or until potatoes are just tender and asparagus and bell peppers are tender-crisp. Drain.

Meanwhile, combine yogurt, green onions, olives, basil, thyme, vinegar, sugar and ground red pepper in large bowl. Add vegetables; toss to combine. Refrigerate, covered, until well chilled.   ***Makes 4 servings***

NUTRIENTS PER SERVING:			
Calories	153.6	Niacin (B_3)	2.09 mg
Protein	5.66 g	Potassium	680.6 mg
Carbohydrate	29.66 g	Pyridoxine (B_6)	0.5 mg
Dietary Fiber	3.49 g	Sodium	173.4 mg
Fat	2.52 g	Thiamin (B_1)	0.2 mg
Saturated Fat	0.64 g	Vitamin C	86.14 mg
Poly Fat	0.31 g	Zinc	0.96 mg
Mono Fat	1.33 g		
Cholesterol	2.33 mg	DIETARY EXCHANGES:	
Sugar	5.81 g	Veg: 1	Bread: 1.5
Beta-Carotene	112.1 µg	Fat: 0.5	
Calcium	110.4 mg	% OF CALORIES FROM:	
Folate	79.61 µg	PRO: 14%	CARB: 72%
Iron	1.58 mg	FAT: 14%	

Table 1

FOOD AND NUTRITION BOARD, NATIONAL ACADEMY OF SCIENCES–NATIONAL RESEARCH COUNCIL
RECOMMENDED DIETARY ALLOWANCES,[a] Revised 1989

Designed for the maintenance of good nutrition of practically all healthy people in the United States.

Category	Age (years) or Condition	Weight[b] (kg)	Weight[b] (lb)	Height[b] (cm)	Height[b] (in)	Protein (g)	Calcium (mg)	Phosphorus (mg)	Magnesium (mg)	Iron (mg)	Zinc (mg)	Iodine (µg)	Selenium (µg)
Infants	0.0–0.5	6	13	60	24	13	400	300	40	6	5	40	10
	0.5–1.0	9	20	71	28	14	600	500	60	10	5	50	15
Children	1–3	13	29	90	35	16	800	800	80	10	10	70	20
	4–6	20	44	112	44	24	800	800	120	10	10	90	20
	7–10	28	62	132	52	28	800	800	170	10	10	120	30
Males	11–14	45	99	157	62	45	1,200	1,200	270	12	15	150	40
	15–18	66	145	176	69	59	1,200	1,200	400	12	15	150	50
	19–24	72	160	177	70	58	1,200	1,200	350	10	15	150	70
	25–50	79	174	176	70	63	800	800	350	10	15	150	70
	51–	77	170	173	68	63	800	800	350	10	15	150	70
Females	11–14	46	101	157	62	46	1,200	1,200	280	15	12	150	45
	15–18	55	120	163	64	44	1,200	1,200	300	15	12	150	50
	19–24	58	128	164	65	46	1,200	1,200	280	15	12	150	55
	25–50	63	138	163	64	50	800	800	280	15	12	150	55
	51–	65	143	160	63	63	800	800	280	10	12	150	55
Pregnant						60	1,200	1,200	320	30	15	175	65
Lactating	1st 6 months					65	1,200	1,200	355	15	19	200	75
	2nd 6 months					62	1,200	1,200	340	15	16	200	75

[a] The allowances, expressed as daily intakes over time, are intended to provide for individual variations among most normal persons as they live in the United States under usual environmental stresses. Diets should be based on a variety of common foods in order to provide other nutrients for which human requirements have been less well defined.

[b] Weights and heights of reference adults are actual medians for the U.S. population of the designated age, as reported by NHANES II. The median weights and heights of those under 19 years of age were taken from Hamill et al. (1979). The use of these figures does not imply that the height-to-weight ratios are ideal.

Tables 1–4 reprinted with permission from Recommended Dietary Allowances, 10th Edition, ©1989, by the National Academy of Sciences, National Academy Press, Washington, D.C.

Table 1 cont.
FOOD AND NUTRITION BOARD, NATIONAL ACADEMY OF SCIENCES—NATIONAL RESEARCH COUNCIL
RECOMMENDED DIETARY ALLOWANCES,ᵃ Revised 1989

Designed for the maintenance of good nutrition of practically all healthy people in the United States.

Category	Age (years) or Condition	Fat-Soluble Vitamins				Water-Soluble Vitamins						
		Vitamin A (μg RE)^b	Vitamin D (μg)^c	Vitamin E (mg α-TE)^d	Vitamin K (μg)	Vitamin C (mg)	Thiamin (mg)	Riboflavin (mg)	Niacin (mg NE)^e	Vitamin B$_6$ (mg)	Folate (μg)	Vitamin B$_{12}$ (μg)
Infants	0.0-0.5	375	7.5	3	5	30	0.3	0.4	5	0.3	25	0.3
	0.5-1.0	375	10	4	10	35	0.4	0.5	6	0.6	35	0.5
Children	1-3	400	10	6	15	40	0.7	0.8	9	1.0	50	0.7
	4-6	500	10	7	20	45	0.9	1.1	12	1.1	75	1.0
	7-10	700	10	7	30	45	1.0	1.2	13	1.4	100	1.4
Males	11-14	1,000	10	10	45	50	1.3	1.5	17	1.7	150	2.0
	15-18	1,000	10	10	65	60	1.5	1.8	20	2.0	200	2.0
	19-24	1,000	10	10	70	60	1.5	1.7	19	2.0	200	2.0
	25-50	1,000	5	10	80	60	1.5	1.7	19	2.0	200	2.0
	51-	1,000	5	10	80	60	1.2	1.4	15	2.0	200	2.0
Females	11-14	800	10	8	45	50	1.1	1.3	15	1.4	150	2.0
	15-18	800	10	8	55	60	1.1	1.3	15	1.5	180	2.0
	19-24	800	10	8	60	60	1.1	1.3	15	1.6	180	2.0
	25-50	800	5	8	65	60	1.1	1.3	15	1.6	180	2.0
	51-	800	3	8	65	60	1.0	1.2	13	1.6	180	2.0
Pregnant		800	10	10	65	70	1.5	1.6	17	2.2	400	2.2
Lactating	1st 6 months	1,300	10	12	65	95	1.6	1.8	20	2.1	280	2.6
	2nd 6 months	1,200	10	11	65	90	1.6	1.7	20	2.1	260	2.6

ᵃRetinol equivalents. 1 retinol equivalent = 1 μg retinol or 6 μg beta-carotene. To calculate IU: for fruits and vegetables, multiply the RE value by 10; for foods from animal sources, multiply the RE value by 3.3.
ᵇAs cholecalciferol. 10 μg cholecalciferol = 400 IU of vitamin D.
ᶜα-Tocopherol equivalents. 1 mg d-α tocopherol = 1 α-T.E.
ᵈNE (niacin equivalent) is equal to 1 mg of niacin or 60 mg of dietary tryptophan.

Tables 1-4 reprinted with permission from *Recommended Dietary Allowances*, 10th Edition, ©1989, by the National Academy of Sciences, National Academy Press, Washington, D.C.

Table 2
SUMMARY TABLE
Estimated Safe and Adequate Daily Dietary Intakes of Additional Selected Vitamins and Minerals[a]

Category	Age (years)	Vitamins	
		Biotin µg	Pantothenic Acid
Infants	0-0.5	10	2
	0.5-1	15	3
Children and adolescents	1-3	20	3
	4-6	25	3-4
	7-10	30	4-5
	11+	30-100	4-7
Adults		30-100	4-7

Category	Age (years)	Trace Elements[b]				
		Copper (mg)	Man-ganese (mg)	Fluoride (mg)	Chromium (µg)	Molyb-denum (µg)
Infants	0-0.5	0.4-0.6	0.3-0.6	0.1-0.5	10-40	15-30
	0.5-1	0.6-0.7	0.6-1.0	0.2-1.0	20-60	20-40
Children and adolescents	1-3	0.7-1.0	1.0-1.5	0.5-1.5	20-80	25-50
	4-6	1.0-1.5	1.5-2.0	1.0-2.5	30-120	50-150
	7-10	1.0-2.0	2.0-3.0	1.5-2.5	50-200	75-250
	11+	1.5-2.5	2.0-5.0	1.5-2.5	50-200	75-250
Adults		1.5-3.0	2.0-5.0	1.5-4.0	50-200	75-250

[a] Because there is less information on which to base allowances, these figures are not given in the main table of RDA and are provided here in the form of ranges of recommended intakes.

[b] Since the toxic levels for many trace elements may be only several times usual intakes, the upper levels for the trace elements given in this table should not be habitually exceeded.

Table 3
Estimated Sodium, Chloride, and Potassium Minimum Requirements of Healthy Persons[a]

Age	Weight		Sodium (mg)[a,b]	Chloride (mg)[a,b]	Potassium (mg)[c]
	(lb)[d]	(kg)[d]			
Months					
0-5	9.9	4.5	120	180	500
6-11	19.6	8.9	200	300	700
Years					
1	24.2	11.0	225	350	1,000
2-5	35.2	16.0	300	500	1,400
6-9	55.0	25.0	400	600	1,600
10-18	110.0	50.0	500	750	2,000
>18[d]	154.0	70.0	500	750	2,000

[a] No allowance has been included for large, prolonged losses from the skin through sweat.

[b] There is no evidence that higher intakes confer any health benefit.

[c] Desirable intakes of potassium may considerably exceed these values (~3,500 mg for adults).

[d] No allowance included for growth. Values for those below 18 years assume a growth rate at the 50th percentile reported by the National Center for Health Statistics (Hamill et al., 1979) and averaged for males and females.

INDEX

Acesulfame-K, 125
Acidophilus, 197
Acids
  bile, 32, 40, 42, 151-152, 295
  ellagic, 348, 361, 385, 499, 527
  essential fatty, 30
  folic, 58-60, 283, 295, 306,
    319, 340, 342, 357, 401-402,
    446, 453
  nicotinic, 55
  oleic, 444
  oxalic, 502, 522, 533, 545
  pantothenic, 61, 559
  phenolic, 315
  stearic, 175
  trans fatty, 31, 168, 175
  uric, 193
Additives, 98, 156, 254-260
  intolerance to, 150
Adrenaline, 146
Aflatoxin, 98, 263, 265, 435
AIDS, 243
Alar, 260, 278
Alcohol, 52, 56, 58, 60, 86, 159,
    170, 189, 190, 232-233
  calories in, 14, 233
  and cancer, 96, 106, 107, 233
  and headaches, 155
  and heart disease, 165
  and osteoporosis, 205
  in pregnancy, 92, 233
  and stroke, 221
  and ulcers, 227
Alkyl benzene compounds, 264
Allergies, 143-150
  diagnosing, 147-149
  food, 90, 143-150, 158, 268,
    415

Allergies *(continued)*
  milk, 143, 150, 195-196, 415
  symptoms, 145-146, 449
  testing for, 90
  triggers for, 145
Allicin, 380
Allylic sulfide, 236
Aluminum compounds, 257
American Cancer Society, 320
American College of Sports
    Medicine, 274
American Dental Association,
    13
American Diabetes Association,
    125, 128
American Dietetic Association,
    96, 125
American Heart Association,
    32, 215
American Institute for Cancer
    Research, 96
American Medical Association,
    96, 125
Amino acids, 19-22, 54, 155,
    433
Anaphylaxis, 146
Anemia, 81-86, 300, 306
  hemolytic, 76
  iron-deficiency, 74, 76, 83
  megaloblastic, 86
  pernicious, 58, 86
  sickle cell, 56
Aneurysms, 219
Angina, 165
Anorexia nervosa. *See* Eating
    disorders.
Antacids, 67, 113, 160, 161, 203,
    227
Antibiotics, 227
Antibodies, 21